Otosclerosis

Diagnosis, Evaluation, Pathology, Surgical Techniques, and Outcomes

Otosclerosis

Diagnosis, Evaluation, Pathology, Surgical Techniques, and Outcomes

Chris de Souza, MS, DORL, DNB, FACS
Marcos V. Goycoolea, MD, MS, PhD
Neil M. Sperling, MD, FACS

Plural Publishing Inc.

PLURAL PUBLISHING
INC.

5521 Ruffin Road
San Diego, CA 92123

e-mail: info@pluralpublishing.com
Web site: http://www.pluralpublishing.com

Typeset in 10.5/13 Palatino by Flanagan's Publishing Services, Inc.
Printed in Korea by Four Colour Print Group

NOTICE TO THE READER
Care has been taken to confirm the accuracy of the indications, procedures, drug dosages, and diagnosis and remediation protocols presented in this book and to ensure that they conform to the practices of the general medical and health services communities. However, the authors, editors, and publisher are not responsible for errors or omissions or for any consequences from application of the information in this book and make no warranty, expressed or implied, with respect to the currency, completeness, or accuracy of the contents of the publication. The diagnostic and remediation protocols and the medications described do not necessarily have specific approval by the Food and Drug Administration for use in the disorders and/or diseases and dosages for which they are recommended. Application of this information in a particular situation remains the professional responsibility of the practitioner. Because standards of practice and usage change, it is the responsibility of the practitioner to keep abreast of revised recommendations, dosages, and procedures.

Library of Congress Cataloging-in-Publication Data

De Souza, Chris (Surgeon), author, editor of compilation.
Otosclerosis : diagnosis, evaluation, pathology, surgical techniques, and outcomes / Chris de Souza, Marcos V. Goycoolea, Neil M. Sperling.
p. ; cm.
Includes bibliographical references and index.
ISBN-13: 978-1-59756-507-3 (alk. paper)
ISBN-10: 1-59756-507-5 (alk. paper)
I. Goycoolea, Marcos V., author, editor of compilation. II. Sperling, Neil M., author, editor of compilation. III. Title.
[DNLM: 1. Otosclerosis. WV 265]
RF294.5.O76
617.8'822—dc23

2013037916

Contents

List of Videos

Introduction

Worldwide, the number of patients suffering from otosclerosis has declined considerably. Although this is a cause for rejoicing, it places the modern-day otologist in a unique predicament. It leaves him or her with very little surgical experience in dealing with otosclerosis. The patient who has undergone surgery for otosclerosis many years ago and now faces problems as a result of that surgery are among the many challenges that the otologist of today will need to face. The modern-day otologist will need to overcome his or her own learning curve before being able to perform the surgery reliably and deliver consistently good results.

There are still quite a few nuances that need to be learned if the otologist is to successfully and effectively treat patients with otosclerosis. Our book strives to help today's otologist achieve that goal. The references are limited to just a few. The atlas section on the surgical procedures is provided by internationally acknowledged experts. Their experience and techniques have been gleaned through years of performing this amazingly demanding procedure and consistently delivering excellent results. Each beautiful picture and illustration is worth a thousand words. Their surgical videos are priceless.

We hope that the current trends continue where otosclerosis will just be a faded memory in the history of illnesses that affect humanity. But until then, all otologists will still need to be familiar with all the dimensions that the treatment of otosclerosis brings.

We thank the contributors for sharing their valuable experience, their extraordinarily beautiful illustrations, and their videos. We appreciate their unselfishness and their graciousness. It is their hope, as well as ours, that all who read this book will benefit from it and as a result their patients will benefit from it too.

Chris de Souza
Marcos V. Goycoolea
Neil M. Sperling

Contributors

Audrey P. Calzada, MD
Clinical Fellow
Neurotology and Skull Base Surgery
House Ear Clinic
Los Angeles, CA
Chapter 25

Christopher de Souza, MS, DORL, DNB, FACS
Otolaryngologist–Head and Neck Surgeon
Holy Family Hospital, Lilavati Hospital, Tata Memorial Hospital, and Holy Spirit Hospital
Visiting Assistant Professor
Otolaryngology–Head and Neck Surgery
SUNY
Brooklyn, NY
Visiting Assistant Professor
Otolaryngology
LSUHSC
Shreveport, LA
Chapters 1–19

John C. Goddard, MD
Associate
House Ear Clinic
Los Angeles, CA
Director of Education
Director of Temporal Bone
House Research Institute
Los Angeles, CA
Chapter 25

Marcos V. Goycoolea, MD, MS, PhD
Otologist
Director Clínica las Condes
Santiago, Chile
Chapters 1–19

Robert K. Jackler, MD
Sewall Professor and Chair
Otolaryngology–Head and Neck Surgery
Professor Neurosurgery and Surgery
Stanford University School of Medicine
Stanford, CA
Chapter 20

Thomas Linder, PhD, MD
Chairman
Department of Otolaryngology–Head and Neck Surgery
Luzerner Kantonsspital
Luzern, Switzerland
Chapter 23

Ashutosh (A. G.) Pusalkar, MD
Master of Surgery (Otolaryngology, University of Mumbai)
Fach Arzt (Otolaryngology, University Tubingen, Germany)
Professor Emeritus
D. Y. Patil Medical College Hospital
Navi, Mumbai
Senior Consultant and Coordinator
Department of ENT and Head and Neck Surgery
Lilavati Hospital and Research Hospital and Research Centre
Mumbai, India
Chapter 26

Christoph Schlegel-Wagner, MD
Co-Chairman
Department of Otorhinolaryngology–Head and Neck Surgery
Luzerner Kantonsspital
Luzern, Switzerland
Chapter 23

Neil M. Sperling, MD, FACS
Associate Professor
State University of New York Downstate Medical Center
Brooklyn, NY
Chapters 22 and 24

Robert Vincent, MD
Otologic Surgeon
Causse Ear Clinic
Béziers, France
Chapter 22

Richard James Wiet, MD, FACS
Professor
Clinical Otolaryngology and Neurosurgery
Northwestern University Medical School
Chicago, IL
Ear Institute of Chicago
Hinsdale, IL
Chapter 21

PART I

Basic Science

CHAPTER 1

Pathology of Otosclerosis

Chris de Souza and Marcos V. Goycoolea

INTRODUCTION

Otosclerosis is primarily a disease of localized bone remodeling.[1] It is thought to affect only the bony capsule of the middle and inner ear selectively. Otosclerosis is a process occurring in two phases: (1) active phase as characterized by bone resorption (spongiosis), and (2) phase of remission characterized by bone deposition (sclerosis).

It is a disease affecting enchondral bone of the otic capsule characterized by disordered resorption and deposition of bone.

An otosclerotic focus consists of areas of bone resorption, new bone formation, vascular proliferation, and a connective tissue stroma.

AGE OF ONSET

It can range from 10 to 48 years of age, however, the mean age of onset is commonly the age of 30.[2]

DeJuan[3] in his study reported the onset of clinical otosclerosis to be 28% between the ages of 18 and 21 years, 40% between 21 and 30, and 22% between 31 and 40.[4]

PREVALENCE

The exact incidence remains unclear and next to impossible to determine.

However, in one report autopsy studies conducted by Konigsmark and Gorlin[5] revealed an incidence of 5% to 18% of the general population.

Jahn and Vernick[6] report that 10% of Caucasians have histologic otosclerosis, but only 1% of these develop clinical manifestations of otosclerosis.

Many authors have noted that the incidence of patients suffering from otosclerosis has declined steeply in recent times.

RACE

There appears to be a definite racial predisposition. Caucasians are more predisposed than Africans. Asians too are far less affected than Caucasians, and the prevalence in American Indians seems to be extremely low across the continent.[2]

GENDER

Shambaugh[7] noted a female preponderance in his study. Otosclerosis is not a genetically sex-linked characteristic disease. Thus, a ratio of 1:1 would have been expected.

Hueb et al[8] reported a higher incidence of bilateral otosclerosis in women than men. This prompted them to believe that this would more likely cause women to seek medical advice than men. This in turn could likely explain the gender disparity. On the other hand, endocrinological factors predisposing to the appearance of otosclerotic foci is a possibility to be considered.

OTOSCLEROSIS AND PREGNANCY

There are many reports that associate the onset of hearing loss caused by otosclerosis and the onset of pregnancy. Shambaugh[9] found that in an analysis of 475 female patients suffering from otosclerosis that 50% suffered from hearing impairment with the onset of pregnancy. Although he and many authors note a correlation between the onset of hearing loss following pregnancy, they are not clear on why or how this occurs. As mentioned earlier, endocrinologic factors have been suspected for this occurrence.

TYPES OF OTOSCLEROSIS

1. Histologic otosclerosis
2. Fenestral otosclerosis
3. Cochlear otosclerosis
4. Malignant otosclerosis
5. Far advanced otosclerosis

Histologic Otosclerosis (Figures 1–1 and 1–2)

Histologic otosclerosis is a finding on microscopic examination of temporal bones. The location of the otosclerotic changes is such that the patient suffers no symptoms related to the otosclerosic changes. Therefore, it generally does not involve the stapes bone, the stapediovestibular joint, or the cochlear endosteum. It is therefore asymptomatic.

Fenestral Otosclerosis

This refers to an otosclerotic lesion that involves the stapes bone and/or the stapediovestibular joint. This in turn causes a conductive hearing loss. This is

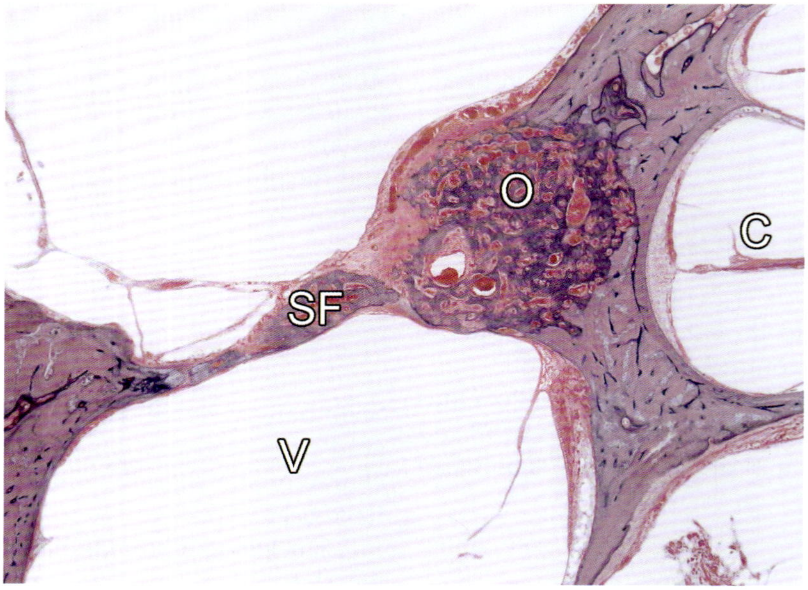

Figure 1–1. Section of human temporal bone demonstrating "histologic otosclerotic" focus. O = "histologic" otosclerotic focus; SF = stapedial footplate; C = cochlea; V = vestibule. Courtesy of University of Minnesota temporal bone collection. Kindly contributed by Dr. Cureoglu and Dr. Paparella.

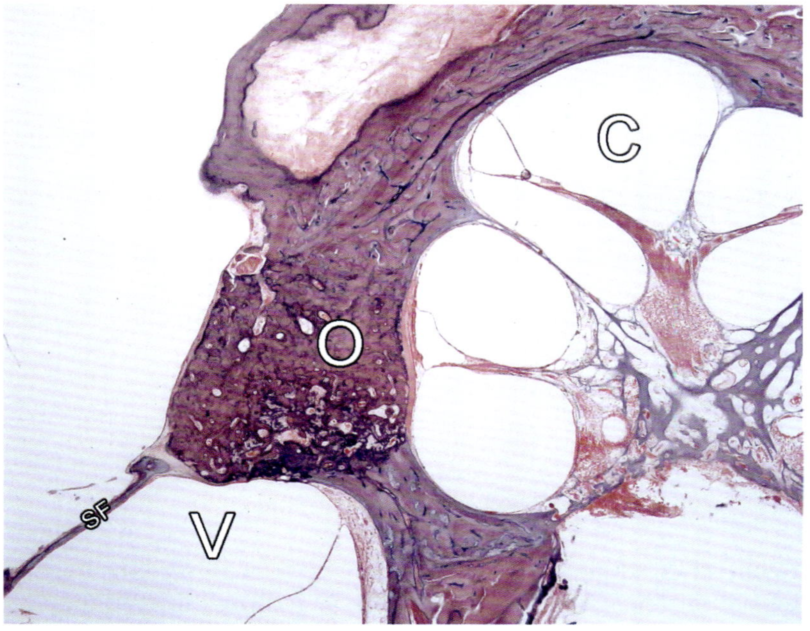

Figure 1-2. Magnified view of histologic otosclerosis. O = otosclerotic focus; V = vestibule; SF = stapedial footplate. Courtesy of University of Minnesota temporal bone collection. Kindly contributed by Dr. Cureoglu and Dr. Paparella.

the most common site of involvement representing 81 to 95% of cases.[10]

Cochlear Otosclerosis (Figure 1–3)

Cochlear otosclerosis is a term used in cases in which the otosclerotic lesion invades the cochlear endosteum and is usually reserved for the occurrence of pure sensorineural hearing loss due to otosclerosis without any conductive component.

"Malignant" (Obliterative) Otosclerosis

This is defined as severely active otosclerosis involving both oval and round windows and most of the bony labyrinth and is manifested initially by mixed hearing loss, which then relentlessly progresses to severe profound sensorineural hearing loss. Both windows are obliterated by the otosclerotic focus. Lamellar new bone is seen in the inner ear of such patients.

Far Advanced Otosclerosis (FAO)

Far advanced otosclerosis is defined as no measurable air or bone conduction or air conduction no better than 95 dB and bone conduction at 55 dB to 60 dB at one frequency only.

A negative Rinne's test result with a 256 Hz magnesium tuning fork is the best way to separate a FAO sensorineural hearing loss from sensorineural hearing losses of other causes.

SITES OF INVOLVEMENT OF THE TEMPORAL BONE BY OTOSCLEROSIS IN ORDER OF FREQUENCY

1. Commonly seen anterior to the oval window
2. The round window niche (Figures 1–4 and 1–5)
3. Posterior to the round window
4. Posterior wall of the internal auditory canal

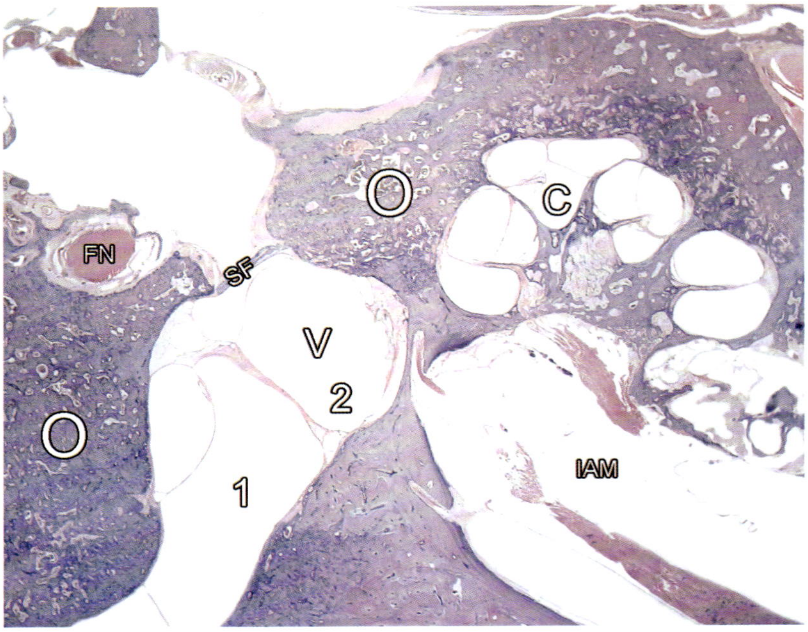

Figure 1–3. Histopathology section of human temporal bone demonstrating cochlear otosclerosis. O = otosclerotic focus; C = cochlea deformed by the otosclerosis; V = vestibule; 2 = saccule; 1 = utricle; SF = stapes footplate; FN = facial nerve. Courtesy of University of Minnesota temporal bone collection. Kindly contributed by Dr. Cureoglu and Dr. Paparella.

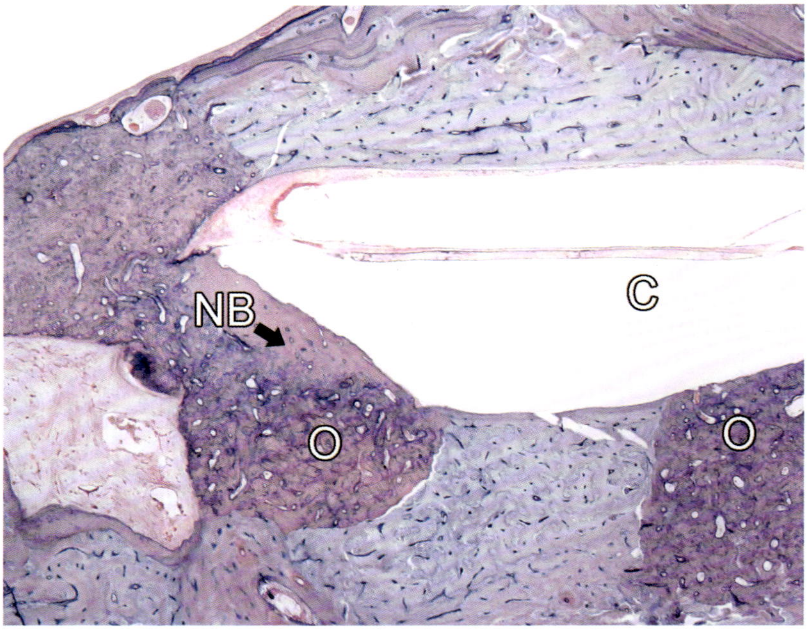

Figure 1–4. HP section demonstrating otosclerotic focus obliterating the round window. O = otosclerotic focus; C = cochlea; NB = new bone formation. Courtesy of University of Minnesota temporal bone collection. Kindly contributed by Dr. Cureoglu and Dr. Paparella.

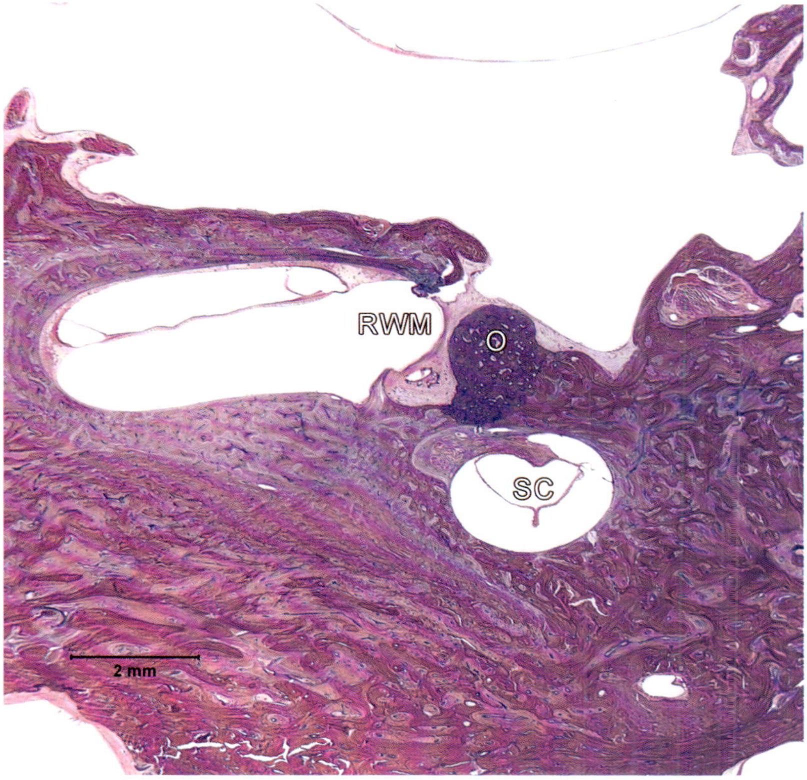

Figure 1–5. HP section demonstrating otosclerotic focus near round window niche. O = otosclerotic focus; RWM = round window membrane; SC = Semicircular canal. Courtesy of University of Minnesota temporal bone collection. Kindly contributed by Dr. Cureoglu and Dr. Paparella.

5. Around the cochlear aqueduct
6. Semicircular canals
7. Totally within the stapedial footplate

HISTOPATHOLOGY OF OTOSCLEROSIS

The otic capsule itself undergoes very little remodeling. The otic capsule contains small regions of immature cartilaginous tissue called the "globuli interossei." This may be the loci of the earliest lesions of otosclerosis.

Otosclerosis is characterized by the following:

1. Bone resorption
2. New bone formation
3. Vascular proliferation
4. Connective tissue stroma.

The very **first** stage of otosclerosis is resorption of enchondral bone around blood vessels.

Second: This results in enlargement of perivascular spaces. Vascular spaces become wider. This is the initial stage characterized by diffuse or patchy demineralization that coincides with preotosclerotic lesions.

Third: This is then followed by deposition of immature (woven) bone.

Fourth: Resorption and deposition of immature bone occurs continuously within an otosclerotic focus with production of more mature (lamellar) bone.

The otosclerotic focus is larger in volume than the bone it replaces and thus it causes thickening of the structure it involves.

Otosclerotic foci may appear as dense mineralized (sclerotic) bone or as an active well-vascularized (spongiotic) bone.

An active focus is characterized by "spongiotic" bone. There is increased vascularity and increased cellularity and bone resorption and new bone deposition.

Schwartz's sign is a reddish blush seen behind an intact tympanic membrane. This is due to vascular shunts between the otosclerotic focus and the vessels on the promontory.

An "inactive" focus is characterized by dense mineralized bone.

An otosclerotic focus can have "active" as well as "inactive" areas.

At the interface of normal and otosclerotic bone two types of changes are seen: (1) a sharply demarcated line between old bone and newly formed active bone that was enzyme mediated, and (2) an advancing front that appeared serrated and appeared to be caused by osteocyte-mediated resorption of ground substance.

ELECTRON MICROSCOPY

Transmission electron microscopy reveals mononuclear cells rich in lysosomes. In the resorption (active) phase histiocytes play an important role. Osteoclasts are rare. Predominant cells noted are osteoblasts, osteoblast precursors, and histiocytes. Increased vascularity and increased osteocyte activity are major factors in otosclerosis.

Criteria for the indication of increased histologic activity in an otosclerotic focus are the following:

1. Nonosseous tissues that demonstrate increased cellularity and vascularity
2. Bone resorption and/or bone deposition
3. Increased vascularity and fibrosis of the overlying mucosa
4. Osseous tissue stained with acidophilic stains.

WHAT IS THE BLUE MANTLE OF MANASSE?

They are islands of basophilic staining normal bone that appears alongside otosclerotic foci. Blue mantles can be found in isolation or in direct continuity with the otosclerotic foci.

REFERENCES

1. de Souza CE, Glasscock ME. Pathology of otosclerosis. *Otosclerosis and Stapedectomy*. New York, NY: Thieme; 2004:3–21.
2. Goycoolea MV. Otosclerosis. In: Paparella MM, Shumrick D, eds. *Otolaryngology*. Philadelphia, PA: W.B. Saunders Co.; 1991:1489–1512.
3. DeJuan P. Consideraciones sobre la otosclerosis. *Acta Otolaryngol Iber Am*. 1960;11(5):389–416.
4. Glorig A, Gallo R. Comments on sensorineural hearing loss in otosclerosis. In: Schuknecht HF, ed. *Otosclerosis*. Boston, MA: Little Brown; 1962:63–78.
5. Konigsmark BW, Gorlin RJ. *Genetic and Metabolic Deafness*. Philadelphia, PA: W.B. Saunders; 1976.
6. Jahn AF, Vernick D. Otosclerosis: diagnosis and treatment. *SIPAC. Am Acad Otolaryngol Head Neck Surg*; 1986:12–20.
7. Shambaugh GE. The diagnosis of otosclerosis. *Prog Otolaryngol*. 1952;1:395.
8. Hueb MM, Goycoolea MV, Paparella MM. Otosclerosis: the university of Minnesota temporal bone collection. *Otolaryngol Head Neck Surg*. 1991;105:396–405.
9. Shambaugh GE. Otosclerosis. *Proceedings of the International Congress of ORL*. Vol 1. Basel: Karger; 1961:367.
10. Goycoolea MV, Hueb MM. Surgery for stapes fixation. In: Goycoolea MV, ed. *Atlas of Otologic Surgery*. New Dehli, India: J.P. Brothers; 2012:863–873.

CHAPTER 2

Genetics of Otosclerosis

Chris de Souza and Marcos V. Goycoolea

INTRODUCTION

Otosclerosis represents a heterogeneous group of genetic disorders in which different genes may be involved. It is postulated that in response to the different gene variants and environmental factors, the physiologic inhibition of bone turnover in the otic capsule is overruled, which then results in otosclerosis.

The first gene responsible for causing otosclerosis is yet to be cloned. It has an autosomal dominant mode of inheritance with incomplete penetrance and variable expressivity, which means that it can skip generations and when it manifests it does not express in the same way in all those that are affected.

THE GENES RESPONSIBLE FOR CAUSATION OF OTOSCLEROSIS

Five genetic loci OTSC1 to OTSC5 have been published to date. This supports the theory that mutations in any number of genes are capable of causing the otosclerosis phenotype.

OTSC1 was mapped to 15q25–q26 in an Indian family. OTSC2 was mapped to 16cM on chromosome 7 (7q34–36) in a family from Belgium. OTSC3 was mapped to a family from Cyprus (6p21.3–22.3).

OTSC4 was located in an Israeli family and OTSC5 was mapped to chromosome 3q22–24 in a Dutch family.

Otosclerosis has long been thought to have a genetic factor. Most genetic studies on families with otosclerosis support a pattern of autosomal dominant transmission with incomplete penetrance.[1] There is growing evidence that suggests that otosclerosis may be a heterogenetic disease, with the typical clinical phenotype arising from more than one possible genetic defect. Evidence that supports a genetic basis comes from studies on monozygotic twins in which evidence of otosclerosis was found in nearly all the cases.[2,3] Linkage studies between otosclerosis and the ABO M:N and Rh blood groups and half the globulin genotypes have failed to demonstrate evidence of linkage.

Recently, linkage analysis of a large kindred from India with a presumptive diagnosis of otosclerosis revealed linkage to a region of chromosome 15q.[4] These investigators suggest that the gene for aggrecan, an extracellular matrix protein found predominantly in cartilage may be a possible candidate gene. However, other families have been examined specifically for evidence of linkage to this region but no evidence supporting this theory was found. This again supports the concept of a heterogenetic disorder. Thalmann and colleagues[5] detected possible alterations in collagenous proteins in otosclerotic tissues. There is recent evidence to suggest that in a small number of cases otosclerosis may be related to gene defects in COL1A1 gene, one of the genes that code for type 1 collagen, the major collagen component of bone. Association analysis has revealed an association between the COL1A1 allelic expression in cultured fibroblasts from individuals with clinical otosclerosis that is either familial or sporadic. Analysis of COL1A1 allelic expression in cultured fibroblasts from individuals with clinical otosclerosis has shown that in a small percentage of cases, ranging from 10% to 20%, one of the COL1A1 alleles is expressed in extremely low reiteration. This is similar to that seen in many cases of mild (type 1) osteogenesis imperfecta. This suggests that in a small percentage of cases the underlying genetic mechanism may be similar to that of osteogenesis imperfect.[6] The hearing loss that occurs in persons with type I osteogenesis imperfecta occurs almost exclusively in association with COL IAI defects and occurs in 50% of affected persons. It shares the same autosomal dominant inheritance with incomplete penetration, as seen with otosclerosis.

Mazzoli, Rosignoli, and Martini[7] examined sporadic and familial (hereditary) patients suffering from otosclerosis and report that in sporadic cases of otosclerosis a genetic cause cannot be excluded because of the possibility of a different mode of inheritance, new mutations, or the absence of expression in family members. They also state that environmental factors may be responsible for the high degree of variability between families.

CONCLUSIONS

1. An autosomal dominant mode of inheritance with incomplete penetrance is seen in familial otosclerosis.
2. Familial otosclerosis displays locus heterogenicity.

REFERENCES

1. Larson A. Otosclerosis: a genetic and clinical study. *Acta Otolaryngol.* 1960;154:1–86.
2. Fowler EP. Otosclerosis in identical twins. *Ann Oto Rhinol.* 1949;56:36.
3. Fowler EP. Otosclerosis in identical twins: a study of 40 pairs. *Arch Otolaryngol.* 1966;83:324–328.
4. Tomek M, Brown MR, Mani SR, et al. Localization of a gene for otosclerosis to chromosome 15q–q26. *Hum Mol Genet.*1998;7:285–290.
5. Thalmann I, Thallinger G, Thalmann R. Otosclerosis: a localized manifestation of a generalized connective tissue disorder? *Am J Otolaryngol.* 1987;8:308–316.
6. McKenna MJ, Kristiansen AG, Bartley ML, et al. Association of COL1A1 and otosclerosis: evidence for a shared genetic etiology with mild ostogenesis imperfecta. *Am J Otol.* 1998;19:604–610.
7. Mazzoli M, Rosignoli M, Martini A. Otosclerosis: are familial and isolated cases different disorders? *J Audiol Med.* 2001;10(1):49–59.

CHAPTER 3

Measles and Otosclerosis

Chris de Souza and Marcos V. Goycoolea

INTRODUCTION

There is increasing evidence that a possible persistent measles virus (MeV) infection is associated with otosclerosis, especially the sporadic variety of otosclerosis. MeV involvement has been demonstrated in morphological, biochemical, and immunological studies in samples of otosclerotic foci. The cause and effect roles of the measles virus are being examined. It is postulated that the widespread immunization against measles has been responsible for the decline in the number of patients presenting with otosclerosis.

HYPOTHESIS

Support for the hypothesis that the measles virus is responsible for being the cause of otosclerosis comes from the detection of ultrastructural and immunohistochemical evidence of measles-like structures and antigenicity in active otosclerotic lesions. Measles RNA has been found in temporal bone collections of specimens in which otosclerosis was found to be present. It was also detected in fresh otosclerotic footplate specimens taken at the time of stapedectomy. Raised levels of antimeasles antibodies have also been reported in the perilymph of otosclerotic patients undergoing stapedectomy as compared to that of normal healthy controls. This hypothesis is further substantiated by the fact that sporadic otosclerosis has dropped significantly. Epidemiological data reveal a steep decline in the incidence of otosclerosis worldwide following the introduction of the measles vaccine.

Chronic inflammation was detected in morphologic investigations of otosclerotic foci and by using immunohistochemical methods. MeV (measles virus) N, P, and F proteins were detected inside the cells of the otosclerotic focus. Thus some authors conclude that otosclerosis is an inflammatory disease with a genetic background.

Filamentous structures resembling the paramyxoviral necleocapsids were detected in otosclerotic samples. The expression of measles virus N, F, and H antigens were found in the osteoclasts and macrophages of otosclerotic tissue.

McKenna and Mills[1] were able to detect MeV RNA in 8 of 11 temporal bones with confirmed otosclerosis. All the negative controls were negative for MeV. Recently, the genotype of MeV has been ascertained. The phylogenetic analysis[2] revealed that the MeV was of genotype A, the type that was present before the vaccination era. McKenna[3] suggests that this would help explain the sporadic nature of the disease as well as the observed incomplete penetrance of the phenotype. McKenna et al[4] suggest that the initial otosclerotic lesion may be initiated by measles infection of the "globuli interossei," which can account for the sole predilection of the temporal bone. The establishment of persistent infection may be related to the relatively quiescent metabolic state or terminal differentiation of the osteocytes or chondrocytes within the "globuli interossei," which results in restricted expression of the measles genomewith little or no expression of late viral genes critical for complete viral assembly and escape.[5] Infected cells produce factors that destabilize the extracellular matrix and lead to activation of the remodeling process. The progression and extension of the abnormal remodeling process is dependent upon an underlying genetic defect in collagen metabolism. There may be multiple different mutations within the COL IAI gene and in other genes within the collagen metabolism pathway that result in the generation of an unstable extracellular matrix with a high propensity for remodeling. Although multiple different mutations in COL IAI may result in null expression of the mutant alleles, the downstream effect on other related factors that are critical determinants in the remodeling process may vary among mutations and produce a varied spectrum in clinical and histologic severity. These are new and interesting theories. Additional studies will be needed to establish which loci and genes are related to the development of otosclerosis. More importantly to substantiate the viral cause of otosclerosis, the virus will need to be isolated from the otosclerotic tissue. Only once the measles virus is isolated from otosclerotic tissue will the measles virus be directly associated with the cause of otosclerosis.

CONCLUSIONS

1. There is strong evidence that MeV is associated with the sporadic form of otosclerosis.
2. Epidemiological data reveals a clear and significant decline in the incidence of otosclerosis following the introduction of the measles vaccine.
3. The measles virus has not been isolated so far from otosclerotic tissue.

REFERENCES

1. McKenna MJ, Mills BG. Ultrastructural and immunohistochemical evidence of measles virus in active otosclerosis. *Acta Otolaryngol.* (suppl) 1990;470:130–140.
2. McKenna MJ, Mills BG. Immunohistochemical evidence of measles virus antigens in active otosclerosis. *Otolaryngol Head Neck Surg.* 1989;101:415–421.
3. McKenna MJ. Polymerase chain reaction amplification of a measles virus sequence from human temporal bone sections with active otosclerosis. *Am J Otol.* 1999;17: 827–830.
4. McKenna MJ, Kristiansen AG, Bartley ML, et al. Association of COL1A1 and otosclerosis: evidence for a shared genetic etiology with mild ostogenesis imperfecta. *Am J Otol.* 1998;19:604–610.
5. Schneider-Schaulies J, Schneider-Schaulies S, ter Meulen V. Differential induction of cytokines by primary and persistent measles virus infections in human glial cells. *Virology.* 1993;195:219–228.

CHAPTER 4

Molecular Biology

Chris de Souza and Marcos V. Goycoolea

INTRODUCTION

Otosclerosis is a process of pathologic remodeling within a bone that is normally resistant to remodeling. The otic capsule is subject to very minimal bone remodeling under normal circumstances. Otosclerosis subjects the otic capsule to frequent bone remodeling

PATHOGENESIS

Osteoprotogerin (OPG), receptor activator of nuclear factor kappa B (RANK), and RANK ligand (RANK-L) play a major role in the remodeling of bone.[1]

RANK-L is expressed in a variety of cells including osteoblasts. RANK-L expressed by osteoblasts that are involved in bone turnover promotes differentiation, activation, and survival of osteoclasts by activation of its specific receptor RANK on osteoclasts. OPG acts as a soluble neutralizing antagonist that binds and inactivates RANK-L. OPG inhibits the differentiation, survival, and fusion of osteoclastic precursor cells, suppresses activation, and promotes apoptosis of osteoclasts.

Osteoclasts are responsible for bone resorption whereas osteoblasts are responsible for bone formation.

WHY IS THE OTIC CAPSULE DEVOID OF POSTDEVELOPMENTAL REMODELING?

Studies have shown that the inner ear itself may play a direct role in the inhibition of remodeling of the otic capsule by producing substances that will prevent remodeling.

The spiral ligament produces OPG, which is secreted into the perilymph.[2] OPG then diffuses into the surrounding otic capsule bone. OPG is a potent inhibitor of bone remodeling and it acts by inhibiting the recruitment, formation, and activity of osteoclasts, which resorb bone. High levels of OPG are found in the otic capsule and this is a significant finding because OPG is a key factor in the final common pathway for regulation of bone metabolism.

Bone remodeling at a local level is very tightly regulated by a delicate balance among the 3 cytokines: (1) OPG, (2) RANK, and (3) RANK-L.

Osteoblasts present the cell surface protein ligand RANK-L, which binds it to the receptor RANK on precursor and immature osteoclasts. The RANK-L and RANK interaction produces mature osteoclasts that set in motion bone resorption. OPG competes with RANK for the RANK-L receptor on osteoblasts and thus becomes a powerful inhibitor of bone remodeling. The ratio of OPG to RANK-L is critical in determining the amount of local bone remodeling.

Overexpression of OPG causes excessive bone formation whereas lower OPG levels cause bone resorption.

Remodeling of the otic capsule is very tightly controlled by the OPG, RANK, RANK-L system and under normal circumstances the otic capsule does not remodel.

In otosclerosis the balance is tipped in favor of remodeling at specific areas within the otic capsule.

REFERENCES

1. Zehnder AF, Kristiansen AG, Adams JC, Merchant SN, McKenna MJ. Osteoprotegrin in the inner ear may inhibit bone remodeling in the otic capsule. *Laryngoscope*. 2005; 115:172–177.
2. Zehnder AF, Kristiansen AG, Adams JC, Kujawa SG, Merchant SN, McKenna MJ. Osteoprotegrin knockout mice demonstrate abnormal remodeling of the otic capsule and progressive hearing loss. *Laryngoscope*. 2006;116:201–206.

PART II

Investigations

CHAPTER 5

Audiological Evaluation of the Patient with Otosclerosis

Chris de Souza and Marcos V. Goycoolea

INTRODUCTION

The audiological signature pattern of fenestral otosclerosis includes the following:

1. Conductive hearing loss with Carhart's notch at 2 kHz
2. Excellent speech discrimination scores
3. Low compliance on impedance (immittance) audiometry (less than 0.3 cc)
4. Normal middle ear pressure
5. Absence of middle ear reflexes.

TUNING FORK TESTS TO EVALUATE HEARING

The first test that should be performed is the tuning fork test using the 512 Hz tuning fork.

Rinne's Test

In the patient with significant conductive hearing loss from otosclerosis, tuning fork testing will indicate that bone conduction is better than air conduction. This is referred to as a negative Rinne's test.[1] Rinne's test is performed by first striking the tines of the 512 Hz tuning fork and then placing it in front of the patient's ear (air conduction testing). Then when the patient can no longer hear the tuning fork, it is placed on the mastoid behind the pinna (bone conduction testing). If the patient can then continue to hear the sound of the tuning fork then it is termed as Rinne's test negative. If it is not heard when placed behind then it is termed as Rinne's test positive. Positive Rinne's tesint is seen in normal hearing and with those who have a sensorineural hearing loss. This test should be done in a soundproof room.

Weber's Test

This is performed by striking the tines of 512 Hz tuning fork and then placing it on the patient's forehead or other midline structure (bridge of the nose, mentum or upper incisors). If the patient hears the sound in the midline, it indicates symmetry of the hearing (normal hearing bilaterally or symmetric hearing loss). If the tuning fork is heard on one side greater than the other, it indicates asymmetric hearing and is said to 'lateralize' to that side. In the presence of a unilateral conductive hearing loss, the tuning fork will lateralize to the side with the conductive hearing loss. If the conductive loss is bilateral, the fork may be midline (when the loss is symmetric) or will lateralize to the side with the greater conductive hearing loss.

Using both the Rinne's and Weber's test the examiner will have a rough idea as to the type of hearing loss and if both ears are involved.

PURE TONE AUDIOMETRY (Figures 5–1 and 5–2)

In the early stages the patient suffering from otosclerosis will demonstrate a low frequency conductive hearing loss. Once the hearing loss reaches the 25 dB stage the patient demonstrates a conductive hearing loss at all frequencies with a dip at 2 kHz known as Carhart's notch.[2]

Carhart's notch is thought to be typical of otosclerosis. It is characterized by depression of bone conduction thresholds of approximately 5 dB at 500 Hz, 10 dB at 1 kHz, 15 dB at 2 kHz, and 5 dB at 4 kHz.

A plausible explanation[3] for this Carhart's notch is that fixation of the stapes disrupts normal ossicular resonance, which in humans is around 2 kHz. It must be understood that Carhart's notch is a mechanical artifact and does not truly represent cochlear reserve. Proof that it is indeed an artifact is seen in overclosure following stapes surgery, defined as improvement of the bone conduction compared to the preoperative levels. It is uncommon to find patients with otosclerosis whose bone conduction thresholds are normal. Surgery improves bone conduction thresholds and Carhart's notch disappears following surgery.

IMPEDANCE (IMMITTANCE) AUDIOMETRY (Figure 5–3)

Impedance tympanometry is the measurement of the tympanic membrane compliance in response to variations of air pressure in the external auditory canal.

The tympanometric peak demonstrates the presence of air in the middle ear space. The location of the peak on the pressure axis serves as an indicator of middle ear pressure relative to ambient air pressure. From it one can figure out the position of the tympanic membrane. Middle ear aeration is not affected in otosclerosis and the middle ear pressure is zero or atmospheric.[4] The height of the peak reflects the mobility of the middle ear apparatus. In the situation of stapedial otosclerosis the tympanometric peak decreases.

STATIC COMPLIANCE

Static compliance is calculated by subtracting the compliance at +200 daPa from the total compliance when the pressure is equilibrated across the tympanic membrane.

Normal static compliance values fall in the range of 0.3 to 1.6 cc. Values lower than 0.3 cc are indicative of stiffness in the conductive mechanism.

If the compliance is around 0.6 cm^3 then the footplate is thin. If it is less than 0.2 cm^3 then it is likely that the footplate is fairly thick and may even be obliterative.

ACOUSTIC REFLEXES (Figure 5–4)

The first sign of otosclerosis is the appearance of a diphasic pattern.[5,6] The diphasic reflex is characterized by brief increases in compliance that occur at the beginning and end of the stimulus when the probe is placed in the affected ear. The explanation for this is that the anterior end of the footplate is fixed by the otosclerotic focus but not the posterior end.

As the otosclerotic process progresses the ipsilateral and contralateral reflexes get affected.

SPEECH AUDIOMETRY

Persons suffering from otosclerosis will present with excellent speech discrimination scores. Speech discrimination scores (SDS) are a measure of word identification accuracy. In the presence of a conductive hearing loss the speech reception coincides with the three frequency pure tone average (500 Hz, 1 kHz, and 2 kHz) within a range of 5 dB. SDS scores fall when there is a sensorineural component to the hearing loss.[7]

Ref. :
Name :
Sex/Age :
History :

Date : 04.06.2013
OPD :
IND:
Receipt No. :
Audio No. :

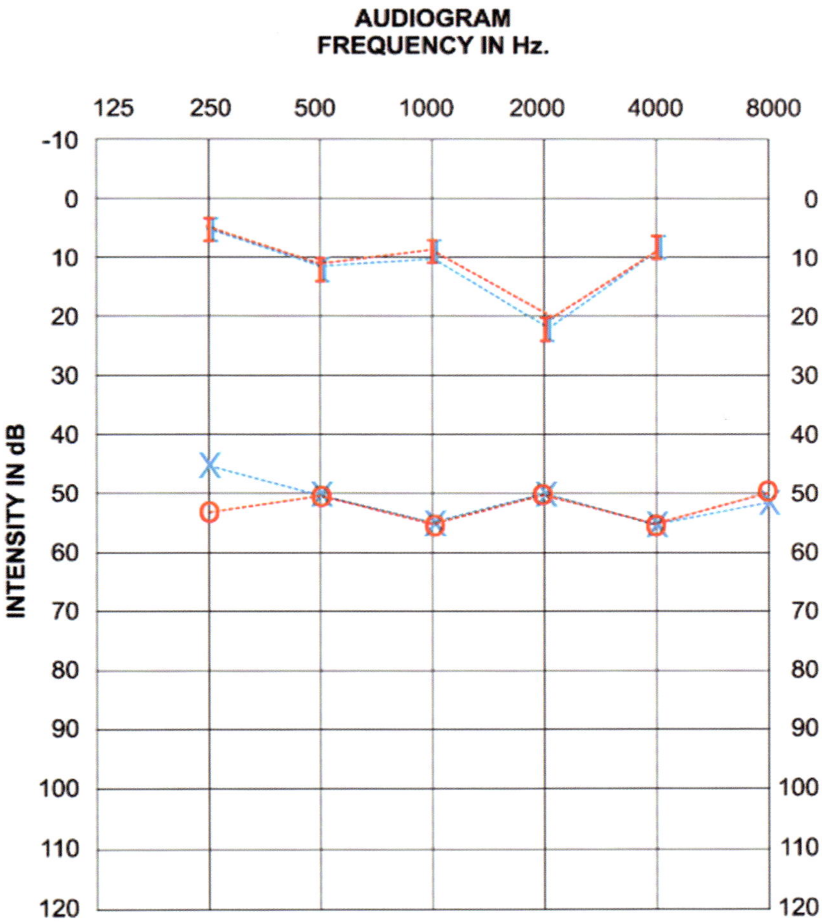

	R. Ear	L. Ear
T. F. Test		
Rinne	-ve	-ve
Weber	⟷	
ABC		
ABLB		
SISI		
TONE DECAY		

Remarks - Bilateral moderate conductive hearing loss.

		SRT	SDS
RT EAR	-	30dB	90%
LT EAR	-	30dB	90%

Audiologist

Figure 5–1. Pure tone audiogram of a patient suffering from otosclerosis. Dip at 2 kHz. Note that the right side of the graph shows Rinne's test as negative and Weber's lateralized in both ears. Speech threshold at the bottom is 30 dB in both ears and speech discrimination scores are 90%. The diagnosis: fenestral otosclerosis.

OTOSCLEROSIS AND STAPEDECTOMY

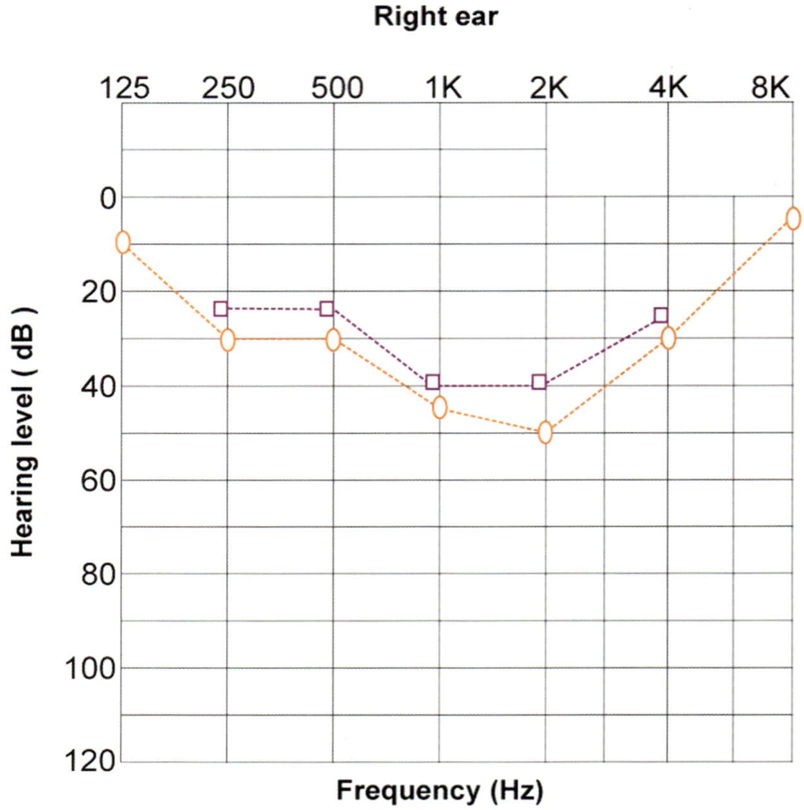

Figure 5–2. Pure tone audiogram shows a typical cookie bite audiogram seen in cochlear otosclerosis.

OTOACOUSTIC EMISSIONS

The measurement of OAE is thought to be helpful in establishing a conductive component to a hearing loss.

OAEs are not present in otosclerosis. Thus the presence will exclude a conductive middle ear component. OAE tests are useful because they are reliable. Transient-evoked OAE are preferable over distortion product (DPOAE) because they are less prone to artifacts.

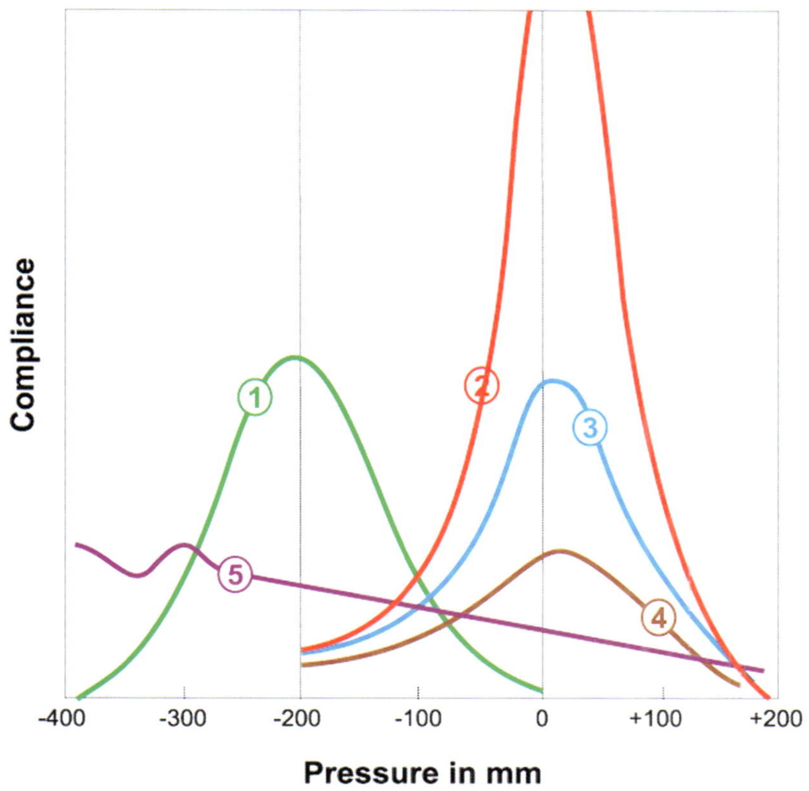

Figure 5–3. Impedance audiometry of various middle ear conditions. Compliance = Excursion of the tympanic membrane. Pressure in mm of water. **Graph Line 1 (Green Graph):** Typical of eustachian dysfunction. There is a shift to the left (negative pressure) but compliance is present. **Graph Line 2 (Red Graph):** Typical of ossicular discontinuity. High compliance but normal pressure. **Graph Line 3 (Blue Graph):** Normal excursion of the tympanic membrane with normal pressure. **Graph Line 4 (Brown graph):** Typical of otosclerosis. Low compliance but normal pressure. **Graph Line 5 (Purple graph):** Typical of fluid in the middle ear. Extreme shift to the left. Very little compliance and negative pressure.

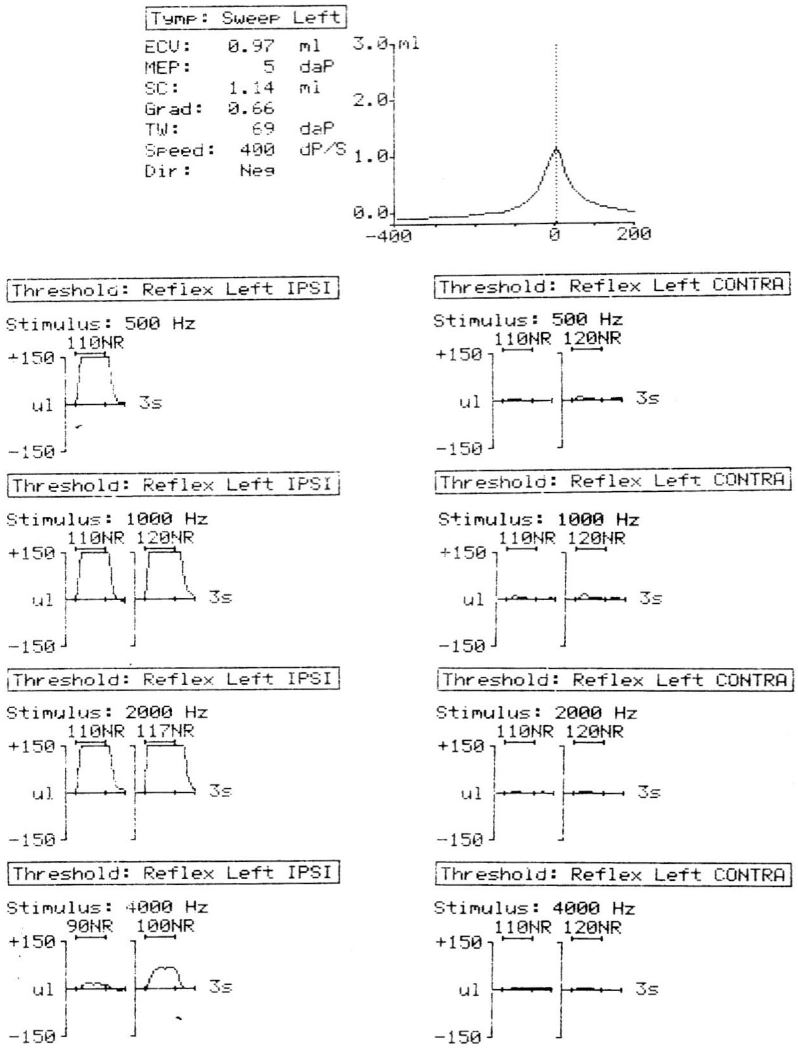

Figure 5–4. Impedance audiometric reading of a patient suffering from otosclerosis demonstrating the following: (1) low compliance, (2) normal pressure, (3) absent stapedial reflexes.

REFERENCES

1. Beales PH. Functional evaluation of hearing. In: *Otosclerosis.* Bristol, UK: John Wright and Sons; 1981:30–50.
2. Carhart R. Clinical applications of bone conduction audiometry. *Arch Otolaryngol.* 1950;51:798–802.
3. Carhart R. Effects of stapes fixation on bone conduction responses. In: Schuknecht HF, ed. *International Symposium on Otosclerosis.* Boston, MA: Little Brown; 1962:175.
4. Jerger J. Clinical experience with impedance audiometry. *Arch Otolaryngol.* 1970;92:311–320.
5. Bel J, Causse JR, Michaux P, et al. Mechanical explanation of the on-off effect (diphasic impedance change) in otospongiosis. *Audiology.* 1976;15:128–130.
6. Flottorp G, Djupesland G. Diphasic impedance change and its applicability in clinical work. *Acta Otolaryngol.* 1970;263:200–205.
7. Hannley MT. Audiologic characteristics of the patient with otosclerosis. *Otolaryng Clin North Am.* 1993;26: 373–387.

CHAPTER 6

Radiological Imaging of Otosclerosis

Chris de Souza and Marcos V. Goycoolea

FENESTRAL OTOSCLEROSIS

Fenestral otosclerosis is fundamentally a clinical diagnosis. It is made on the basis of the history, family history, tuning fork tests, and audiometry. In recent times with the continued refinement of CT scanning the round window can be clearly visualized. Therefore, pathologies in and around the oval window can also be visualized.

In fenestral otosclerosis CT scanning was found to have a sensitivity of 91% where the slice thickness of the CT scans was 1 mm.

Active otosclerotic foci were more likely to be identified than inactive foci. This is because in active otosclerotic foci the bone is perceived as "hypodense" (Figure 6–1). The most important area to be visualized is the area anterior to the footplate.

For the otosclerotic focus to be detected on CT scanning the following should be present:

1. The focus must be greater than 1 mm in diameter.
2. The density of the focus must differ from the rest of the otic capsule. That is why active foci (areas of demineralization) are easier to detect than inactive (sclerotic) foci.
3. The normal otic capsule is very dense. Sclerotic foci can be detected only when they are very close to the periosteal or endosteal surfaces of the otic capsule.

The radiographic appearance of the otosclerotic lesion varies with the stage of the disease. The otosclerotic focus can only be visualized when the otosclerotic focus is more than 200 Hounsfield units.

Typical of cochlear otosclerosis is the formation of a double ring effect due to multiple foci coalescing with each other. A mosaic picture characterized by areas of decreased and increased density occurring simultaneously can occasionally be found.

WHAT IS THE ROLE OF CT SCANNING IN OTOSCLEROSIS?

1. It can detect active foci provided they are more than 1 mm.

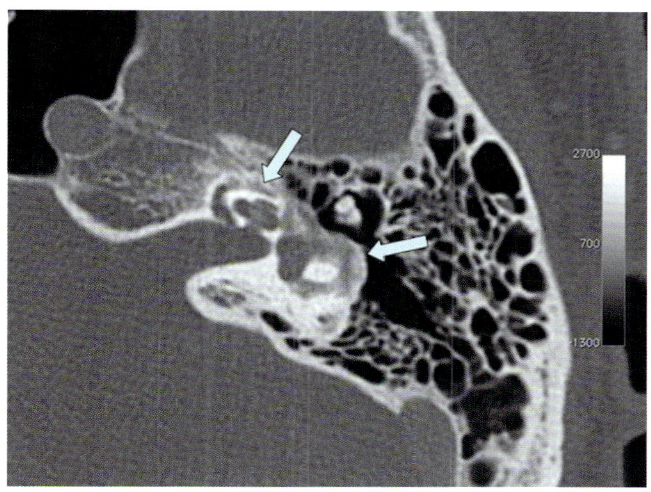

Figure 6–1. CT scan of temporal bone of a patient suffering from cochlear otosclerosis. The cochlea and semicircular canals are demineralized (arrows). This is the active phase of otosclerosis. Photo courtesy of Dr. Neil Sperling.

2. It is useful in the case of cochlear otosclerosis especially when the patient presents with bilateral sensorineural hearing loss.
3. Postoperatively. In the situation where the patient experiences good hearing initially and then at a later stage develops a hearing impediment. It is possible to visualize the oval window and the location of the prosthesis.
4. CT scanning can help identify the possibility of a large cochlear aqueduct and thus prepare for the possibility of a potential perilymph gusher.
5. CT scanning is mandatory in far advanced otosclerosis especially when cochlear implantation is considered.
6. CT can be valuable when a diagnosis other than otosclerosis is suspected as the cause for conductive hearing loss. Other middle ear or temporal bone anomalies can be demonstrated.

CT DENSITOMETRY

Quantitative data of the involvement of the otic capsule is plotted using CT densitometry. The cochlea is identified in the scout digitalized image. Six to eight axial sections at 1-mm increments are taken. Densitometry data are then collected from two CT scan sections (two axial CT scans) taken at different levels. The lower section passes through the basal turn of the cochlea and the round window niche. The upper section crosses the modiolus exposing all three coils of the cochlea. Readings are taken as the cursor moves along the various areas of the cochlea just described.

Readings are taken from normal patients' CT scans and compared with those in whom otosclerosis is suspected.

Variations exceeding standard deviations of 10 to 15% for each point indicate cochlear involvement. It can thus be seen that CT densitometry studies depend on comparisons between normal patients and those suffering from otosclerosis. CT densitometry is useful where cochlear otosclerosis is suspected.

Usefulness of CT densitometry:

1. Identification of otosclerotic focus in the otic capsule.
2. Helps discern if disease is active or inactive.
3. Useful in evaluating response to fluoride therapy.

It should be noted that densitometric curves of otosclerosis are undistinguishable from that occurring in Paget's disease, osteogenesis imperfecta.

THE ROLE OF MRI IN OTOSCLEROSIS

CT scanning is far superior to MRI in providing information when the possibility of otosclerosis is considered. However, it must be noted that Valvassori[1] came up with a protocol for using MRI where otosclerosis is considered. This is to be used only in very limited situations where Schwartz's sign is positive. He observed a faint blush of enhancement within demineralized areas of the capsule.

MRI may be contraindicated in the postoperative stage if a ferro-magnetic metallic prostheses is used. MRI has the potential to cause vibration, which could result in dislodgement or heating of the prosthesis. Most modern prosthesis are compatible with today's magnet strengths.

SINGLE PHOTON EMISSION COMPUTED TOMOGRAPHY (SPECT) IN OTOSCLEROSIS

In CT scanning the density of the otosclerotic focus is variable and the active otosclerotic focus can only be visualized when the density loss is more than 200 Hounsfield units, whereas the inactive or sclerotic focus being isodense with the normal osseous tissue is detectable when the apposition of new otosclerotic focus causes irregularity or thickening of the otic capsule.

Tympanocochlear scintigraphy (TCS) was used by Ross et al[2] In this technique the bone turnover caused by the otosclerotic focus can be detected using a radiopharmaceutical agent such as 99m Tc diphosphonate, which undergoes higher adsorption on immature (hydrated) than on mature (crystalline) hydroxyapatite. A major limitation of this technique is the absence of clear anatomic landmarks, so it does not enable the distribution of the radioactive agent to be precisely located. Single photon emission computed tomography (SPECT) scintigraphy is a dynamic technique that allows the study of bone metabolic activity by detecting the distribution of diphosphonate in petrous bone while also providing quantification of the radioactivity. In addition to providing a semiquantitative analysis of metabolic activity as in tomographic techniques, it also improves image contrast because it focuses on a thin slice of the structure and thus provides better location of anatomic landmarks. This allows the distribution of the radioactive agent to be located precisely.

To improve the ability of TCS to detect and localize otosclerotic foci a correlation study must be performed between metabolic patterns and conventional radiographs or high-resolution CT scans. To date experimental and clinical studies of TCS have examined some temporal bones and only restricted and often undefined groups of otosclerotic patients without control groups.

A study was conducted by Berrettini et al[3] on the sensitivity of SPECT in 36 patients with surgically confirmed otosclerosis using controls. A cutoff value of 1.35 scintigraphic uptake index (UI) was used and only 2 out of 72 ears in the otosclerotic group gave a false negative outcome. Although the otosclerotic disease was bilateral in both patients, the UI was above the cutoff value in only one ear of each patient. Only 1 of 24 ears in the control group gave a false positive result. They therefore conclude that SPECT appears to be very sensitive in differentiating otosclerotic bone from normal bone.

It was noted that the uptake index (UI) values of the otosclerotic patients had a varied range. This was attributed to the different stages of the disease. Lower values were associated with low bone turnover indicating inactive disease whereas higher values were associated with high bone turnover associated with active disease. The mean UI value was 2.214 in otosclerotic patients whereas in the control group it was 1.131. This difference was found to be statistically significant.

In bilateral disease no statistical difference was found between the UI values for both the ears of the same subject. The authors found that this confirmed that otosclerosis is indeed a bilateral disease. It was interesting to note that in this study they found three patients with clinical impairment also had high UI values on the side with normal hearing. They concluded that such findings could be explained that SPECT allows the detection of pathologic increases of bone metabolism even in the absence of clinical manifestations of the underlying process.

When the UI values were considered in relation to gender, no significant differences could be found. However, when age and gender findings were correlated they noted that women under 45 years had a mean UI value that was higher than that of men in that age group. Whereas for women and men above the 45-year age group the values were almost the same. They found this to be in keeping with the observations found on histopathology.

The uptake of the bony labyrinth in relation to age revealed a higher uptake in younger patients. Again these findings were consistent with that of literature where active foci are more likely to be associated with younger patients.

Comparison of SPECT alterations with the severity of sensorineural hearing loss in younger versus older patients revealed a statistically significant correlation in the younger patients. This was found to indicate an increase in bone turnover, increased metabolic activity, and increased incidence of sensorineural hearing loss.

Berrettini[3] thus concluded that SPECT presented a valid imaging technique that detected and localized otosclerotic foci. Another advantage was that it helped quantify the disease. It was also a cost-effective method.

The primary disadvantage was the length of the examination. This was because an interval of 3 hours was required between the injection of the isotope and the acquisition of data on the accumulation of radioisotope in the bone.

SPECT was found to have a sensitivity of 97.2%. At this time it is the only method that provides structural as well as functional data of the labyrinth of otosclerotic patients.

REFERENCES

1. Valvasorri GE. Imaging of otosclerosis. *Otolaryngol Clin North Am.* 1993;26:359–371.

2. Ross UH, Trinhardt MJ, Berlis A. Localization of active otosclerotic foci by tympanocochlear scintigraphy (TCS) using corelative imaging. *J Laryngol Otol.* 1995;109:1051–1056.

3. Berrettini S, Ravecca F, Volterrani D, et al. Single photon emission computed tomography in otosclerosis: diagnostic accuracy and correlation with age, sex and sensorineural involvement. *Otol Neurotol.* 2002;23:431–438.

PART III

Cochlear Otosclerosis and Conservative Management of Otosclerosis

CHAPTER 7

Cochlear Otosclerosis

Chris de Souza and Marcos V. Goycoolea

INTRODUCTION

Otosclerosis exists as a spectrum of disease. On one end is histologic otosclerosis, which is discovered accidentally on postmortem examination and is silent, asymptomatic, and never seems to progress. In the middle is fenestral otosclerosis, which involves the footplate and presents with a conductive hearing loss. At the far end of the spectrum exists cochlear otosclerosis, presenting with rapidly progressive sensorineural hearing loss. Cochlear otosclerosis differs from fenestral otosclerosis in that the sensorineural component of hearing loss is the dominant factor. There may or may not be a mild conductive component, but the chief finding is a sensorineural hearing loss. Surprisingly, speech discrimination scores are good. This helps the clinician decide if the sensorineural hearing loss is caused by cochlear otosclerosis or not. Sensorineural hearing losses caused by other problems are usually associated with poor discrimination scores.

DEFINITION

Cochlear otosclerosis is a gradually progressive sensorineural hearing loss caused by the direct or indirect enzymatic action of the otosclerotic microfoci in the otic capsule. The sensorineural hearing loss is bilateral and symmetrical and may undergo periods of activation and remission.

Pure tone and speech audiometry usually shows either a pure sensorineural hearing loss or mixed type hearing loss.

INCIDENCE

Pure cochlear otosclerosis without stapedial involvement is a difficult condition to identify. The incidence of cochlear otosclerosis is greater than generally believed. Linthicum et al[1] found in a double-blind study on histologic and polytomographic correlations in cochlear otosclerosis that two-thirds of cases were found to have cochlear otosclerosis. However, the clinical incidence of cochlear otosclerosis is much more difficult to determine. Causse and Causse[2] in an evaluation of 11,062 cases found a similar percentage of 22.9% of cases suffering from cochlear otosclerosis. They feel that this percentage would have been higher if polytomography was used systematically. They state further that the incidence of cochlear otosclerosis in progressive sensorineural hearing loss occurs frequently enough to warrant that such patients be evaluated thoroughly to eliminate the possibility of cochlear otosclerosis.

Females are more affected than males and the age of onset is similar to that of stapedial otosclerosis.

The clinical development of cochlear otosclerosis depends on the progression of otosclerotic focus. This in turn depends on other factors such as the genetic predisposition of the patient, endocrine factors such as puberty, pregnancy, and so forth. Because the progress of cochlear otosclerosis depends on wide-ranging factors the disease process itself undergoes periods of activation and periods of remission.

SIGNS AND SYMPTOMS

1. Dominant family history and the patient usually has relatives who have suffered from proven otosclerosis.
2. The hearing loss may have started or increased during pregnancy or following the use of oral contraceptives.
3. Examination of the tympanic membrane can demonstrate a positive Schwartz sign.
4. The patient usually experiences tinnitus and vertigo.

SPECIALIZED HEARING TESTS

1. The commonest pattern of pure-tone audiogram is the "cookie bite" audiogram (Figure 7–1). In cochlear otosclerosis the audiological pattern is one of end organ disease.
2. The Békésey audiogram is usually a type 2.

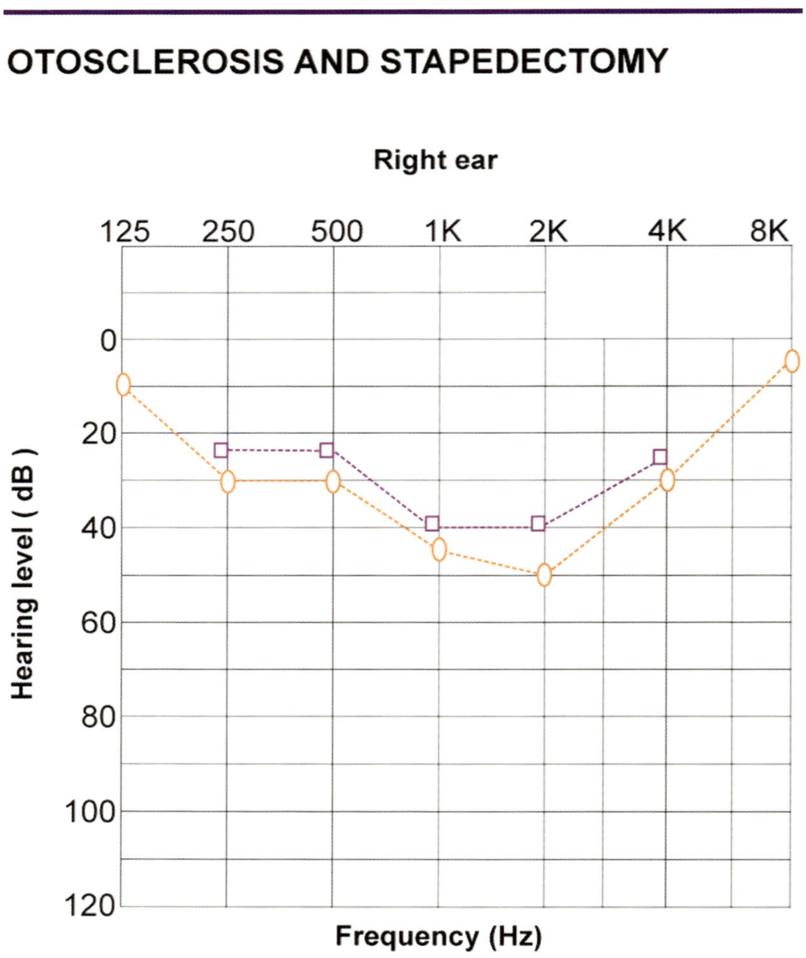

Figure 7–1. Pure tone audiogram demonstrating typical cookie bite pattern.

3. There is a moderate tone decay of up to 20 dB. Speech discrimination scores of 80 to 90% are typical of cochlear otosclerosis.
4. The SISI scores are high (60 to 100%).
5. Loudness discomfort may be present at 10 to 110 dB.
6. The stapedial reflex is usually present. This differs from fenestral otosclerosis where the reflexes are absent.

TINNITUS

This symptom is encountered in the older age group. In pure cochlear otosclerosis tinnitus is usually the dominant symptom.

VERTIGO

With otosclerosis compromising the otic capsule it is reasonable to assume that in some cases there should be involvement of the vestibular system as well. Clinical evidence has shown otosclerotic patients to have symptomatic vestibular involvement in 27% of cases, with 28.8% prevalence when electronystagmographic studies are included and 27.7% when caloric testing is done. Histological changes in the vestibular endosteum has been observed in 63% of temporal bones with otosclerosis.[3]

Vertigo secondary to endolymphatic hydrops is a somewhat frequent symptom. Benign paroxysmal positional vertigo is also commonly seen. Transient episodes of positional vertigo are also commonly encountered.

HOW TO MAKE A DIAGNOSIS OF COCHLEAR OTOSCLEROSIS

Beales[4] has suggested parameters that help identify the patient suffering from cochlear otosclerosis.

1. Sensorineural hearing loss with very good speech discrimination.
2. Recruitment is present, high SISI scores with a Békésey type II audiogram.
3. Progression of a sensorineural hearing loss from early adulthood.
4. The sensorineural hearing loss should be bilateral and symmetrical.
5. The audiometric pattern should be unusual (cookie bite) in configuration.
6. The patient should have a history of successful use of a hearing aid before the hearing loss progresses to a severe degree.
7. A negative Rinne's test.

Causse et al[5] described three criteria for making a diagnosis of cochlear otosclerosis

1. **Criteria of presumption**
   a. Slow progressive sensorineural hearing loss since childhood that gets aggravated at puberty. There should be a family history of progressive sensorineural hearing loss.
   b. Sensorineural hearing loss in a woman aggravated by pregnancy, menstruation, menopause, or following the use of oral contraceptives or following treatment with estrogens.
   c. The patient should have good speech discrimination for a patient who is using a hearing aid and who has a sensorineural hearing loss especially during conversations in noisy surroundings.
2. **Criteria for probability**
   a. A positive Schwartz sign should be present in one or both ears.
   b. A sensorineural hearing loss with a "cookie bite" audiogram.
   c. Positive findings on radiological imaging for otosclerosis.
3. **Criteria of certainty**
   a. The appearance of an "on-off" impedance effect (diphasic impedance change) indicating impending fixation of the stapes in a case of slowly progressive pure sensorineural hearing loss.
   b. An air–bone gap (even a small gap) in one ear in a case of slowly progressive symmetrical pure sensorineural hearing loss and the replacement of the on-off effect by the disappearance of the stapedius reflex.
   c. CT densitometry demonstrating cochlear otosclerosis.

HISTOPATHOLOGICAL CORRELATES

Lindsay and Beale[6] found sensorineural hearing losses in temporal bones with extensive and multifocal otosclerosis. Linthicum[7] demonstrated a relationship between the degree of cochlear endosteal involvement, with hyalinization of the spiral ligament and sensorineural hearing loss. Hueb and Goycoolea[8] in their study found that the otosclerotic focus expands from the anterior margin of the oval window toward the apex of the cochlea and involved the endosteum of the upper half of the basal turn sometimes without stapedial fixation. Cochlear otosclerosis (Figure 7–2) can occur without stapedial fixation though any otosclerotic focus large enough to cause sensorineural hearing loss invariably causes stapedial fixation. They also note that in cochlear otosclerosis the cochlea endosteum was involved only in the area of the basal turn, sometimes with atrophy and hyalinization of the spiral ligament and atrophy of the stria vascularis. Johnsson et al[9] note that this area of the basal turn becomes a target for possible toxic substances released by the otosclerotic focus, which result in sensorineural hearing loss when it involves the endosteum of the scalae, especially when the lesion is active.

MECHANISMS BY WHICH SENSORINEURAL HEARING LOSS IS THOUGHT TO OCCUR IN COCHLEAR OTOSCLEROSIS

1. Toxic metabolites are thought to be liberated by the active otosclerotic focus into the inner ear fluids.
2. Vascular compromise and hypoxic lesions of the structures of the inner ear. The presence of

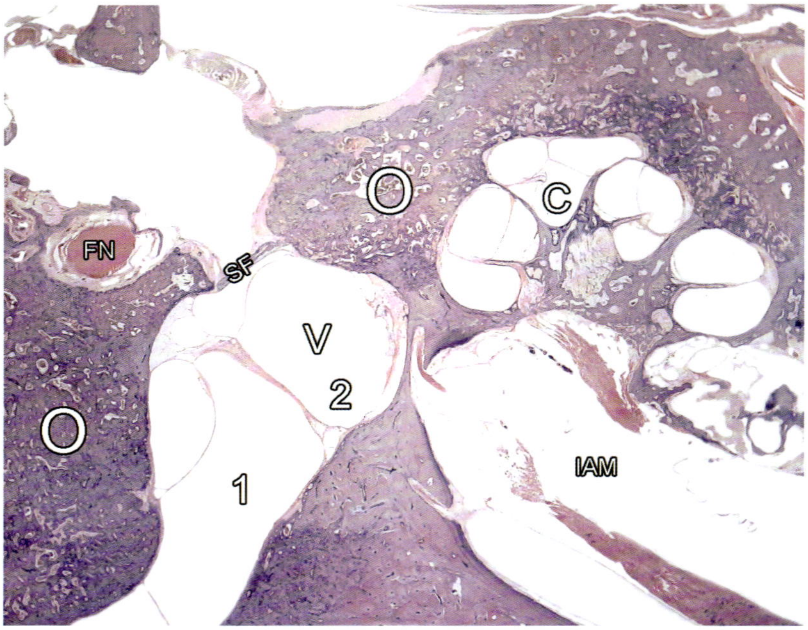

Figure 7–2. Histopathology section of human temporal bone demonstrating cochlear otosclerosis. O = otosclerotic focus; C = cochlea deformed by the otosclerosis; V = vestibule; 2 = saccule; 1 = utricle; SF = stapes footplate; FN = facial nerve. Photo courtesy of University of Minnesota temporal bone collection. Courtesy of Dr. Cureoglu and Dr. Paparella.

venous shunts have been demonstrated between the otosclerotic focus and the vessels of the inner ear that caused venous congestion which resulted in hypoxia of the cochlea.

RADIOLOGICAL DEMONSTRATION OF COCHLEAR OTOSCLEROSIS (Figure 7–3)

Conventional radiography is of little value in otosclerosis especially in the case of cochlear otosclerosis. Linear tomography is of limited value. CT scanning is the only imaging modality that is of some value in otosclerosis. For the otosclerosis focus to be picked up on CT scanning the focus has to be bigger than 1 mm. Otic capsule bone is the densest bone in the body and cannot become more dense. It can, however, increase in thickness. Thus otosclerotic deposits can be picked up in the inactive phase. In the active phase where bone resorption occurs the otic capsule appears roughened or scalloped, its outlines becoming irregular. Derlacki and Valvassori[10] have demonstrated that otic capsule changes can be demonstrated in 65% of patients with fenestral otosclerosis and in 30% of patients in whom cochlear otosclerosis has been suspected.

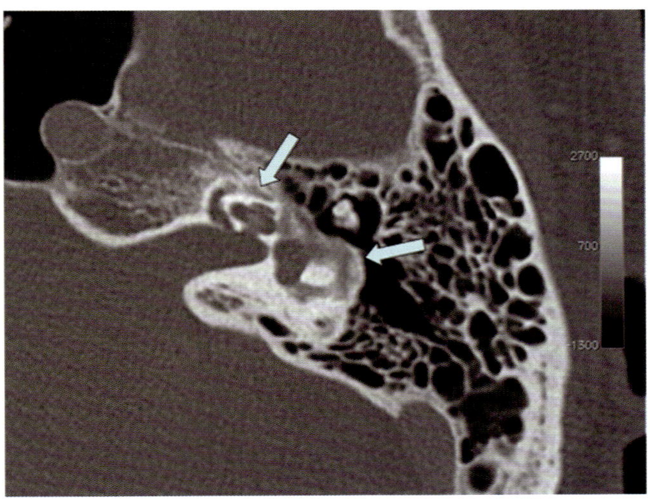

Figure 7–3. CT scan of temporal bone of a patient suffering from cochlear otosclerosis. The cochlea and semicircular canals are demineralized (*arrows*). This is the active phase of otosclerosis. Photo courtesy of Dr. Neil Sperling.

TREATMENT OF COCHLEAR OTOSCLEROSIS

There have been numerous publications on the efficacy of sodium fluoride in the treatment of cochlear otosclerosis. All claim to have arrested the progress of sensorineural hearing loss. In a study by Derks et al[11] CT scanning and audiometric evaluation was used to monitor the progress of 19 patients treated with fluoride for 1 to 5 years and were matched with 22 untreated controls. They found that fluoride was more effective for higher frequencies in cases of sensorineural hearing loss of less than 50 dB. They also found that fluoride treatment for 4 years did not seem to be superior to a shorter treatment. They also noted that CT scanning did not provide reliable information as to the efficacy of fluoride treatment. Hearing loss stabilized and did not progress when on treatment. However, once treatment was stopped six patients experienced minimal deterioration in sensorineural hearing loss. The medical management of cochlear otosclerosis includes sodium fluoride in association with calcium, vitamin D, and diphosphonates.

ROLE OF SURGERY IN PATIENTS SUFFERING FROM COCHLEAR OTOSCLEROSIS

Surgery in patients with cochlear otosclerosis may be useful in those patients presenting with a hearing loss so profound that bone threshold cannot be evaluated and a gap between air and bone conduction cannot be excluded. In such circumstances stapes surgery can improve hearing to a level that may provide a useful application for a hearing aid.

It should be remembered that surgery to be effective must be combined with the administration of sodium fluoride.

SUMMARY

Cochlear otosclerosis is an aggressive and progressive manifestation of otosclerosis characterized by sensorineural hearing loss that is symmetrical and bilateral. Speech discrimination scores are better than one would associate with such a kind of sensorineural hearing loss. Treatment consists mainly of sodium fluoride, calcium, vitamin D, and diphosphonates. Surgery can be beneficial in certain situations. The purpose of surgery is to bring up the hearing to an amplifiable level, which will then benefit from a hearing aid.

REFERENCES

1. Linthicum FH, Ruenas R, Belal A. Histologic and polytomographic correlation in cochlear otosclerosis. In: Shambaugh GE Jr, Shea JJ, eds. *Shambaugh-Shea International Workshop on Microsurgery.* Huntsville, AL: Strode Publishers; 1981:468–471.
2. Causse JR, Causse JB. Prognosis: sensorineural deterioration and cochlear otosclerosis. In: Wiet RJ, Causse JB, Shambaugh GE, Causse JR, eds. *Otosclerosis (Otospongiosis).* Washington, DC: American Academy of Otolaryngology–Head and Neck Surgery Foundation Inc.; 1991: 87–96.
3. Goycoolea MV. Otosclerosis. In: Papàrella MM, Shumrick D, eds. *Otolaryngology*. Philadelphia, PA: W.B. Saunders Co. 1991:1489–1512.
4. Beales PH. Diagnosis of sensorineural deafness. In: *Otosclerosis*. Bristol, UK: John Wright and Sons; 1981:68–75.
5. Causse J, Shambaugh GE, Chevance LG, Bretlau P. Cochlear otospongiosis: etiology, diagnosis and therapeutic implications. *Ann Otorhinolaryngol.* 1975;22:43–47.
6. Lindsay JR, Beals DD. Sensorineural deafness in otosclerosis: observations on histopathology. *Ann Otol, Rhinol Laryngol*. 1966;75:436–457.
7. Linthicum FH. Pathology and pathogenesis of sensorineural deafness. *ENT Digest*. 1967;29:51–56.
8. Hueb MM, Goycoolea MV, Papàrella MM. Otosclerosis: the University of Minnesota temporal bone collection. *Otolaryngol, Head Neck Surg*. 1991;105:396–405.
9. Johnsson LG, Hawkins JE, Linthicum FH. Cochlear and vestibular lesions in capsular otosclerosis as seen in microdissection. *Ann Otol, Rhinol Laryngol*. 1978;87(suppl 48):1–40.
10. Derlacki E, Valvassori G. Clinical and radiological diagnosis of labyrinthine otosclerosis. *Laryngoscope*. 1965;75: 1293–1306.
11. Derks W, de Groot JA, Raymakers JA, Veldmann JE. Fluoride therapy for cochlear otosclerosis? An audiometric and computerized tomography evaluation. *Acta Otolaryngol*. 2001;121:174–177.

CHAPTER 8

Medical Treatment of Otosclerosis

Chris de Souza and Marcos V. Goycoolea

INTRODUCTION

Can medical treatment arrest or reverse the problems caused by otosclerosis? So far, medication has been directed at arresting the progress of otosclerotic lesions. More specifically, medications arresting the progress of sensorineural hearing loss have been reported. There are no reports on medical treatment erasing otosclerotic lesions.

Medical management of otosclerosis is directed at the active phase of fenestral otosclerosis, presumed cochlear otosclerosis, and has also been reported to be given poststapedectomy to prevent an otosclerotic focus from becoming active. This serves to stabilize hearing following a stapedectomy.

HISTORICAL PERSPECTIVE

It was Shambaugh and Scott[1] who first suggested that sodium fluoride in moderate dosages would promote recalcification and reduce bone resorption in an active otosclerotic focus.

In humans fluoride is very effective only when the otosclerotic focus is active and is ineffective when it is not.

WHAT IS FLUORIDE?

Fluoride is a trace element and is found in varying concentrations in ground water. And it varies between 0.1 and 16 parts per million. Some local authorities add fluoride to drinking water to bring the concentration to 1 part per million, and this has proven very effective in preventing dental caries.

Daniel[2] compared the incidence of stapedial fixation in an area of low fluoride concentration with that in an area of high fluoride concentration in drinking water. He found that stapedial fixation was four times higher in the low fluoride concentration than in high fluoride concentrations.

HOW DOES SODIUM FLUORIDE ACT?

Fluorides act by:

1. Reducing bone resorption.
2. Increasing osteoblastic bone formation.
3. Fluorides prevent the release of proteolytic enzymes that are cytotoxic to the cochlea.
4. Sodium fluoride reduces osteoclastic bone resorption and at the same time promotes osteoblastic bone formation. In new bone the fluoride ion replaces the hydroxyl radical in hydroxyapatite; the resulting flucrapatite is harder, of better quality, and more resistant to bone resorption than hydroxyapatite.
5. Sodium fluoride promotes maturation of active otosclerosis by reducing its vascularity and its bone resorption activity and by increasing its new bone formation to eventually produce inactive otosclerosis.

WHAT DOES SODIUM FLUORIDE DO?

It causes the active otosclerotic focus to become inactive. It does not eradicate or erase the otosclerotic focus.

RATIONALE FOR THE USE OF SODIUM FLUORIDE IN OTOSCLEROSIS

The rationale for the use of sodium fluoride for the treatment of otosclerosis is based on the following evidence in the literature:

1. Daniel[2] has demonstrated that there is an increase of stapedial otosclerosis in areas where the levels of fluoride were low.
2. Changes of reversal from active to inactive in the clinical and radiological conditions of patients suffering from cochlear or active fenestral otosclerosis occurs when administered sodium fluoride.

CLINICAL DATA ON THE EFFECTIVENESS OF SODIUM FLUORIDE (NAF)

Bretlau et al[3] conducted a double-blind trial to determine the effectiveness of NaF on otosclerosis. They used calcium/phosphate ratio as an indication of bone maturity. They judged the efficacy of NaF in stabilizing otosclerosis by the retention of calcium levels relative to phosphorous. The clinical double-blind placebo controlled study of 95 patients showed a statistically significant worse deterioration of the hearing loss in the placebo group than in the active treated group (40 mg NaF daily). They state that NaF can change otospongiotic active lesions to more dense inactive otosclerotic lesions.

Causse et al[4] in a study presented their findings taken from 648 perilymph samples taken during stapedectomies performed from February 1976 to September 1980. They studied microdosages of three selected enzymes: trypsin, alpha 1 antitrypsin, and alpha 2 macroglobulin. In each of the samples their relationship with cochlear deterioration expressed in dBs of bone conduction decreased in pure tone audiometry testing. They discovered that NaF not only inhibits direct trypsin inhibition but also an overall reduction in enzymatic values in the perilymph of otosclerotic patients.

INDICATIONS FOR THE USE OF SODIUM FLUORIDE

1. Patients with otosclerosis who demonstrate rapidly progressive sensorineural deafness.
2. Patients who present with sensorineural deafness (cochlear otosclerosis) and have a family history of otosclerosis. Their age of onset should be early with an audiometric pattern suggestive of otosclerosis with good speech discrimination.
3. Patients with radiological changes on CT scanning compatible with that of otosclerosis. These patients should also have a positive Schwartz sign.
4. Patients who have otosclerosis and simultanous hydrops.
5. Stapedial otosclerosis, without sensorineural hearing loss, when surgery has been refused by the patient and the patient seeks alternative forms of treatments.

CONTRAINDICATIONS TO SODIUM FLUORIDE THERAPY

1. Patients who have chronic nephritis with nitrogen retention that could lead to a toxic buildup of fluoride.
2. Patients who suffer from chronic rheumatoid arthritis.
3. Pregnant women and lactating mothers should not receive sodium fluoride.
4. Very young children.
5. Those patients who have an allergy to fluoride.
6. Patients with skeletal fluorosis.

DOSAGE AND ADMINISTRATION OF SODIUM FLUORIDE

In fenestral otosclerosis when the lesion is thought to be active, a daily dose of 50 mg of sodium fluoride can be given.

When the Schwartz sign is positive and a sensorineural hearing loss is present then the dose may be increased to 75 mg daily.

When the hearing stabilizes, Schwartz sign fades, and there is radiological evidence of recalcification, then a maintenance dose of 25 mg can be given for the rest of the patient's life.

A single large dose of 5,000 mg can be fatal.

Fluorical is used as a dietary supplement in the United States and it contains 8.3 mg of sodium fluoride and 364 mg of calcium carbonate. Two capsules of fluorical taken three times a day will supply approximately 50 mg sodium fluoride with 2,184 mg of calcium carbonate. This is sufficient to provide the calcium needed for new bone formation that the sodium fluoride has induced.

Four hundred units of vitamin D is given from time to time to ensure intestinal absorption of calcium.

It is interesting to note that in the United States the Food and Drug Administration has forbidden the sale of sodium fluoride preparations. It is regarded as an unapproved medication despite the fact that sodium fluoride has been used since 1960 for the treatment of osteoporosis and has been given to over 20,000 patients without a single instance of permanent harm.[5]

RESULTS OF TREATMENT WITH SODIUM FLUORIDE

Hearing Loss

Shambaugh and Causse[6] reported the results of treatment with sodium fluoride in over 4,000 patients. Eighty percent of patients who had a sensorineural hearing loss had their hearing stabilized.

This study included a smaller control group that did not receive treatment. This group experienced a more rapid progression of hearing loss.

Clinical proof of the effectiveness of NaF in optimum dosage to promote maturation of active otosclerosis (converting an active otosclerotic focus to an inactive focus) has been very clearly demonstrated.

Shambaugh and Causse[6] demonstrated in a case controlled study of 575 patients that 80% of these patients when treated with NaF exhibited stabilization of their sensorineural hearing loss. Their hearing stabilized and they did not exhibit further deterioration in hearing. Another 3% of these patients demonstrated an improvement in hearing whereas 17% experienced deterioration in hearing despite receiving NaF. In 8% of patients when the sodium fluoride was stopped the sensorineural hearing loss that had stabilized started to progress further, necessitating continued administration of NaF.

Several double-blind prospective studies[7] have confirmed that sodium fluoride does stabilize hearing in sensorineural hearing loss whereas the controls who do not receive treatment continue to experience a deterioration in their hearing.

STAPEDIAL REFLEX

In a study conducted by Colletti and Fiorino[8] the stapedial reflex was evaluated in 93 relatives of those patients suffering from otosclerosis, which was confirmed surgically. The subjects were divided into two groups, the first group was treated with sodium fluoride for 2 years. The second group served as controls. Before the start of the study all subjects (groups 1 and 2) had abnormalities in the reflex morphology as evidenced by a partial to complete on–off effect in one or both ears. Changes in stapedial reflex morphology (from partial to complete on–off and from complete on–off to absence of the reflex) were evaluated at 1 and 2 years. Both groups did not develop significant differences at 1 year. At the second year, however, the incidence of stable stapedius reflex findings was 91.5% in the treated ears and 77% in the control group. The difference was significant (p less than 0.05) and indicated the stabilizing effect of sodium fluoride on the otosclerotic disease process.

CONTROL OF VESTIBULAR SYMPTOMS

Freeman[9] demonstrated that sodium fluoride was effective in reversing symptoms of vestibular dysfunction.

RADIOLOGICAL EVIDENCE OF IMPROVEMENT

Radiological evidence of arrest of otosclerosis is not in itself sufficient evidence that otosclerosis has been arrested. Radiological evidence must be combined with audiological evidence that the progress of otosclerosis has been halted.

Radiological studies have demonstrated that the otosclerotic focus did mature with the administration of sodium fluoride.

ENZYMATIC EVIDENCE

Small doses of sodium fluoride are found to be effective in inhibiting protein metabolism.[10] Sodium fluoride was found to be essential in protecting the hair cells of the labyrinth from toxic damage by the enzymes of bone resorption produced by active otosclerosis.

SIDE EFFECTS OF SODIUM FLUORIDE THERAPY

Those patients who have received sodium fluoride therapy should receive a skeletal survey every 2 years. A skeletal survey should be done before the administration of sodium fluoride. Causse et al[10] has observed radiological evidence of early fluorosis of the spine in 0.25% of patients and this condition is reversible when treatment was discontinued.

Gastric disturbances are a common side effect. This occurs because of the production of hydrofluoric acid in the stomach. This is prevented by enteric coating of the tablet.

Those patients suffering from chronic arthritis may experience an increase in arthralgia in their joints. However, this stops when treatment is stopped.

OTHER MEDICATIONS THAT ARE USED IN THE MEDICAL MANAGEMENT OF OTOSCLEROSIS

Biphosphonates (Diphosphonates)

In case sodium fluoride is not well tolerated then biphosphonates can be given. Biphosphonates are alternatives to NaF that can be used in the treatment of otosclerosis. They are administered orally. Their mechanism of action is that they are incorporated into bone and inhibit osteoclastic activity. Other postulated mechanisms of action are primary enzymatic inhibition and promoting stable secondary new bone formation. They are well tolerated and are effective. Newer biphosphonates have negligible effects on bone formation. Brookler and Tanyeri[11] discovered that etidronate appeared to halt the progression of otosclerotic foci as observed with high-resolution CT scanning. In this past decade biphosphonates like etidronate and alendronate have been used widely for the treatment of osteoporosis with well-documented beneficial effects with no accompanying adverse effects. However, there were a few reports[12, 13] that claim sensorineural hearing loss in otosclerotic patients who were treated with first-generation bisphosphonates, aminohydroxypropylidene, and etidronate. But in the literature the widespread use of alendronate has not been associated with sensorineural hearing loss. The most promising biphosphonates are those potent inhibitors of bone resorption, such as third-generation biphosphonates such as alendronate, residronate, and zolendronate.

Cytokine Inhibitors

Cytokine antagonists may suppress the resorption seen in otosclerosis. Interleukin 1 receptor antagonist and TNF-binding protein have been shown to halt bone resorption that invariably occurs following ovariectomy. It is thought to be quite likely that these factors inhibit bone modeling as well. Cytokine inhibitors are thought to be promising because it is likely that these compounds would halt the progress of otosclerosis. However, it is thought that these would be best used when the otosclerotic focus is in its active phase.[14]

SUMMARY

The medical management of otosclerosis is limited to converting active otosclerotic foci to inactive ones. By doing so the toxins liberated in the active phase of otosclerosis are prevented from being released into the inner ear. This protects the hair cells from the damaging effects of these toxins. This in turn preserves hearing.

Sodium fluoride is the preferred medication of choice, though biphosphonates are also available. NaF has been found to be effective, and can be given for prolonged periods of time without any major side effects.

REFERENCES

1. Shambaugh GE, Scott A. Sodium fluoride for the arrest of otosclerosis. *Arch Otolaryngol.* 1964;80:263.
2. Daniel HJ. Stapedial otosclerosis and fluorine in the drinking water. *Arch Otolaryngol.* 1969;90:585–587.
3. Bretlau P, Causse J, Causse JB, Hansen HJ, Johnsen NJ, Salomon G. Otospongiosis and sodium fluoride. A blind experimental and clinical evaluation of the effect of sodium fluoride treatment in patients with otospongiosis. *Ann Oto Rhinol Laryn.* 1985;94(2 pt 1):103–107.
4. Causse JR, Uriel J, Berges J, Shambaugh GE, Bretlau P, Causse JB. The enzymatic mechanism of the otospongiotic disease and NaF action on the enzymatic balance. *Am J Otol.* 1982;3(4):297–314.
5. Beales PH. Medical treatment. *Otosclerosis.* Bristol, UK: John Wright and Sons; 1981:76–84.
6. Shambaugh GE, Causse JR. Ten years experience with fluoride in otosclerotic (otospongiotic) patients. *Ann Otol Rhinol Laryngol.* 1974;83:635–637.
7. Bretlau P, Salomon G, Johnsen NJ. Otospongiosis and sodium fluoride. A clinical double blind placebo controlled study on sodium fluoride treatment in otospongiosis. *Am J Otol.* 1989;10(1):20–22.
8. Colletti V, Fiorino FG. Effect of sodium fluoride on early stages of otosclerosis. *Am J Otol.* 1991;12(3):195–198.
9. Freeman J. Otosclerosis and vestibular dysfunction. *Laryngoscope.* 1980;90(9):1481–1487.
10. Causse JR, Causse JB, Uriel J, Berges J, Shambaugh GE, Bretlau P. Sodium fluoride therapy. *Am J Otol.* 1993;14(5): 482–490.
11. Brookler KH, Tanyeri H. Etidronate for the neurotologic symptoms of otosclerosis: preliminary study. *Ear Nose Throat J.* 1997;76:371–376, 379–381.
12. Boumans LJ, Poublon RM. The detrimental effect of aminohydroxypropylidene biphosphonate (APD) in otospongiosis. *Eur Arch Oto-Rhino-Laryngol.* 1991;248: 218–221.
13. Yasil S, Comlekci A, Guneri A. Further hearing loss during osteoporosis treatment with etidronate. *Postgrad Med J.* 1998;74:363–364.
14. Chole RA, McKenna M. Otophysiology of otosclerosis. *Otol Neurotol.* 2001;22(2) 249–257.

CHAPTER 9

Hearing Aids and Otosclerosis

Chris de Souza and Marcos V. Goycoolea

INTRODUCTION

Patients suffering from otosclerosis present with a hearing loss. This hearing loss may be conductive, purely sensorineural, or mixed. The unusual characteristic is that, whatever the type of hearing loss in otosclerosis, speech discrimination scores are usually good.

THE ROLE OF HEARING AIDS IN OTOSCLEROSIS

Amplification via hearing aids or assistive listening devices as an authentic alternative to surgical intervention needs to be presented to patients as a viable alternative.[1] It is now a medicolegal responsibility to present these alternatives in an unbiased manner. On occasion there are a number of patients who may be adequately managed with amplification either alone without surgical intervention or following surgery, especially following surgery for far advanced otosclerosis.

SITUATIONS IN WHICH AMPLIFICATION (HEARING AIDS) MAY BE CONSIDERED

Patients who can be managed in such a way include patients with the following conditions:

1. Cannot undergo surgery because of major systemic illnesses.
2. The only hearing ear.
3. Inadequate hearing reserve or poor speech discrimination scores or both.
4. Congenital fixation of the stapes with the real risk of it developing into a nonhearing ear if surgery is contemplated.
5. Surgery is not elected for by the patient.
6. Early (mild) conductive hearing loss.
7. Unsuccessful surgery for otosclerosis upon the other ear.
8. The patient has otosclerosis and Ménière's disease.
9. Those patients who have undergone stapedectomy for far advanced otosclerosis.

CONTROVERSIES

In a paper that generated many rebuttals, Howard[2] states that hearing aids need to be offered to patients as an alternative to surgery to patients who have otosclerosis. O'Connor and Wiet[3] state that when presenting management alternatives to the otosclerotic patient, amplification via hearing aids or assistive listening devices or both must be offered as a viable alternative to surgical and/or medical intervention. This is necessary not only from the medicolegal point of view but also from the ethical point of view as well. This is because a significant number of patients can be managed appropriately solely with amplification.

Lundy[4] in his letter to the editor in response to Howard's paper notes that his reason for advising stapedectomy over a hearing aid is because hearing aids are expensive ($800 to $2,500) per hearing aid, which needs to be replaced every 3 to 4 years. Batteries also need to be changed every 2 weeks. In addition repair costs need to be included, which further pushes up the costs of a hearing aid. He further notes that hearing aids are not covered by Medicare or the vast majority of insurers. He considers that unless hearing aids become a covered benefit of Medicare and insurers, then hearing aids are not truly an equal alternative for the patients who have otosclerosis.

Are the prescriptions of hearing aids a viable, risk-free alternative for the management of conductive hearing losses? Lundy[4] agrees that hearing aids are essentially risk-free. They are risk-free because when used the patient is not subjected to the risk of a possible irreversible, profound sensorineural hearing loss that can occur poststapedectomy. Lundy cautions that hearing aids are not always reliable or available and that the value of treatment is more than just the risks involved.

Most of the authors in response to Dr Howard's paper concede that the major impediment to advocating a hearing aid lies in the problem that they are expensive and are not covered by Medicare and most health insurers in the United States.

Gauthier[5] in a letter to the editor regarding Dr Howard's paper raises the following points:

1. Stapedectomy is covered by most insurance plans, whereas a hearing aid is not.
2. Would not an ethical situation demand that the patient have similar cost and benefit for both options (for hearing aids as well as for stapedectomy surgery)?
3. Is it ethical that only the rich can afford the low-risk option of hearing aids?

REBUTTAL

Gianoli et al[6] raise several points in which he disagrees with the premise that hearing aids are an equal alternative to a successful stapedectomy. They specify that hearing aids are not an equivalent to a successful stapedectomy. They add that the quality of sound produced by a hearing aid is nowhere close to the sound produced by a successful stapedectomy. A successful stapedectomy patient never has trouble with acoustic feedback, never runs out of batteries, and never has to take out his hearing aid while bathing, swimming, and so forth. A successful stapedectomy patient is less prone to accumulation of wax and otitis externa and has less problems with word discrimination in the presence of background noise.

In premise 5, that hearing aids are complication free, Gianoli et al[6] note that they witnessed a patient lose his job because of discrimination caused by a hearing impairment.

Miller,[7] an audiologist, notes in his reply to the editor that he offers hearing aids as an alternative modality of treatment to otosclerotic patients. However, he "tilts" in favor of surgery when there is a large air–bone gap, good to excellent word recognition scores, and good cochlear reserve.

Finally, in his reply to the editor, Howard[8] concedes that hearing aids are not covered by Medicare insurers. This would then cause patients to opt for surgery because stapedectomy is covered by insurance whereas hearing aids are not.

All the authors of the letters to the editor quoted above discuss not the ethicality of the procedure but the ethics of the surgeon who will do the procedure.

The important question they ask is this: "Has the patient been offered amplification as an alternative modality?"

Our view is that amplification must be offered as an alternative modality not just from the aspect of compliance of medicolegal regulations but also from an ethical point of view. That being said it must be stated that everything should be placed in perspective. We feel that the patient should be allowed to meet and discuss with other patients who have undergone a successful stapedectomy as well as those who wear a hearing aid. This will help them appreciate the pros and cons of both modalities.

WHAT IS INFORMED CONSENT?

Informed consent is a sine qua non of any procedure. It is incumbent upon the surgeon to make it clear to the patient the real, albeit low, risk of a permanent irreversible sensorineural hearing loss that may accompany an apparently uneventful and for all practical purposes, successful stapedectomy. And that the permanent irreversible sensorineural hearing loss could be immediate or delayed.

The surgeon should be in a position to indicate to the patient in a language that the patient understands the complications, results, and effects of the surgery that the surgeon has encountered himself while performing this procedure. The figures quoted by the operating surgeon should be from the surgeries that he has performed and not from papers or books published by other authors.

CONCLUSION

The stapedectomy surgeon should discern which patients he feels would genuinely benefit from amplification and those from surgery. He should also be in a position to decide that the patient may still need amplification in situations like far advanced otosclerosis where the hearing is brought up to amplification levels.

REFERENCES

1. Johnson EW. Hearing aids and otosclerosis. *Otolaryngol Clin North Am*. 1993;26:491–502.
2. Howard ML. Is stapedectomy ever ethical? *Am J Otol*. 1998;19:541–543.
3. O'Connor C, Wiet RJ. Hearing aid use: an alternative to surgery. In: Wiet RJ, Causse JB, Shambaugh GE, Causse JR, eds. *Otosclerosis (Otospongiosis)*. Alexandria, VA: American Academy of Otolaryngology–Head & Neck Surgery Foundation Inc. 1991;129–133.
4. Lundy LB. "Ethics" of stapedectomy. *Am J Otol*. 1999;20(1):137–138.
5. Gauthier MG. Never say "ever." *Am J Otol*. 1999;20(1):138.
6. Gianoli GJ, Gonsoulin T, Amedee R, Tabb H, Mann W. Is stapedectomy ever ethical? Faulty premise, faulty conclusion. *Am J Otol*. 1999;20(1):138–139.
7. Miller M. An audiologist replies (letters to the editor). *Am J Otol*. 1999;20(1):140–141.
8. Howard ML. Authors reply in letters to the editor. *Am J Otol*. 1999;20(1):141.

PART IV

Surgical Management of Otosclerosis

CHAPTER 10

Stapedectomy

Chris de Souza and Marcos V. Goycoolea

INTRODUCTION

Stapedectomy represents one of the most demanding surgeries in the entire human body. It demands precision. There is no room for error and it is unforgiving. At the same time, it is one of the most rewarding and satisfying surgical procedures available with a greater than 98% chance of changing somebody's quality of life for the better. Stapedectomy has also undergone a revolution in the way in which it is done. Total stapedectomy has evolved to small fenestra stapedectomy. Lasers have added safety and have reduced complications. The stapedectomy surgeon must be familiar with middle ear anatomy and all the nuances and variations the otosclerosis can bring.

INDICATIONS FOR STAPEDECTOMY

1. The patient should be suspected of having otosclerosis and a bone conduction level of 0 to 25 dB in the speech range and an air conduction loss of 45 dB to 65 dB. The air–bone gap should be at least 15 dB. If the air–bone gap is less than 20 dB the disease may be early and actively growing and the patient's hearing not significantly impaired. The surgeon will likely encounter a floating footplate if surgery is attempted.
2. Far advanced otosclerosis. Patients with hearing losses in the 90 to 100 dB range may be suitable for stapedectomy; surgery might enable them to use a hearing aid.

CONTRAINDICATIONS

Absolute Contraindications

1. The only hearing ear.
2. Active middle ear or external ear infections.
3. When the otosclerotic patient presents with symptoms of hydrops and has vertigo and tinnitus. These should be completely controlled. Only when the patient is symptom-free for a minimum period of 6 months can the patient be considered a suitable candidate for stapedectomy.
4. Stapedectomy is contraindicated in middle ear atelectasis, especially if the atelectasis is severe.

Relative Contraindications

1. General medical diseases that cause the patient to be unfit to undergo surgery.
2. When the patient presents a positive Schwartz sign stapedectomy should not be done at that time. The patient should be given sodium fluoride and observed. Only once the Schwartz sign has receded and the patient disease has stabilized can the patient be considered fit to undergo surgery.
3. Surgery is contraindicated during pregnancy.
4. Surgery is contraindicated in those whose professional activities put them at risk. Patients such as boxers, professional wrestlers, and those who indulge in severe physical strain should avoid having a stapedectomy done until they have given up such activities.

PREOPERATIVE COUNSELING

All patients who are about to undergo a stapedectomy should be told about the pros and cons of stapedectomy. They should be offered the opportunity to seek alternative measures such as hearing aids to help manage the problem.

Patients should be told about the real risk of permanent sensorineural hearing loss, no matter how small the chance is of such an event occurring.

The patient should be given detailed instructions that should be followed in the postoperative period. The patient should be advised against lifting heavy weights, to cough or sneeze without straining, and to avoid instrumenting the ear.

The patient should be instructed to be alert and to report immediately symptoms that might herald complications like vertigo, tinnitus, and hearing loss.

ANESTHESIA

Most surgeons prefer local anesthesia with the patient lightly sedated. This gives the surgeon a chance to check if the patient's hearing improves immediately once the prosthesis has been inserted. The surgeon can check intraoperatively if the patient has any other symptoms such as vertigo or tinnitus immediately. In this way the surgeon can be alerted immediately and take corrective action.

General anesthesia—which used to have a higher risk than local anesthesia—avoids the situation of a struggling patient. The surgical steps can be gone through smoothly. The surgeon is unable to check on the immediate impact of the surgery. The potential disadvantage of this situation is that of using a prosthesis that is too long, with the utriculosacular risks that this involves. However, in our day, general anesthesia is quite safe and it is unlikely that an experienced surgeon will place an excessively long prostheses without realizing it.

Endaural Incision

Endaural incisions are useful if the canal is small or tortuous. Endaural incisions help widen the canal in such circumstances.

Endomeatal Incision

Endomeatal incision is a good incision for a large canal allowing the surgeon to look comfortably into the middle ear while giving the surgeon a good exposure to the structures in the middle ear.

A local anesthetic (1 to 10,000 epinephrine solution in 2% xylocaine) is used to anesthetize the outer ear.

THE TEN STEPS THE SURGEON SHOULD OBSERVE TO PERFORM A STAPEDECTOMY FLAWLESSLY

1. Adequate exposure: The surgeon should be able to get an unhindered view of all the contents and landmarks of the middle ear.
2. Hemostasis. Bleeding should be controlled. Because the surgeon is working in a small space, bleeding can compromise vision of important structures.
3. The bony overhang over the stapedius muscle and stapes should be curetted away to allow the surgeon complete exposure of the footplate. The overhang should be removed until the pyramidal eminence is seen clearly. Both the oval and round window should be clearly seen in their entirety. The chorda tympani is identified, preserved, and gently pushed out of the operative field.
4. Check the mobility of the stapes and the mobility of the malleus. Check if the otosclerotic focus involves the oval window and the round window. Check for other anomalies/ abnormalities.
5. Control hole in posterior part of the footplate is created with the laser.
6. Gentle disarticulation of the stapes from the incus. The anterior and posterior crurae of the stapes superstructure are lysed with the help of the laser. Slight widening (stapedotomy) of the control hole to allow insertion of the prosthesis of choice. Eversion of mucosa over footplate to avoid a perilymphatic fistula
7. Measuring the correct length of prosthesis.
8. Correct placement of the vein/perichondreal seal over the fenestra.

9. Atraumatic insertion of prosthesis into the stapedotomy fenestra over the vein graft/perichondrial seal. This is the most important step because it will determine the result of the stapedectomy. The surgeon must check if the prosthesis is inserted correctly into the fenestra. The seal should be checked. The round window reflex occurs when a drop of saline is placed over the round window. The prosthesis is gently pressed down. If the drop of saline over the round window shimmers or moves then the prosthesis has been placed correctly. The prosthesis is then crimped to avoid excessive movement. The surgeon checks for hemostasis.
10. Correct and careful repositioning of the tympanomeatal flap (TMF). The surgeon makes sure that there is no debris. The TMF if replaced incorrectly can impede an otherwise flawless stapedectomy. If there is a tear in the TMF then the surgeon needs to repair it at this time to avoid a perforation.

SHOULD THE STAPEDIAL MUSCLE BE PRESERVED?

This is an attempt to try to replicate the physiological protective stabilizing effect of the stapes muscle on the prosthesis. Most conventional techniques do not reconstruct the stapedius muscle. Necrosis of the long process of the incus does not occur with reconstruction of the stapedius muscle. This is known as stapedioplasty. The incidence of perilymph fistula is reported to be low with this technique. The disadvantage of this technique is that reclosure of the oval window is higher.

TYPES OF PROSTHESES AVAILABLE

Robinson-Type Prosthesis

The advantage of this prosthesis is that it does not require crimping, and it is relatively easy to insert. The prosthesis is also self-centering. A narrow stem prosthesis is also available that can be used for posterior half footplate removal. This is a metal stem prosthesis designed to fit under the lenticular process of the incus.

Causse-Type Prosthesis

This is made of Teflon and is designed to attach to the long process of the incus. The Teflon ring is spread open and the prosthesis is snapped onto the incus. Teflon has a long memory and it does not require crimping. The prosthesis can be adjusted easily. This prosthesis can be used in small fenestra stapedectomy

Fisch/McGee-Type Piston Prosthesis

It consists of a malleable ribbon-like crook connected to a metal or Teflon stem. The crook is attached to the long process of the incus and must be crimped into position. One advantage of the prosthesis is that the distal end of the prosthesis is scored. This makes checking the exact length of the prosthesis that is required easy. This prosthesis can be used in small fenestra stapedectomy.

House-Type Wire Prosthesis

On one end is a shepherd crook-like arrangement. At the other end is a loop. The crook is attached and crimped to the long process of the incus. This prosthesis is technically more difficult to attach than other prostheses. This prosthesis is used in total stapedectomy.

- Following placement of the prosthesis the malleus is palpated and the movement of the prosthesis inspected. The tympanomeatal flap is repositioned.
- The patient is gently aroused and asked if hearing has improved. The patient is also asked if vertigo or tinnitus is experienced. If the patient experiences sudden vertigo this means that the prosthesis is too long and the prosthesis may need to be replaced with one of an appropriate length. Some doctors check the patient's hearing with a 512 Hz tuning fork.
- The external auditory canal is packed with Gelfoam® or with antibiotic ointment. A stitch is taken over the tragus from where the perichondrium has been harvested.

POSTOPERATIVE CARE

The patient is advised against violent movement in the first 24 hours. Slight dizziness may be experienced, but this usually settles down. Analgesics and antiemetics may be given. The patient is advised against straining. The following day the patient is encouraged to be ambulatory.

Hearing should be checked only a month after the stapedectomy to allow the middle ear to recover from the surgery.

CHAPTER 11

Stapedectomy Versus Stapedotomy

Chris de Souza and Marcos V. Goycoolea

INTRODUCTION

When stapedectomy was in its infancy, total stapedectomy was considered to be the procedure of choice. As time went by it was discovered that total stapedectomy led to a lot of problems, principally, that of perilymph fistulae with resulting sensorineural hearing loss. This then led to the development of the partial stapedectomy, which then evolved to the stapedotomy technique.

Improvement of speech discrimination scores, time tested stable hearing results, and fewer complications have been cited as justification for small fenestra as the technique of choice.

A LOOK AT A STUDY COMPARING TOTAL STAPEDECTOMY, PARTIAL STAPEDECTOMY, AND STAPEDOTOMY

Persson, Harder, and Magnuson[1] examined the hearing results in 407 patients who had undergone partial stapedectomy, total stapedectomy and stapedotomy as primary surgeries. The comparison between the three groups 1 year postoperatively showed the following:

1. The air–bone gap was smaller for partial and total stapedectomy than stapedotomy for all frequencies except at 4 kHz.
2. Partial and total stapedectomy also showed larger improvements of bone conduction thresholds compared with stapedotomy for all frequencies except 4 kHz
3. At the 3-year follow-up the hearing gain for all frequencies (250 to 8 kHz) was larger for partial and total stapedectomy as compared to stapedotomy.
4. Yet when comparing the decline of hearing from 1 to 3 years postoperatively, the hearing gain achieved with partial and total stapedectomy was much more rapid than stapedotomy.
5. Their results therefore showed that in the short term partial or total stapedectomy gives better hearing results even at high frequencies.
6. Stapedotomy on the other hand yielded more stable hearing results over time.

Conclusions

They concluded that all things considered good stable hearing results are seen with stapedotomy.

WHY IS STAPEDOTOMY THE PREFERRED TECHNIQUE FOR OTOSCLEROSIS?

1. Complications are reduced.
2. Hearing results are good.
3. Hearing results are stable for many years.

A tissue seal using vein or perichondrium must be used with this technique.

RATIONALE FOR THE PREFERRED USE OF THE STAPEDOTOMY TECHNIQUE

1. Marquet et al[2] describes the surface tension of perilymph to be an important factor in the protection of the labyrinth. Following stapedectomy the surface tension of the perilymph together with the contact angle of the perilymph on the prosthesis determines the shape of the reparative soft tissue that will close the fenestra. The shape of the meniscus, which is concave, protects the labyrinth by preventing footplate particles from entering the vestibule. In a small fenestra footplate the particles are very minimal and are thus far less traumatic to the contents of the vestibule. This procedure produces complete closure of the air–bone gap in high frequencies.
2. The middle ear is an impedance-matching device that changes sound energy into mechanical energy. In stapedectomy the prosthesis attempts to simulate the action of the footplate and the annular ligament complex.
3. Causse et al[3] have suggested that a small fenestra in the footplate provides adequate energy in the tip of the piston but does not provide adequate energy further distal in the cochlea. Consequently, the high pitched tones in the basal part of the cochlea give successful hearing results from stapedotomy.
4. Causse et al[3] report that the annular ligament of the stapes footplate has significant elastic fibers that add resistance as a mode of protection from excessive vibration. Vein grafts have more elastic fibers even 2 years after being transplanted into the middle ear. The prosthesis and the vein graft act as a single unit, mechanically stimulating the vestibule. The vein graft acts as a trampoline where distortion of the undersurface of the trampoline is not related to small changes in the width of the vibrating body (diameter of the prosthesis) especially if the size of the vibrating body is small compared to the overall surface of the trampoline (fenestra). The vein dampens or attenuates the effect of the prosthesis on the basal turn so no hearing ability is lost.
5. Causse, Causse, and Wiet[4] provide additional reasons for a small fenestra. The fenestra should be approximately 0.8 mm and should be placed in the posterior half of the footplate. Their rationale is the following:
   a. The utricle and saccule are located under the anterior two-thirds of the footplate and thus will not be traumatized by the prosthesis.
   b. Small fenestra avoids release of proteolytic enzymes into the labyrinth by rupture of the otosclerotic focus, which is located anteriorly.
   c. This procedure avoids rupture of neovessels in the otosclerotic focus.
   d. This procedure allows reconstitution of good impedance and compliance around the piston. If the portion of the vein graft located between the rim of the footplate fenestra and the piston edge is approximately 0.2 mm in size there will be sufficient anatomophysiologic reconstitution of a pseudoannular ligament. This behaves in the same manner as the annular ligament would. Explained simply, the seal over the small fenestra acts as a trampoline, exerting pressure equally in all directions. Furthermore, the labyrinth is not traumatized in this situation.

WHAT ARE THE IDEAL DIMENSIONS OF THE STAPEDOTOMY?

The recommended dimensions of the small fenestra are approximately 0.8 mm to 0.6 mm. The prosthesis is generally 1 mm to 2 mm smaller than the fenestration, keeping in mind that an interposed tissue graft can account for 1 mm to 2 mm. A recent meta-analysis studying only cases that did not use an interposed tissue graft, concluded that a 0.6-mm diameter piston prosthesis is associated with significantly better results than a 0.4-mm prosthesis.[5]

WHERE SHOULD THE FENESTRA BE PLACED?

The fenestra should be placed in the posterior half of the footplate in order to avoid trauma to the saccule.

WHAT IS THE INSTRUMENT OF CHOICE WITH WHICH THE FENESTRA SHOULD BE CREATED?

Lasers are the preferred instrument of choice to create a fenestra.

STAPEDECTOMY

Advantages

1. Relatively easier to perform.
2. Good closure of the airborne gap.

Disadvantages

1. Relatively more traumatic to the inner ear.
2. Hearing results (in most reports) decline over time.
3. Relatively more complications like floating footplate, subluxation, and perilymph fistula occur with this technique.

STAPEDOTOMY

Advantages

1. Less traumatic to the inner ear.
2. Stable hearing results over time.[6]
3. Fewer complications like perilymph fistula are associated with this procedure.

Disadvantages

1. Technically more difficult to perform.
2. Closure of air–bone gap not as good as with partial stapedectomy.

WHAT TECHNIQUE SHOULD THE SURGEON EMPLOY? STAPEDECTOMY (PARTIAL OR TOTAL) OR STAPEDOTOMY?

1. The surgeon should employ the technique that consistently and reliably brings about the best possible results in his hands.
2. The results should be able to withstand the tests of time and hearing should be stable.
3. Should the surgeon start out to perform a small fenestra stapedotomy but is unable to do so, he should then settle for a safe, atraumatic, and reliable procedure as the circumstances demand. The operating surgeon should be flexible enough to adapt to the needs of the situation.
4. At all times the procedure should be done in as atraumatic a manner as possible with correct positioning of the prosthesis.

AFTER STAPEDOTOMY WHAT NEXT?

Stapedioplasty is a new technique being advocated by Poe,[7] which represents a laser version of the traditional stapes interposition technique described by Portmann[8] for cases with anterior fixation and a healthy posterior crus. Using a laser Poe vaporized the anterior crus and mobilized the posterior portion of the footplate. This eliminated the need for the use of a stapedial prosthesis. However, this technique was found useful only when the otosclerotic focus was limited to the anterior portion of the footplate. Similarly, Silverstein et al[9] have reported on laser stapedotomy minus prosthesis (Laser STAMP). This is in essence the same technique described by Poe.[7] Silverstein in particular looks at refixation of the newly mobilized footplate. Silverstein et al conclude that laser STAMP is a minimally invasive procedure that over the follow-up period has a low incidence of refixation as evidenced by a lack of progressive conductive hearing loss. The success of this procedure depends upon correct selection of patients. Only those who have an otosclerotic focus limited to the anterior portion of the footplate are considered suitable candidates for this procedure. The final conclusion was that Laser STAMP was a viable alternative to conventional stapedotomy, yielding good results without evidence of refixation of the footplate as seen over an extended period of time.

SUMMARY

Small fenestra stapedotomy provides better hearing results especially in the high-frequency range and is associated with fewer complications.[10] Equally important as the creation of the small fenestra is atraumatic technique using a laser,[11] a good seal using connective tissue rather than Gelfoam® and a good prosthesis.

REFERENCES

1. Persson P, Harder H, Magnuson B. Hearing results in otosclerosis surgery after partial stapedectomy, total stapedectomy and stapedotomy. *Acta Otolaryngol.* 1997;117(1):94–99.
2. Marquet J, Creten WC, Van Camp KI. Consideration about the surgical approach in stapedectomy. *Acta Otolaryngol.* 1972;74:406–411.
3. Causse JB, Gherini S, Lopez A, Juberthie L, Oliver JC, Bastianelli G. Impedance transfer: acoustic impedance of the annular ligament and stapedial tendon reconstruction in otosclerosis surgery. *Am J Otol.* 1993;14:613–617.
4. Causse JB, Causse JR, Wiet RJ. Surgical treatment. *Otosclerosis (Otospongiosis).* Alexandria, VA: American Academy of Otolaryngology–Head and Neck Surgery. 1991;107–126.
5. Laske RD, Röösli C, Chatzimichalis MV, Sim JH, Huber AM. The influence of prosthesis diameter in stapes surgery: a meta-analysis and systematic review of the literature. *Otol Neurotol.* 2011;32:520–528.
6. Levy R, Shvero J, Hadar T. Stapedotomy technique and results: ten years' experience and comparative study with stapedectomy. *Laryngoscope.* 1990;100(10 pt 1):1097–1099.
7. Poe DS. Laser assisted endoscopic stapedectomy: a prospective study. *Laryngoscope.* 2000;110(5 pt2 suppl 95):1–37.
8. Portmann M. Stapes surgery for otosclerosis. In: *The Ear and Temporal Bone.* New York, NY: Masson Publishing; 1979:101–137.
9. Silverstein H, Jackson LE, Conlon WS, Rosenberg SI, Thompson JH. Laser stapedotomy minus prosthesis (Laser STAMP): absence of refixation. *Otol Neurotol.* 2002;23(2):152–157.
10. Goycoolea MV, Hueb MM. Surgery for stapes fixation. In: Goycoolea MV, ed. *Atlas of Otologic Surgery and Magic Otology.* New Dehli, India: JP Brothers; 2012:863–895.
11. Posada R., Fisch U. Stapedotomy and malleo stapedotomy: the Fisch technique. In: Goycoolea MV, ed. *Atlas of Otologic Surgery and Magic Otology.* New Dehli, India: JP Brothers; 2012:897–922.

CHAPTER 12

Lasers in Otosclerosis

Chris de Souza and Marcos V. Goycoolea

INTRODUCTION

The introduction of lasers for the use of carrying out a stapedectomy has significantly improved the results of stapedectomy and reduced complications of this procedure. They offer precision, and cause far less mechanical trauma. Lysis of the crurae, creation of a fenestra are precise and do not subject the footplate to manual mechanical force that could cause subluxation, floating footplate, and all the other complications that occur when the stapes superstructure and footplate are subjected to mechanical force. They also offer excellent hemostasis. Lasers are particularly useful in revision stapedectomy. The laser is used to lyse adhesions and thus avoid avulsing them. Before the advent of lasers adhesions were dissected and this resulted in inadvertent trauma to the contents of the vestibule, which resulted in permanent, irreversible sensorineural hearing loss.[1]

The word laser is an acronym for **L**ight **A**mplification by **S**timulated **E**mission of **R**adiation.

IDEAL QUALITIES REQUIRED IN A LASER FOR USE DURING A STAPEDECTOMY

1. Precision. Precise optics in order to focus the laser beam at the place required.
2. It should be able to vaporize either the bone or the collagen at the oval window in a predictable and controlled manner.
3. The thermal footprint of the laser should not be beyond (deeper) than the site of application. If it penetrated deeper than the site of application it would cause thermal damage to the utricle and the saccule below.
4. The laser should not heat the perilymph.
5. It should be cost effective.

ADVANTAGES OF THE CO_2 LASER

The CO_2 laser has near ideal tissue absorption characteristics.[2] The CO_2 laser energy is absorbed by water. The water component of bone is approximately 60%. At the high power density setting the pulsed laser vaporizes bone and releases heat and tissue into the vapor plume. Because the CO_2 laser energy is absorbed by water, it does not penetrate.

DISADVANTAGES

1. The laser apparatus formerly was quite cumbersome. This has now been overcome by the use of a flexible cable-delivered CO_2 laser.
2. Increased working distance between the microscope and the operative site.
3. Diminished light through the microscope because of the use of the beam splitter.
4. The aiming beam and the working beam do not have the same wavelength, and so it became difficult to focus both together at the same spot.

In short, the CO_2 laser can be said to have optimal tissue characteristics but suboptimal optical characteristics for use in stapedectomy.[1]

ADVANTAGES OF VISIBLE LASERS

1. Convenience of handheld probe for use of lasers during surgery.
2. Spot size can be chosen accurately.

DISADVANTAGES

The visible light lasers depend on char formation to begin creation of a rosette (fenestra) on the footplate. The char absorbs laser energy and creates heat. The laser energy can pass through either directly or by scatter and injure the neural tissue of the utricle or saccule.

CHOICE OF LASER FOR STAPEDECTOMY

The visible lasers, especially the argon Endo-Otoprobe has excellent optical precision and is superior to the CO_2 laser. However, the CO_2 laser has superior interaction of laser energy with bone, collagen, and perilymph.

Fluency threshold studies confirm that 15 to 20 times more argon or KTP energy is required to ablate bone.[2]

Thermocouple experiments demonstate that should correct energy parameters and surgical care during surgery be taken, then both visible and invisible (infrared) lasers can be used safely for stapedectomy.[3]

A pulsed CO_2 laser beam is ideal for revision stapedectomy.

IDEAL SITUATIONS FOR USING THE LASER FOR STAPEDECTOMY

1. Primary (virgin) stapedectomy. The laser offers precision, a controlled manner of how big and where the fenestra should be created, and it avoids the use of manual mechanical force for the removal of the stapes superstructure and creation of a fenestra. Laser offers excellent hemostasis.
2. Revision stapedectomy. Adhesions between the prostheses, the neomembrane, and the contents of the vestibule are lysed in a precise, atraumatic way. The chief cause of failures when the adhesions were mechanically avulsed/dissected was that the saccule and utricle were traumatized resulting in profound irreversible sensorineural hearing losses.
3. Obliterative footplate. Lasers are far better than even a drill-out as they offer precision, control, and no mechanical force and hemostasis.

ADVANTAGES OF LASER STAPEDECTOMY

1. Precision.
2. It avoids the use of manual mechanical force.
3. Good hemostasis.

Lasers are just a tool, and when used correctly and intelligently they offer the surgeon the opportunity to carry out the stapedectomy flawlessly.

SUMMARY

All recent literature overwhelmingly provides evidence that the laser has improved results and lowered complications when used for stapedectomy. The single most important factor is that the laser does away with the use of manual mechanical force. As stated over and over again in this article it offers precision especially when lysing the crurae of the stapes superstructure and in the creation of a fenestra in the footplate. The laser is only a tool and is only as good or as bad as the hand that wields it.

REFERENCES

1. Poe DS. Laser assisted endoscopic stapedectomy: a prospective study. *Laryngoscope*. 2000;95(suppl 110):1–37.

2. Lesinski SG, Newrock R. Carbon dioxide lasers for otosclerosis. *Otolaryng Clin North Am.* 1993;26:417–441.
3. Perkins R. Laser stapedotomy for otosclerosis. *Laryngoscope.* 1980;90:228–241.

CHAPTER 13

The Stapedectomy Prosthesis

Chris de Souza and Marcos V. Goycoolea

INTRODUCTION

The stapedectomy prosthesis has undergone evolution since the first stapedectomy was performed.

There are still issues that face the stapedectomy surgeon. The issues related to the choice of prosthesis are discussed here.

THE IDEAL CHARACTERISTICS OF A STAPEDECTOMY PROSTHESIS?

1. The ideal prosthesis should mimic the function of the stapes as closely as possible.
2. It should be biocompatible.
3. It should not cause problems with the incus or with the neomembrane.
4. It should be of similar weight to the human stapes.
5. The shaft should be long enough to prevent scar tissue from reaching the platform.
6. It should be corrosion resistant and it should not cause allergic reactions.
7. It should be easy to see on radiological imaging modalities especially on MRI without posing a danger of hearing loss.

The material that fits these requirements is titanium. Titanium prostheses are easy to handle; titanium has no spring when it is crimped; it does not bend easily and allows radiological studies with magnetic resonance imaging.[1]

DOES THE WEIGHT OF THE PROSTHESIS INFLUENCE HEARING OUTCOMES?

Bruijn et al[2] compared the individual audiometric hearing results obtained when using gold and Teflon prostheses. He found that the heavier gold prostheses gave more gain in the lower and midfrequency range, whereas the lighter Teflon prosthesis gave more gain in the high-frequency range.

Although changing the weight of the prosthesis has a relatively small effect on the final hearing result, this effect may be significant if it contributes approximately 5 dB gain over other prostheses.

This in turn can be an influential factor in deciding which prosthesis is to be used in patients with mixed hearing losses because a gain of even 5 dB can change the result from a nonserviceable hearing level to a serviceable one.

Robinson[3] too found better hearing results with the Robinson stainless steel prosthesis over the Robinson Teflon prosthesis.

IS THE DIAMETER OF THE PROSTHESIS IMPORTANT?

Fucci et al[4] used a 0.4-mm prosthesis in one ear and a 0.6-mm prosthesis in the other ear. Audiological results were evaluated at 1 month, 6 months, and 1 year postoperatively. All patients underwent partial stapedectomy and vein graft and by the same surgeon. They concluded that a difference of 0.2 mm in the diameter of the prosthesis had no significant effect on hearing. A recent meta-analysis, however, studying only cases that did not use an interposed soft tissue graft, concluded that a 0.6-mm diameter piston prosthesis is associated with significantly better results than a 0.4-mm prosthesis.[5]

WHAT IS THE OPTIMUM LENGTH OF THE PROSTHESIS THAT SHOULD BE IN THE FENESTRA?

The ideal length of the prosthesis that should be in the vestibule in partial stapedectomy is 0.1 mm to 0.2 mm below the fenestra. This allows for excellent hearing, minimizing vestibular symptoms and preventing migration of the prosthesis.

HOW DO PATIENTS VIEW THEIR OUTCOMES FOLLOWING STAPEDECTOMY?

Meyer and Megerian[6] conducted a retrospective study of patients who had undergone stapedectomy. Patients were evaluated by completing two versions of the Hearing Disability and Handicap Scale (HDHS). Their findings revealed that a significant difference between audiometric findings and HDHS scores are useful in identifying patients who might benefit from additional counseling and/or auditory rehabilitation. This is useful in helping patients and surgeon decide to choose any other modality over surgery.

STAPEDECTOMY AND HIGH-FREQUENCY HEARING

Meyer[7] conducted a retrospective study and found statistically significant improvement ($p < .05$) in closure of the air–bone gap between 500 Hz and 4 kHz. Stapedectomy failed, however, to influence hearing above 4 kHz. Age appeared to be an important variable with poorer results in the high-frequency range in older patients.

CAN STAPEDECTOMY BE PERFORMED AS AN OUTPATIENT PROCEDURE?

Corvera and colleagues[8] examined small fenestra stapedectomy as an outpatient procedure. They concluded that it could be done. It should be understood that these were small fenestra procedures.

REFERENCES

1. Goycoolea MV, Hueb MM. Surgery for stapes fixation. In: Goycoolea MV, ed. *Atlas of Otologic Surgery*. New Dehli, India: JP Brothers; 2012:863–895.
2. Bruijn AJG, Tange RA, Dreschler WA. Comparison of stapes prostheses. A retrospective analysis of individual audiometric results obtained after stapedectomy by implantation of a gold and Teflon piston. *Am J Otolaryngol*. 1999;20:573–580.
3. Robinson M. Stapes prosthesis. Stainless steel vs Teflon. *Laryngoscope*. 1974;84:1982–1995.
4. Fucci MJ, Lippy WH, Schuring AG, Rizer FM. Prosthesis size in stapedectomy. *Otolaryngol Head Neck*. 1998;118(1):1–5.
5. Laske RD, Röösli C, Chatzimichalis MV,Sim JH, Huber AM. The influence of prosthesis diameter in stapes surgery: a meta-analysis and systematic review of the literature. *Otol Neurotol*. 2011;32:520–528.
6. Meyer SE, Megerian CA. Patients perceived outcomes after stapedectomy for otosclerosis. *Ear Nose Throat J*. 2000;79(11):846–848.
7. Meyer SE. The effect of stapes surgery on high frequency hearing patients with otosclerosis. *Am J Otolaryngol*. 1999;20(1):36–40.
8. Corvera G, Cespedes B, Ysunza A, Arrieta J. Ambulatory vs in patient stapedectomy: a randomized twenty patient pilot study. *Otolaryngol Head Neck*. 1996;114:355–359.

CHAPTER 14

Bilateral Otosclerosis

Chris de Souza and Marcos V. Goycoolea

INTRODUCTION

Otosclerosis is usually a bilateral phenomenon.

When a patient presents with otosclerosis in both ears, the surgeon is confronted with the decision of whether both the ears should be operated upon. If so, then what are the factors that will help the surgeon decide if and when the contralateral ear should be operated upon? The reason this question presents itself is because stapedectomy carries the risk of profound, irreversible sensorineural hearing loss even if the procedure has been initially uneventful and performed by experts. The other nonoperated ear is considered the reserve ear. Should the ear that has undergone stapedectomy experience problems then the nonoperated ear should not be operated upon.

This is a controversial subject with many for and against.[1]

It has been found that even with the best techniques permanent cochlear hydrops can result from surgery.[2] Causse, Causse, and Wiet[3] have found that 1 patient of 7,000 can develop profound sensorineural hearing loss.

SITUATIONS THAT ARE CONSIDERED A CONTRAINDICATION FOR SECOND EAR STAPEDECTOMY

1. If the patient develops complications following the first surgery then the second ear should not be operated upon.
2. If the patient develops tinnitus and/or persistent vertigo following surgery upon the first ear then stapedectomy should not be carried out on the second ear.

ARGUMENTS AGAINST SECOND EAR STAPEDECTOMY

1. It is impossible to guarantee a long-term successful result.
2. The second ear should be preserved as a reserve ear should the operated ear develop complications.
3. The actual figures reported of sensorineural hearing loss may be higher than those reported because many patients are lost to follow-up.
4. An initial successful stapedectomy can fail many years later, resulting in profound sensorineural deafness.
5. Today there is a marked decrease in the number of patients undergoing stapedectomy, leaving younger surgeons with less experience in dealing with these complicated and technically challenging problems.
6. An inexperienced surgeon should never operate upon the second ear.

HOW LONG SHOULD ONE WAIT BEFORE OPERATING ON THE OTHER EAR?

Causse, Causse, and Wiet[3] recommend that the second ear be operated upon after a minimum period of 1 year if the other ear is doing well in terms of hearing as well as in terms of vestibular symptoms. The reason cited is that surgically induced severe cochlear deterioration (profound irreversible sensorineural hearing loss) usually occurs within the first year postoperatively. If any hearing loss occurs after that it usually manifests itself as a conductive hearing loss.

In predicting success to patients who are to undergo surgery upon the second ear the surgeon should consider the following:

1. If the first ear was anatomically normal and the procedure was successful, there is a 95% chance that the procedure in the second ear will be successful too. Most abnormalities occur at a bilateral rate of approximately 25% in the other ear.
2. The abnormalities that can occur include promontory overhang, malleus fixation, and a dehiscent or overhanging facial nerve.

Abnormal middle ear findings during stapedectomy occur in a significant percentage of patients.[4] Reasonable rates of success and overclosure can still be expected, but this is findings-specific. Understanding this, the percentage of bilateral abnormalities and their impact on predicting rates of success can help the surgeon counsel the patient correctly.

It should not be the patient's request for second ear surgery that should direct the surgeon regarding his decision whether to perform surgery on the second ear. Instead it should be the surgeon's opinion regarding the patient's general health and otological health as to whether to go through surgery upon the other ear with a good chance for a successful outcome that should dictate his decision regarding surgery.

With this goal in mind the surgeon should be familiar with all the nuances of stapedectomy, should be very experienced, and should have the best possible equipment for performing the surgery.

REFERENCES

1. Porter MJ, Zeitoun H, Brookes GB. The Glasgow benefit plot used to assess the effect of bilateral stapedectomy. *Clin Otolaryngol.* 1995;20:68–71.
2. Smyth GD, Kerr AG, Singh KP. Second ear stapedectomy: a continued controversy. *J Laryngol Otol.* 1975;89:1047–1056.
3. Causse JB, Causse JR, Wiet RJ. Special conditions in otosclerosis surgery. In: Wiet RJ, Causse JB, Shambaugh GE, Causse JR, eds. *Otosclerosis (Otospongiosis).* Alexandria, VA: American Academy of Otolaryngology–Head and Neck Surgery; 1991:134–152.
4. Daniels RL, Krieger LW, Lippy WH. The other ear: findings and results in 1,800 bilateral stapedectomies. *Otol Neurotol.* 2001;22:603–607.

CHAPTER 15

Revision Stapedectomy

Chris de Souza and Marcos V. Goycoolea

INTRODUCTION

Revision stapedectomy is one of the most demanding surgeries in otology. The causes of failure are many and the operating surgeon must be familiar with all the nuances of stapedectomy. If the surgeon is revising a surgery that he has done he will be at an advantage because he will be familiar with the anatomy he encountered. Revising a surgery performed by someone else is a challenge especially if it was done some time ago.

THE DANGERS THAT ACCOMPANY REVISION STAPEDECTOMY

Histopathologic studies on stapedectomy patients conducted by Schuknecht[1] have shown adhesions between the prosthesis or the oval window neomembrane and the utricle and saccule. Surgical manipulation of the prosthesis or neomembrane could rupture these delicate inner ear structures resulting in permanent profound sensorineural hearing loss, which is accompanied by vertigo.

This being so, the surgeon must discover the reason why a stapedectomy has failed, and this will entail manipulating the various structures in the middle ear. This runs the risk of a permanent sensorineural hearing loss.

The introduction of lasers for revision stapedectomy has significantly contributed to improvement in results in hearing while at the same time lessening the incidence of complications. The argon, KTP, and carbon dioxide lasers have all been reported to be very useful in revision stapedectomy.[2]

WHAT ARE THE CAUSES OF THE REAPPEARANCE OF A CONDUCTIVE HEARING LOSS FOLLOWING STAPEDECTOMY?

Most authors[3,4] report that the most common causes for residual conductive hearing loss or the reappearance of a conductive hearing loss following stapedectomy are the following:

1. Migration (displacement) of the stapes prosthesis.
2. Erosion of the incus causing the prosthesis to be displaced.
3. Fibrous adhesions.
4. Regrowth of the otosclerotic focus or the appearance of postoperative reparative new bone formation.
5. Obliteration of the round window by otosclerosis that went unrecognized at the primary surgery.
6. Incorrect placement of the prosthesis.

INCUS EROSION (RESORPTIVE OSTEITIS = RO)

The cause of RO of the incus is thought to be due to:

1. Pressure necrosis, due to medial fixation of the strut, a loose crimp, or damage to the mucosa

enveloping the incus, which is presumed to provide anastomotic blood supply to the incus.[5,6]
2. Postoperative inflammation as a common etiology.
3. Biological bone vibrating against a fixed inert prosthesis. A loosely crimped wire loop prosthesis was usually the cause of incus erosion. Over crimping was never a factor. The erosion invariably began on the undersurface of the incus. The longer the duration of the conductive hearing loss the greater the degree of erosion.

Nadol[7] postulates that RO of the incus could well be caused by the differential motion of the incus at the junction of its attachment to the prosthesis. Thus, if motion of the prosthesis is limited by fibrosis this would in turn lead to movement of the attachment portion of the prosthesis with reference to the incus. This in turn leads to friction between the prosthesis and the incus, which could likely result in resorptive osteitis.

OBLITERATION OF THE ROUND WINDOW BY OTOSCLEROSIS

Nadol[7] comments that in his series the incidence was high (5 out of 22 cases) and notes that in literature such a finding is not common. He goes on to state that in the operative notes the operating surgeon had neglected to mention the condition of the status of the round window. He therefore advocates that all otosclerosis surgeons carefully inspect the round window and check for its patency at the time of primary stapedectomy. If round window obliteration by otosclerosis is present then it should be dealt with during the primary surgery. This would help reduce unnecessary revision procedures.

PROSTHESIS ABUTTING THE BONY MARGIN OF THE OVAL WINDOW OR ON RESIDUAL FOOTPLATE FRAGMENTS

Meticulous technique prevents this from occurring. Blood can obscure complete visualization of the footplate, which in turn can lead to creation of an inadequate fenestra, which could lead to the prosthesis migrating to the remnants of the stapedial footplate resulting in a postoperative conductive hearing loss. To prevent this from occurring excellent hemostasis and proper magnification can help visualize the footplate. Creation of a clean and adequate fenestra will then minimize the chance of such an event from occurring.

MALLEUS FIXATION

This should be recognized as far as possible in the preoperative period. Briefly, it may be stated that with the pneumatic otoscope it is possible to determine if malleus fixation is present. If the excursion of the tympanic membrane is shallow during the inflation of the bulb then malleus fixation is more likely to be present. Intraoperatively, the surgeon must check the mobility of each individual ossicle independently. When mallus fixation has been detected it has to be dealt with in the appropriate manner. This will usually entail a malleovestibularpexy described elsewhere in this book.

NEW BONE FORMATION IN THE OVAL WINDOW

In Nadol's series new bone formation occurred when a drill out technique for oval window obliteration was used. He notes that the new bone that appeared was different from otosclerotic bone. The bone appeared to be consistent with reparative bone rather than otosclerotic bone. This was seen exclusively in the patients who required a drill-out for an obliterated oval window. The clinical implication of this finding is that when a drill is used to drill out an extensively obliterated oval window the surgeon should expect the formation of new bone and thus should make the final fenestra much larger than the piston prosthesis to accommodate the occurrence of new bone formation without it resulting in a postoperative conductive hearing loss. Nadol finally concludes his report by stating that there are possibly other etiologies at work that could cause a conductive hearing loss, notably piston diameter. A piston diameter of 0.8 mm is adequate. However, a piston diameter of 0.3 mm would be more likely to result in a conductive hearing loss.

LASER: THE TOOL TO BE USED IN REVISION STAPEDECTOMY

The laser is the instrument of choice in performing a revision stapedectomy. Revision stapedectomy should be performed by an experienced surgeon.

CRITERIA FOR REVISION STAPEDECTOMY

1. Revision stapes surgery is generally reserved for patients who continue to have a conductive hearing loss after initial hearing improvement.
2. Progressive, fluctuating sensorineural hearing loss or incapacitating vertigo will need exploration. A perilymphatic fistula should be anticipated.
3. Since revision stapes surgery is fraught with difficulties a larger air–bone gap is needed as an indication for surgery. Horn et al[8] use a 20 dB air–bone gap as a minimum hearing loss for revision surgery.

SUMMARY

1. Only an experienced otosclerosis surgeon should perform a revision stapedectomy.
2. A laser should be used when performing a revision stapedectomy.
3. Revision stapedectomy should be performed at the earliest as the commonest cause is migration of the prosthesis and the incus may not be that extensively eroded.
4. Attaching the prosthesis to the incus has a better chance of improving hearing.
5. Some authors recommend waiting for 6 weeks after the primary surgery before revising the stapedectomy. This time interval will allow the postoperative reaction to resolve. Otherwise, bleeding and edema will impede surgery.
6. Local anesthesia should be used when operating on a revision in order to better monitor vertigo and hearing losses.
7. A tissue seal (vein or perichondrium) should be used over the oval window. As this: (a) prevents a perilymphatic fistula from forming. (b) If fistulas of the oval window are present they may not always be evident. A tissue seal (vein or perichondrium) will close even those fistulas that are not apparent. (c) Absorbable gelatin sponge should never be used to create the neomembrane as it will not safely support a rigid piston.
8. There is controversy as to whether the neomembrane interfacing between the prosthesis and the vestibule should be opened. In cases of doubt or difficulty the neomembrane should be left alone. If manipulated blindly this can cause a profound sensorineural hearing loss.
9. When otosclerosis regrowth is encountered the growth should be left alone.
10. If the problem cannot be identified (negative findings) those cases with the tissue seal should be left undisturbed.

REFERENCES

1. Schuknecht H. *Pathology of the Ear.* Cambridge, MA: Harvard University Press; 1974.
2. Palva T, Ramsey H. Revision surgery for otosclerosis. *Acta Otolaryngol.* 1990;110:416–420.
3. Ayache D, El Kihel M, Eetsch C, Bou Malhab F, Elbaz P. Revision surgery of otosclerosis: a review of 26 cases. *Annales d'Oto-laryngologie et de Chirurgie cervico faciale.* 2000;117(5):281–290.
4. Fisch U, Acar GO, Huber AM. Malleostapedotomy in revision surgery for otosclerosis. *Otol Neurotol.* 2001; 22(6):776–785.
5. Anson BJ, Harper DC, Winch TR. Intraosseous blood supply of the auditory ossicles in man. *Ann Oto Rhinol Laryngol.* 1964;73:645–653.
6. Sttot C. Stapedectomy revision. In: Goycoolea MV, ed. *Atlas of Otologic Surgery.* New Delhi, India: JP Brothers; 2012:939–942.

7. Nadol JB. Histopathology of residual and recurrent conductive hearing loss after stapedectomy. *Otol Neurotol.* 2001;22:162–169.

8. Horn KL, Gherini SG, Griffin GM. Revision stapes surgery using the fiberoptic argon laser. *Oper Techn Otolaryngol Head Neck.* 1998;9(2)88–93.

PART V

Complications of Stapedectomy

CHAPTER 16

Post-Stapedectomy Perilymph Fistula

Chris de Souza and Marcos V. Goycoolea

INTRODUCTION

Perilymph fistula is one of the common causes of sensorineural hearing loss following stapedectomy.

Perilymph fistulae have been observed with all types of stapes prostheses and with all techniques.

SIGNS AND SYMPTOMS OF PERILYMPHATIC FISTULA

1. Fluctuating sensorineural hearing loss
2. Roaring tinnitus
3. Vertigo
4. Fullness in the ear

If it occurs immediately following surgery the diagnosis of perilymphatic surgery is obvious and is termed as "primary" or "early" perilymphatic fistula. However, if symptoms occur long after stapedectomy then establishing a diagnosis of perilymphatic fistula may not be that easy. This fistula is termed as "delayed" or "secondary" perilymphatic fistula.

INCIDENCE

Perilymph fistulas account for 9% to 10% of failures of stapedectomies.

"EARLY" (PRIMARY) PERILYMPH FISTULA

The primary perilymph fistula occurs when the fistula created at the time of surgery persists and fails to seal off the vestibule from the middle ear. This can occur immediately following surgery and symptoms can persist for days and weeks following surgery.

SIGNS AND SYMPTOMS

The typical symptoms consist of fluctuating hearing loss, tinnitus, and vertigo.

The signs and symptoms vary with the size of the leak. Large fistulas result in rapid hearing loss, tinnitus, and vertigo. Morrison[1] notes that such large fistulae accompanied technical difficulties by the operating surgeon at the time of stapedectomy. Fluctuation in hearing loss is unlikely to be a feature in such a situation. In early perilymph fistulas when the leak is small the hearing loss may initially appear as a conductive hearing loss and then has a sensorineural component and then progresses to a total sensorineural hearing loss. When such a fistula is repaired late the hearing does not improve, though vertigo may resolve. When a minute fistula is present the only evidence of the fistula is failure of a good closure of an air–bone gap, mild fluctuation in hearing, and small decrease in speech discrimination scores.

CAUSE OF PRIMARY PERILYMPH FISTULA

Improperly sealed oval window fenestras are the cause of such fistulae. Goodhill[2] states that if a mucosal seal does not hermetically seal off the vestibule from the middle ear at the time of surgery then the chances of such a fistula forming are high. Failure to reflect the mucoperiosteal flaps may allow the lacerated edges of tissue to extend down into the vestibule and prevent formation of a new endosteal membrane at the level of the oval window. A prosthesis that is too long will also prevent the fistula from sealing off.

Numerous studies[3] have shown that the use of gelatin sponge (Gelfoam®) as a seal for the oval window fenestra is associated with a high incidence of perilymph fistula. Sheehy and Perkins[4] compared gelatin sponge fat and fascia as seals for the fenestra and found that the incidence of perilymph fistula was 3.5% when gelatin sponge was used, 1.9% when fat was used, and 0.6% when fascia was used. Lippy and Schuring[5] compared the incidence of perilymph fistula formation with the use of gelatin sponge versus that of the Robinson vein graft prosthesis. They report a significant difference: 50% for gelatin sponge and 4% for tissue seals. Gelatin sponge is found to be inadequate as an oval window seal because: (1) it may be resorbed before the neomembrane has formed, (2) the gelatin sponge will get softened by the perilymph and the prosthesis will penetrate through the gelatin sponge causing a perilymph fistula, and (3) the neomembrane that forms with a gelatin sponge is very thin and gets perforated repeatedly by the prosthesis leading to the formation of a perilymph fistula.

LATE (DELAYED OR SECONDARY) PERILYMPHATIC FISTULA

Such a fistula can occur long after a successful stapedectomy. Morrison[1] states that this is often the cause of sensorineural deafness that sometimes occurs long after a successful stapedectomy. Most authorities state that the longer stapedectomy patients are followed up the greater the chances of perilymphatic fistula occurring. He found that in 50% of late perilymphatic fistulae no obvious cause could be discerned. In the other patients pressure changes (barotrauma) from flying, mountaineering, lifting heavy objects, coughing, sneezing, and head injury. Otitis media following stapedectomy is not likely to cause a perilymph fistula.

CLINICAL FINDINGS

Clinical examination of the ear will appear normal to external appearances. Occasionally, the tympanic membrane will be retracted.

AUDIOMETRIC EVALUATION

Pure tone audiometry usually reveals sensorineural hearing loss in the low frequencies followed by a flat sensorineural hearing loss that fluctuates. Recruitment will be present in the initial stages and short increment sensitivity index (SISI) scores are often above 75%. In the early stages speech discrimination scores fluctuate with the pure tone thresholds. Later on they may lower disproportionately. A variable conductive hearing loss may be seen.

VESTIBULAR TESTS

1. Hallpike caloric tests
   Canal paresis or a hypoactive response is a likely finding. However, it must be appreciated that there is a high incidence of diminished caloric response. Thus, it becomes difficult to assess the true value of its significance in using it to diagnose the presence of a perilymph fistula.
2. Electronystagmography (ENG)
   ENG may reveal a direction fixed positional nystagmus. But again this cannot be used to diagnose a perilymph fistula.

3. Fistula test
   Fistula tests with a pneumatic otoscope have been found to be negative in one-third of the cases. However, fistula tests with ENG give a higher degree of accuracy.

RESULTS OF THE ENG FISTULA TEST

Beales[6] reports that 16 patients who had a negative fistula test but in whom a fistula was suspected were reoperated on to rule out a fistula. Only one had a perilymph fistula. Although out of six patients with a positive ENG fistula test five were found to have a fistula. Thus, the incidence of false positive and false negative findings was low enough to make this test reasonably reliable.

RADIOLOGICAL EVALUATION

There have been reports on the use of high-resolution CT scanning to detect the presence of perilymphatic fistula. High-resolution CT scans 1 mm slice thickness in the axial and coronal planes were taken. Reports of an air bubble (in the vestibule) at the end of the prosthesis were considered to be an indirect sign of the presence of a perilymphatic fistula. This was the finding in six patients and all were found to have perilymphatic fistula. This was found to be quite a sensitive finding. Thus, a CT scan was found to be of value in detecting the presence of perilymphatic fistula poststapedectomy.

HOW CAN A PERILYMPH FISTULA BE PREVENTED?

Following are what the surgeon should keep in mind to avoid a perilymph fistula:

1. Reflect the mucosa off the footplate completely before making a fenestra.
2. Stapedotomy technique is less likely to result in perilymph fistula formation.
3. Tissue graft seal (vein or perichondrium) over the fenestra can act as a barrier between the perilymph (vestibule) and the prosthesis.
4. The prosthesis should be securely placed on the incus to prevent it from migrating.
5. Do not use Gelfoam® as a seal.

Postoperatively the patient should be instructed to carry out the following:

1. Avoid trauma to the head.
2. Cough and sneeze with the mouth wide open.
3. Do not strain against a closed glottis.
4. Avoid the possibility of barotrauma for at least a month following stapedectomy.
5. Avoid lifting heavy weights.
6. Report immediately if symptoms like vertigo, tinnitus, or hearing loss manifest themselves.

MANAGEMENT OF A PERILYMPH FISTULA

Surgical closure of the fistula is the treatment of choice. Many surgeons consider this to be a surgical emergency. It is important that the field be kept dry to inspect the oval window area to see if perilymph oozes out. If the leak is not visible then the patient's head should be lowered and the internal jugular vein on the same side should be compressed in an effort to make the leak visible. Causse, Causse, and Wiet[7] devised a test to help detect a perilymph fistula intraoperatively. They use a 1.0-mm diamond bur to remove fibrous adhesions from the oval window. This can now be replaced by lasers.

To confirm that a fistula is present they place a small piece of Gelfoam® at the site of the suspected fistula. They then test it on Clinitest glucose test paper. If the paper turns red then perilymphatic fluid is present, indicating the presence of a perilymphatic fistula.

Once the leak is detected then the fistulous tract is excised and the prosthesis removed. Lasers have proved immensely helpful and are excellent working tools in such a situation. The mucosa over the footplate is elevated completely.[8] A fresh soft tissue seal is placed over an adequately created fenestra. A new adequate prosthesis is placed over the seal. The patient is advised total rest in bed for 48 hours.

RESULTS OF TREATMENT OF PERILYMPH FISTULAS

Improvement of hearing especially once sensorineural hearing loss is present is low. By then usually serous labyrinthitis has been well established.

However, early repair of perilymph fistulas help symptoms like vertigo resolve. Tinnitus may not resolve completely. Thus, the treatment of choice is to diagnose perilymph fistulas early and to treat them as a surgical emergency.

REFERENCES

1. Morrison WW. Otosclerosis: diseases of the otic capsule. In: Ballantyne J, Groves J, eds. *Diseases of the Ear, Nose and Throat*. Vol 2. New York, NY: Appleton-Century-Crofts, Inc.; 1984:405–464.
2. Goodhill VH. The conductive hearing loss phenomenon in poststapedectomy perilymphatic fistulas. *Laryngoscope*. 1967;77:1179–1190.
3. Sheehy JL, Nelson RA, House HP. Revision stapedectomy: a review of 258 cases. *Laryngoscope*. 1981;91:43–51.
4. Sheehy JL, Perkins JH. Stapedectomy: Gelfoam® compared with tissue grafts. *Laryngoscope*. 1976;86:426–443.
5. Lippy WH, Schuring AG. Stapedectomy revision following sensorineural hearing loss. *Otolaryngol Head Neck*. 1984;92:580–582.
6. Beales PH. The perilymph fistula after stapedectomy. *Otosclerosis*. Bristol, UK: John Wright and Sons Ltd.; 1981:148–168.
7. Causse JB, Causse JR, Wiet RJ. Special conditions in otosclerosis surgery. *Otosclerosis (Otospongiosis)*. Alexandria, VA: American Academy of Otolaryngology–Head and Neck Surgery Foundation Inc.; 1991:134–152.
8. Goycoolea MV, Hueb MM. Surgery for stapes fixation. In: Goycoolea MV, ed. *Atlas of Otologic Surgery and Magic Otology*. New Dehli, India: JP Brothers; 2012:863–895.

PART VI

Miscellaneous

CHAPTER 17

Obliterative Otosclerosis

Chris de Souza and Marcos V. Goycoolea

INTRODUCTION

Obliterative otosclerosis is a condition where the oval window is totally obscured by the otosclerotic focus and cannot be delineated from its surroundings.

CLINICAL FEATURES

It is associated with:

1. Very advanced otosclerosis.
2. Teenage: Develops at around puberty.
3. The oval window is affected. The round window is usually spared total obliteration.
4. It is bilateral.
5. Drilling out the obliterated footplate is accompanied by a sensorineural hearing loss.
6. Reclosure of the drilled away footplate occurs in 50% of cases.
7. Some consider obliteration to be a contraindication for stapedectomy.

PATHOLOGY

The same aggressive immunoenzymatic process seen in cochlear otosclerosis is responsible for causing obliteration. The stapes superstructure and its crura are buried by the obliterative otosclerotic focus.

INCIDENCE

Gristwood[1] reports a 12.5% incidence of obliterated footplates, most were adolescents. Gristwood and Venables[2] report that they have no evidence that pregnancy increases the progression of obliterative otosclerosis.

The male-to-female ratio was 1.48 males compared to 1 for females. The mean age at onset was 19 years.

TYPES OF OBLITERATED FOOTPLATES

A. Truly obliterated footplate
The boundaries of the footplate cannot be identified and there is no delineation present to indicate the margins of the footplate. The crura of the footplate are covered and sometimes buried by the massive otosclerotic focus. The otosclerotic bone may be up to 2.5 mm thick.

B. Partly obliterated footplate
The footplate is diffusely thickened. However, a rim of delineation can be identified.

C. Spuriously delineated footplate
It only becomes clear that the delineation (rim surrounding the footplate) is false when the

surgeon tries to remove the footplate and fails because the surgeon finds the footplate thicker than expected.

D. Biscuit footplate
This has been called the *"biscuit"* or *"rice grain"* footplate in literature. This footplate is diffusely thickened while retaining a clear, well-delineated rim and an intact annular ligament. This "biscuit" footplate is more likely to get dislodged and get subluxed during surgery. This would either result in a floating footplate or a subluxed footplate.

E. Crowded oval window niche
In this situation the oval window is crowded by the otosclerotic focus. A slit-like opening is all that is seen. The footplate is not truly obliterated. The overhanging bone should be removed with care in order to fully visualize the footplate.

ROUND WINDOW OBLITERATION

The round window is the second most common site at which otosclerosis occurs. But it is still uncommon to get total obliteration of the round window. Obliteration of the round window has a sensorineural component as opposed to a conductive element seen with obliteration of the oval window. Hearing loss occurs only when the round window niche is totally obliterated. Even if there is a small opening it is thought to be adequate for vibratory motion of the cochlear fluids between the round and oval windows. Obliterated round windows should not be drilled out as this leads to profound sensorineural hearing losses. Delayed round window closure can occur following stapedectomy for far advanced otosclerosis. Should round window obliteration occur some surgeons consider this an indication for sodium fluoride therapy.

CAN AN OBLITERATED FOOTPLATE BE DETECTED BEFORE SURGERY?

Obliterative otosclerosis cannot be diagnosed on the basis of clinical and audiometric evaluation. It is usually diagnosed during surgery. However, recently high-resolution CT scanning can help diagnose an obliterated footplate.

MANAGEMENT OF THE OBLITERATED FOOTPLATE

Medical Treatment

Sodium fluoride therapy has been found to be useful in slowing down the progression of obliteration of the footplate, especially when Schwartz sign is positive. The treatment of choice of an obliterated footplate is surgery (stapedectomy). A dosage of 25 mg to 50 mg is advised for 6 months prior to surgery.

Should an obliterated footplate be discovered during surgery, sodium fluoride can still be given in the postoperative period. Postoperatively the dosage given is usually 25 mg and can be tapered off to 5 mg.

SURGERY

Nadol[3] recommends a large fenestra so that this will accommodate the possibility of new bone formation and thus prevent failure of the primary stapedectomy. If the footplate is soft and friable it is possible to make an opening of at least 1 mm in diameter. If the bone is hard then it may be necessary to use a micromotor and drill out the bone. At times these thick "chalky type" footplates cannot be fractured and come out in one large piece, leaving a seemingly extremely wide oval window opening. In these cases the window is to be sealed completely with perichondrium and the prostheses placed over the perichondrium. Lasers have added a new dimension of safety and convenience to surgery on an obliterated footplate.

If the footplate is to be drilled out then the drill bit should be turned slowly so as not to generate heat or prematurely enter the vestibule. The vestibule should be blue-lined where a thin shelf of bone covers the vestibule. When the vestibule is blue-lined the fenestra can be created in the usual way.

SELECTION OF PISTON

The piston must be long enough to extend beyond the otosclerotic focus. Gristwood[1] noted that the thickness of the obliterated footplate varied from 0.5 mm to over 2.00 mm. If over 2.00 a longer piston was needed. He also used a slim piston and sealed the fenestra with a connective tissue seal. Causse, Causse, and Wiet[4] find the long piston without the use of a vein graft seal to be risky having as its attendant risk a perilymphatic fistula. They also report that a longer piston may actually reach the saccule and traumatize it. There is also increased risk of reclosure if only a small channel is created in the foci on a large piece of bone. Furthermore, there is a great risk of bleeding into the vestibule if there is no seal interposed between the contents of the vestibule and the prosthesis.

Nadol[3] in his report notes that obliteration of the round window is the cause of failure of primary stapedectomy. He notes that in none of the cases of his series was there mention of the status of the round window at the time of surgery. The surgeon likely overlooked this possibility. Therefore, Nadol[3] recommends that at the time of stapedectomy, whether it be primary or revision stapedectomy, the patency of the round window should be noted and documented. If noted it should be drilled out carefully.

RECLOSURE (REOBLITERATION OF THE FOOTPLATE AND OTHER ASSOCIATED COMPLICATIONS)

Sensorineural hearing loss is significantly higher in obliterated footplates especially when a drillout procedure is required as compared to those that do not require a drillout. Regrowth or reclosure of the footplate occurs because of new bone growth. This new bone is different from otosclerotic bone and is not an otosclerotic focus. Nadol[3] considers it to be reparative bone.

Sheehy et al[5] reports an incidence of 9% of reclosure by this reparative bone that returns to obliterate the footplate once again, thus resulting in failure of stapedectomy. There are reports that if sodium fluoride is given at the time of primary stapes surgery when the obliterated footplate is first discovered, it serves to prevent regrowth.[4]

WHAT SHOULD THE SURGEON DO WHEN A RECLOSURE OF THE FOOTPLATE OCCURS AFTER PRIMARY STAPES SURGERY WHEN AN OBLITERATED FOOTPLATE HAS BEEN ENCOUNTERED IN THE FIRST SURGERY?

Sheehy et al[5] report that when they attempted to drill out the reclosure a significant number of patients developed a sensorineural hearing loss. Wiet et al[6] recommends getting a high-resolution CT scan when a reclosure of an obliterated footplate is suspected following primary stapes surgery. This is to confirm if reobliteration has recurred.

Gherini et al[7] reported excellent results with the use of the fiberoptic hand-held argon laser when dealing with an obliterated footplate. Literature has proven that lasers for revision surgery, especially in conditions like reobliteration, are an effective way to get good results and avoid sensorineural hearing losses that accompany revision surgery.

Cases of reclosure by new bone should be treated with caution. If surgical intervention is considered then it should be performed by an experienced surgeon who will use a laser. Hearing aids are definitely a viable alternative and should be given serious consideration.

CONCLUSIONS

1. Even when the surgeon resorts to total footplate removal the otosclerotic focus can likely regrow causing reobliteration.
2. In obliterated footplates following stapedectomy the new bone that grows once again to obliterate the footplate is not otosclerotic bone but new bone that regrows probably in reparation

to surgical trauma. Thus, a large fenestra stapedectomy is the better option when faced with an obliterated footplate.

3. Reclosure of the footplate can occur even if a small fenestra stapedectomy is performed.
4. Obliterated footplates are likely found in young adults and in the teenage group.
5. Rapid and early onset hearing loss in very young patients is usually indicative of an obliterated footplate.
6. Obliteration is usually associated with bilateral otosclerosis.
7. Obliterated footplates are usually discovered during surgery.
8. In the active phase sodium fluoride can be prescribed.
9. The introduction of lasers has served to provide a relatively atraumatic (as compared to a microdrill) tool when dealing with this problem.
10. Redrilling of the footplate that has undergone reclosure following primary stapedectomy is associated with a high incidence of sensorineural hearing loss. Sodium fluoride therapy is indicated for these patients.

CONGENITAL FOOTPLATE FIXATION

1. Congenital footplate fixations are usually unilateral and are diagnosed in late childhood or adolescence.
2. Unlike adolescent otosclerosis the hearing loss is nonprogressive and has been present since birth.
3. If the condition is bilateral then speech acquisition will be affected and the cause detected early.
4. The audiometric configuration, however, can be identical to that of otosclerosis including the presence of Carhart's notch.
5. A perilymphatic fistula (CRF/perilymph gusher) may be anticipated in patients with congenital footplate fixation.
6. Minor congenital abnormalities of the stapes superstructure may be associated with congenital fixation of the footplate.
7. Most otologists recommend leaving a congenital fixed footplate alone because of the high association of CSF/perilymph gushers and the accompanying profound sensorineural hearing loss that results.

REFERENCES

1. Gristwod RE. Obliterative otosclerosis: an analysis of the clinical and audiometric findings. *J Laryngol.* 1966;80:115–120.
2. Gristwood RE, Venables WN. Pregnancy and otosclerosis. *Clin Otolaryngol.* 1983;8:205–210.
3. Nadol JB. Histopathology of residual and recurrent conductive hearing loss after stapedectomy. *Otol Neurotol.* 2001;22(2):162–169.
4. Causse JB, Causse JR, Wiet RJ. Special conditions in otosclerosis surgery. *Otosclerosis (Otospongiosis).* Alexandria, VA: American Academy of Otolaryngology–Head and Neck Surgery Foundation Inc. 1991:134–139.
5. Sheehy JL, Nelson RA, House HP. Revision stapedectomy: a review of 258 cases. *Laryngoscope.* 1981;91:43–51.
6. Wiet RJ, Harvey SA, Bauer GP. Complications in stapes surgery. *Otolaryng Clin North Am.* 1993;26(3):471–490.
7. Gherini SG, Horn KL, Bowman CA, Griffin G. Small fenestra stapedectomy using a fiberoptic hand-held argon laser in obliterative otosclerosis. *Laryngoscope.* 1990;11(2):1276–1282.

CHAPTER 18

The Learning Curve

Chris de Souza and Marcos V. Goycoolea

WHO SHOULD PERFORM STAPEDECTOMIES?

This is a question being asked all over the world. Concerns regarding a decline in patients suffering from otosclerosis have left residents in training with very little exposure in surgical technique of the treatment of this problem. Many reports acknowledge a learning curve in residency and among junior stapedectomy surgeons and a diminishing pool of patients suffering from otosclerosis. A surgeon with a special interest and a fellowship in otology no matter how junior will obviously be at an advantage over the casual stapedectomy surgeon. Many experts acknowledge that stapedectomy can be successfully performed early in surgical experience, but the learning curve should be acknowledged and discussed with the patient.

Yung and Oates[1] discuss this in a very enlightening paper. They state that for a relatively uncommon surgery like stapedectomy the learning curve may take years to complete. They define the end point of the learning curve as the time the "curve reaches the plateau." Hughes[2] defined his learning curve as a 10 dB closure in the postoperative air–bone gap in 90% of his stapedectomies. There is international concern that with the rapidly declining amount of stapedectomy work there will be few who can provide authentic training in this area of expertise. Yung and Oates[1] conclude that with the current decline in otosclerosis it will take an entire working life of an otologist to complete the learning curve. The era of see one, do one, teach one is over. The transition where students become teachers is blurred because of the lack of experience.

All those who undertake stapedectomy should be familiar with all the possible findings and nuances of stapedectomy surgery. Should they encounter difficulties, they should acknowledge their limitations and abandon surgery rather than proceed and cause a calamity.

Revision stapedectomies should always be done by an experienced stapedectomy surgeon.

FAR ADVANCED OTOSCLEROSIS

Far advanced otosclerosis (FAO) is defined as no measurable air or bone conduction, or air conduction no better than 95 dB and bone conduction at 55 dB to 60 dB at one frequency only. A negative Rinne's test result with a 256-Hz magnesium tuning fork is the best way to separate FAO sensorineural hearing loss from other causes. Stapedectomy benefits patients who have FAO by bringing their hearing to levels that will benefit from amplification. Some experts believe that cochlear implantation is not the best treatment for FAO because some are better off with stapedectomy.

STAPEDECTOMY IN CHILDREN

There is a gathering body of evidence that children can be included as candidates for stapedectomy. Two groups of patients are identified: those with congenital fixation of the stapes and those who have juvenile otosclerosis. Some authors state that although good results are rewarding, complications can be devastating.

The principal concern in children undergoing stapedectomy was that stapedectomy would impede their sporting activities. A similar concern was that middle ear infections and effusions would prove a problem. Despite these concerns it was found that stapedectomy was a safe procedure in children. Nonetheless children and their families are cautioned about avoiding trauma to the head and the importance of treating all infections promptly and effectively.

STAPEDECTOMY IN THE ELDERLY

Experts report that hearing results and complication rates show no difference between the elderly and younger age groups. Stapedectomy serves not only to reduce a handicap but to also improve the quality of life in the elderly. Furthermore, amplification following successful stapedectomy in which a mixed hearing loss is present can prove to be of greater benefit.

STAPEDECTOMY IN COMBAT PILOTS

Some authors have reported stapedectomy on fighter pilots with full return to active duty (full flight status) without any vestibular symptoms. Full flight status can be given around 3 months following successful stapedectomy without endangering flight safety.

Some experts conclude that stapedectomy does not appear to increase the risk of inner ear barotrauma in scuba divers, skydivers, and pilots. They add that normal eustachian tube function needs to be established first.

STAPEDECTOMY FOLLOWING TYMPANOPLASTY

Patients who suffer from chronic otitis media (COM) are not common. Patients with COM and otosclerosis have a larger air–bone gap. Closure of the air–bone gap in these patients is significant but less than those who have only otosclerosis. The results of stapedectomy in patients who have had surgery for COM are durable and reliable but not as good as those who have only otosclerosis but not COM.

Stapedectomy can be performed in those patients who have had COM with a perforation. It should not be performed in those who have cholesteatoma. These surgical procedures are always sequential and never simultaneous as any contamination of the vestibule will quite likely result in profound a sensorineural hearing loss. The surgeon should wait for at least 24 months following successful repair of the perforation. The ear that needs stapedectomy should be stable, free from infection, and the eustachian tube should be functioning normally.

REFERENCES

1. Yung MW, Oates J. The learning curve in stapes surgery and its implication for training. In: Arnold W, Hausler R, eds. *Otosclerosis and Stapes Surgery. Advances in Otorhinolaryngology*. Basel: Karger; 2007:361–369.
2. Hughes GB. The learning curve in stapes surgery. *Laryngoscope*. 1991;101:1280–1284.

CHAPTER 19

Special Conditions and Complications in Otosclerosis Surgery

Chris de Souza and Marcos V. Goycoolea

A. CEREBROSPINAL FLUID (CSF) GUSHER ALSO KNOWN AS A PERILYMPH GUSHER

The term perilymph gusher is a misnomer as in reality it is a CSF gusher. A stapes gusher is the result of an inner ear anomaly and an abnormal patent communication between the intracranial cavity and the vestibule. This is most commonly associated with congenital fixation of the footplate. To identify a potential CSF gusher the physician should have a strong index of suspicion. The parameters that will lead the physician to suspect this condition are as follows:

1. A conductive hearing loss or a mixed progressive hearing loss. The hearing loss present in childhood and no obvious cause for the hearing loss can be determined. Over time the hearing loss gets progressive.
2. A history may reveal a history of a stapes gusher in the family.
3. A high-resolution CT scanning will reveal the abnormal widening of the vestibule and internal auditory canal.
4. The mother of the patient is the obligate carrier. Genetic testing of the X chromosome will likely confirm the clinical diagnosis of the X-linked stapes gusher syndrome. This is known as the DFN3 gene and it was mapped to the Xq21 region by genetic linkage analysis.[1] The underlying gene POU3F4 is identified. POU3F4 mutations or deletions are responsible for a majority of stapes gushers. Deletions located far upstream of the POU3F4 gene are very likely to disrupt a transcriptional regulatory element. Most cases of CSF gushers are associated with congenital fixation of the footplate in the pediatric population rather than adults. However, Suzuki[2] has shown that as age increases so does the incidence of patency of the cochlear aqueduct.

Can the Surgeon Be Alerted Prior to Surgery About the Presence of a Possible CSF Gusher?

CT scan of the temporal bones can demonstrate the presence of an abnormally patent cochlear aqueduct or if a defect of the fundus exists.

Two other clues can help alert the surgeon to the presence of a gusher.[3] They are:

1. An avascular congenital middle ear.
2. An abnormal anterior insertion of the posterior crus to the footplate.

Management of a CSF Gusher

1. Elevation of the head.
2. Lumbar spinal drain to remove as much CSF as possible.
3. Small fenestra stapedotomy.

4. Tissue seal over the fenestra is mandatory, and some recommend that a prosthesis be placed to keep the seal over the fenestra in place.

Complete control of the CSF gusher is needed as this complication has the potential to cause meningitis. The patient's hearing is likely to deteriorate following such a complication. Some surgeons recommend creating a small control hole in the footplate prior to creating an actual fenestra for stapedotomy. This is done to avoid a "cork in a bottle" effect when the vestibule is suddenly opened.

B. MALLEUS FIXATION

Malleus fixation may result from ossification of the superior and anterior suspensory ligaments. The malleus head may be fixed congenitally. Approximately three-fourths of malleus fixation are associated with stapedial otosclerosis. The incidence of malleus fixation is approximately 1% as reported[4] by most centers.

Can Malleus Fixation Be Diagnosed Prior to Surgery?

Moon and Hahn[5] offer several clues to diagnose the presence of malleus fixation:

1. Lack of movement of the manubrium and umbo on pneumatic otoscopy.
2. Palpation of the malleus. However, on occasion this may prove painful.
3. Audiologic findings seldom reveal an air–bone gap of more than 30 dB.
4. Acoustic reflexes with isolation of the tensor tympani on impedance audiometry. A jet of air is blown across the cornea or the tragus is stroked. If no readings are detected or if they are faint then it is likely that malleus fixation is present.

Vincent, Lopez, and Sperling[6] present the following features by which malleus ankylosis may be suspected. The features are:

1. Unilateral mixed hearing loss that is usually nonprogressive.
2. Small air–bone gap predominantly in the low frequencies.
3. Association with sensorineural impairment in the high frequencies.
4. Acoustic reflex absent on the impaired side but present in the contralateral ear.

Moon and Hahn[5] describe an atrophic tympanic membrane that becomes flaccid while continuing to function against a fixed malleus handle. Many of these tympanic membranes return to normal once the ankylosis is repaired. Primary malleus fixation occurs late in life whereas otosclerosis occurs mainly in young or middle-aged adults. A conductive hearing loss of 10 or 15 dB is more commonly seen with isolated malleus fixation. A Carhart notch that is typical of stapedial otosclerosis can also be seen in malleus fixation as a result of ossicular inertia.

Management

If the ossified ligaments are fractured it is likely that they will get refixed.

An incus bypass procedure using either an incus replacement prosthesis (IRP) or a total ossicular replacement prosthesis (TORP) has been advocated. The treatment lies in amputating the head of the malleus after removing the incus. The tympanic membrane is dissected off the handle of the malleus and an incus replacement prosthesis (IRP) is crimped over the handle and placed into the fenestra of the footplate.

C. INCUS PROBLEMS ENCOUNTERED DURING PRIMARY STAPES SURGERY

These include fusion of the incus to the malleus, accidental dislocation of the incus during surgery, congenital anomalies, and incudal necrosis.

Incus malleus fixation has a 1% reported incidence in association with otosclerosion. Fused malleus and incus are seen in congenital abnormalities of the ear. Postinflammatory changes such as tympanosclerosis, fibrosis, adhesions can lead to fixation of the incus. An abnormally short incus or malformed incus may make it difficult to attach the prosthesis to the incus. Overall incus problems (fixation, dislocation, congenital abnormalities) are common indications for a bypass technique. When a bypass technique is undertaken an IRP or a TORP is used most commonly. It is therefore necessary for the otolaryngologist to be able to perform such bypass techniques.

Management

If the incus is accidentally dislocated it can be replaced without further problems and the stapedectomy can proceed as usual. Alternatively, the incus can be removed and an incus bypass procedure undertaken. An IRP or a TORP can be used in this situation.

D. POSTOPERATIVE REPARATIVE GRANULOMA

Postoperative reparative granuloma has been defined as an exaggeration of the normal reparative process and is well known to cause sensorineural hearing loss following stapedectomy.

Incidence

Kauffman and Schuknecht[7] found an incidence of 1.3% of cases that developed granuloma formation.

Clinical Presentation

Sudden deterioration in hearing 1 to 6 weeks following surgery is suggestive of reparative granuloma. On inspection the tympanic membrane appears reddish in color especially at the posterior superior quadrant. Bone conduction and speech discrimination scores are affected. Kauffman and Shucknecht[7] report that in the majority of cases symptoms occurred in the first 3 weeks following surgery. Hearing loss is a typical finding. Vertigo was also found to occur in 20% to 35% of such patients.

In some patients vertigo and tinnitus are present.

Some granulomas may occupy the middle ear without invading the vestibule and these usually heal without catastrophic sequelae. Even though they may extend into the vestibule they are generally not adherent to the saccule or utricle and can be safely removed. However, those that invade the vestibule are accompanied by sensorineural hearing loss. Serous labyrinthitis is usually an accompanying feature. Such invasive granulomas are usually associated with fat or gelatin sponge being used as a seal on the fenestra created by the surgeon.

Reparative granulomas are often found to engulf the prosthesis and long process of the incus often in direct contact with the tympanic membrane.

Audiological Findings

A pure-tone threshold loss for bone conduction is a typical finding. A simultaneous conductive hearing loss may also be present, partly due to the mass effect of the granuloma and partly due to the fluid in the middle ear.

There is a marked decrease of speech discrimination scores usually with a score of 60% or less.

Appearance of the Tympanic Membrane

The tympanic membrane is thickened especially in the posterior half. On occasion the tympanic membrane may even be edematous.

Etiology

The exact cause of granuloma formation is not clear. Some authors[8] attribute it to the possible aspiration of gastric acid into the middle ear via the eustachian tube in the postoperative phase. Another author attributes it to the possible leakage of either CSF or perilymph into the middle ear.[9] Granuloma formation is associated with total removal of the footplate and the use of gelatin sponge. It is rarely associated with small fenestra stapedotomy. Gacek[10] associated gelatin sponge as an oval window seal with the formation of granuloma. They found no evidence of infection. Infection is not a common cause.

Microscopic examination of granuloma demonstrates fibroblastic proliferation in numerous capillaries, chronic cell infiltrate, and foreign body giant cells.

Harris and Weiss[11] demonstrated bone spicules, foreign body material such as cotton fibers and keratin, and postulated that these might have been the cause of granulomas.

Granuloma formation has been associated with the following: fat wire prosthesis, gelatin sponge (Gelfoam®), and large fenestra stapedectomy.

Management

Early surgery with removal of the granuloma with regrafting of the oval window and a change of the prosthesis is recommended. Early recognition along with prompt removal of the granuloma offers the best chance to cure the ear of this problem especially if it is removed before serous labyrinthitis has occurred. When a granuloma has occurred the results may not be favorable.

E. PERSISTENT STAPEDIAL ARTERY

The stapedial artery is a primitive vessel structure that normally atrophies during the third month of human fetal life. Hyrtl first reported persistence of the stapedial artery 1836. The stapedial artery arises from the internal carotid artery, enters the middle ear in the anteroinferior quadrant, passes over the promontory, proceeds through the obturator foramen of the stapes, and turns anteriorly into the horizontal portion of the facial canal through a bony dehiscence. Subsequently, it enters the middle cranial fossa and terminates into the middle meningeal artery. The stapedial artery has two major divisions: the dorsal (supraorbital) and ventral (maxillomandibular) divisions. The supraorbital division undergoes anastamosis with the ophthalmic artery and is incorporated into the anterior branch of the middle meningeal artery. The maxillomandibular division undergoes anastamosis with the internal maxillary branch of the external carotid artery, supplying the lower face, inferior alveolar, and infraorbital regions.

Usually, the stem of the stapedial artery atrophies and the anastamosis with the external carotid artery takes over the blood supply of both divisions. If the transition fails to take place the middle meningeal artery will be supplied by the ophthalmic artery or a persistent stapedial artery.

Incidence

The reported incidence of persistent stapedial artery is 1 in 5,000 to 10,000 ears.[12]

Can a Persistent Stapedial Artery Be Diagnosed Before Surgery?

A persistent stapedial artery can cause pulsatile tinnitus. It may also present with a conductive hearing loss by limiting stapes movement. Sensorineural hearing loss, probably caused by erosion of the bony otic capsule, has been reported.

A persistent stapedial artery can be associated with internal carotid artery or middle ear anomalies, especially with anomalies of the stapes and facial nerve. It has been infrequently associated with trisomy 13, 15 syndrome, second branchial arch anomaly, Paget's disease, otosclerosis, and thalidomide deformities.

Treatment

The most important clinical significance of persistent stapedial artery is the possibility of bleeding from injury to the vessel during the course of stapedectomy.

However, treatment of a persistent stapedial identified during the course of stapedectomy is not well established. There is a theoretical risk of hemiplegia if the vessel is clamped. In fact the embryonic origin has caused surgeons in the past to fear complications like contralateral hemiplegia. This fear has led to surgeons abandoning stapedectomy. If a persistent stapedial artery is identified then as atraumatic surgery as possible should be performed with due care being accorded to the vessel.

In 12 reported cases of persistent stapedial artery with associated footplate ankylosis, 11 underwent stapedectomy. In 9 cases in which a prosthesis was placed there were no postoperative complications. In 5 of these cases the artery was sectioned or clipped without complication. Horn and Visvanathan[13] thus conclude that successful stapedectomy can be performed even in the presence of a persistent stapedial artery.

The persistent stapedial artery causes horizontal obscuring of the oval window. The first important step is removal of the stapes superstructure without damaging the artery. The laser is a suitable tool for this step. Fenestration of the footplate should also be accomplished with minimal trauma. Again the laser is a suitable tool for this. Horn and Visvanathan[13] note that the artery lies closer to the anterior crus than to the posterior crus. They recommend the Causse prosthesis as the prosthesis of choice in this situation because it is smooth and less likely to traumatize the artery.

F. FLOATING FOOTPLATE

This can occur when the footplate is not properly fixed and gets mobilized. It is most likely to occur if a fenestra is placed in the center. Some authors advise creating a control hole in the footplate before removal of the arch of the stapes. If it is not possible to remove the footplate atraumatically or efficiently surgery should be abandoned. A soft tissue seal should be placed over the oval window and the surgery abandoned. Some reports in literature advocate applying a vein graft above the floating footplate and then attaching a prosthesis from the incus to the floating footplate if it remains hinged inward. Good results have been reported with this technique. If the mobilized footplate is mostly blue with diffuse otosclerosis then the success rate is 95%.[14] If the footplate is thick, white, or biscuit-shaped the hearing success rate is approximately 52%. Should the footplate mobilize again during revision surgery no further surgery should be planned. Lippy[14] states that when he followed this protocol none of the 147 cases who developed a floating footplate in a series of 8,000 cases developed a sensorineural hearing loss.

Should it not be possible to proceed with surgery and if further attempts are made to remove the footplate this could result in further submerging the footplate with resulting sensorineural hearing loss. Surgery in such cases should be abandoned.

A floating footplate is less likely to be encountered when a laser is used to create a fenestra. Should a floating footplate be encountered and no laser is available then Perkins[15] recommends that the procedure be halted and reoperation considered after a period of 4 months. This should be adequate time to allow the footplate to get refixed. Laser is best used for such a condition and a vein-clad prosthesis is used for this condition.

Other surgical procedures advocated for a floating footplate include creating a pothole in the promontory near the footplate and then lifting and removing the submerged footplate.

In a poll conducted by Wiet et al[16] on a strategy regarding a floating footplate, the majority (45%) of respondents advocated removal of the footplate whereas the minority (12%) stated that they would terminate the procedure. One-third stated that they would place a prosthesis with or without a seal on the oval window. When polled about a submerged footplate 71% stated that they would leave the footplate alone whereas 29% stated that they would attempt removal.

G. DEHISCENT (PTOTIC) FACIAL NERVE

Proctor and Nager[17] have summarized the course of the facial nerve and its variations within the temporal bone. A common anomaly is failure of osseous closure of the fallopian canal by the otic capsule. An incidence of 55% of bony dehiscence of the fallopian canal has been reported. A minor dehiscence of the fallopian canal does not lead to a ptotic facial nerve.

Durcan et al[18] hypothesize that inferior displacement of the facial nerve is likely due to an arrest or anomaly of Reichert's cartilage. They also describe three anomalies of the facial nerve in relationship to the oval window. These include an overhanging facial nerve, a bifid facial nerve, and a facial nerve coursing over the promontory. They postulate that failure of Reichert's cartilage to make contact with the lateral wall of the cartilaginous otic capsule leads to a ptotic facial nerve. This results in an anomalous stapes arch that does not contact the otic capsule. The absence of the normal stapes superstructure allows the facial nerve to develop at the level or below the level of the oval window. The bifid facial nerve is due to late union of Reichert's cartilage to the otic capsule. Usually, under these circumstances, the stapes crura are atrophic and the anterior crura is frequently absent. Welling et al[19] state that when facial nerve anomalies are present they do not occur alone but are part of a continuum of anomalies. Horn and Viswanathan[13] offer the options of abandoning the procedure, fenestration, facial nerve decompression with displacement from the oval window, or cochleotomy as for dealing with the ptotic facial nerve when treating otosclerosis. In cases where there is partial ptosis of the facial nerve, the nerve may be gently retracted and the surgeon can proceed with stapedectomy. However, if there are a severe degree of anomalies present it is advisable that the surgeon terminate the procedure immediately.

Dysgeusia and Ageusia

Most surgeons try to preserve the chorda tympani. Once the annulus of the tympanic membrane is elevated and the middle ear is entered the next step should be to try and locate the chorda tympani. It is then elevated out up to the handle of the malleus. Care should be taken not to stretch the nerve. If the chorda is allowed to dry out taste disturbances last approximately 4 to 5 months. And they generally disappear without treatment. Should the chorda tympani obstruct vision (in very rare instances) then it is better to section the nerve rather than stretch it. Should taste disturbances persist and prove a problem to the patient following stapedectomy long after then the nerve should be sectioned.

Facial Paralysis

This can occur even in the most experienced hands. If the facial nerve is dehiscent and the surgeon is experienced and confident that he has not damaged the nerve, the nerve can be expected to recover. If the nerve has been damaged then decompression may be required. On occasion, the facial palsy may be a result of the local anesthetic affecting a dehiscent facial nerve, in which case the facial nerve recovers within hours.

Cholesteatoma Formation Poststapedectomy

This fortunately is a rare occurrence. The surgeon needs to take proper care to prevent implantation of stratified keratinizing squamous epithelium in the middle ear. If the cholesteatoma is small it can be removed without affecting the stapedectomy. However, if the cholesteatoma is large then it needs to be attended to. The prosthesis may need to be removed after weighing the risks with the patient.

Mechanisms by which cholesteatoma can occur following stapedectomy are chronic Eustachian tube dysfunction and negative middle ear pressures. Fergusson et al[20] report on how cholesteatoma can occur. They report that if the prosthesis extrudes then it provides a portal through which keratinizing stratified squamous epithelium can enter the middle ear. On occasion an attic retraction pocket can grow into a cholesteatoma. Cholesteatoma can also occur if unrecognized stratified squamous epithelium has been inadvertently implanted into the middle ear. An inverted tympanomeatal flap that was not positioned correctly and from a disrupted annulus marginal perforation. Once cholesteatoma formation has occurred it has to be dealt with appropriately because it has the potential not only to destroy hearing but also to cause life-threatening meningitis.

TYMPANIC MEMBRANE PERFORATION

The tympanic membrane may be perforated during surgery. This can be repaired immediately and simultaneously with perichondrium or with a vein graft. This is done by underlay technique and is nearly always successful.

Perforation of the tympanic membrane nearly always occurs when elevating the tympanomeatal flap. Careful identification of the annulus will help avoid this complication. Damage to the tympanic membrane has been reported in 1.9% of cases.[21]

REFERENCES

1. Cremers CWRJ. How to prevent a stapes gusher. In: Arnold W, Hausler R, eds. *Otosclerosis and Stapes Surgery: Advances in Otorhinolaryngology.* Vol 65. Basel: Karger; 2007:278–284.
2. Suzuki T. A study on the communication between labyrinth and cerebrospinal space through cochlear aqueduct in human body. *J Otolaryngol (Japan).* 1960;63:2298–2312.
3. Causse JB, Causse JR, Wiet RJ, Yoo TJ. Complications of stapedectomies. *Am J Otol.* 1983;4:275–280.
4. Lippy WH, Schuring AG. Stapedectomy for otosclerosis with malleus fixation. *Arch Otolaryngol.* 1978;98:80–81.
5. Moon CN, Hahn MJ. Primary malleus fixation: diagnosis and treatment. *Laryngoscope.* 1981;91:1298–1306.
6. Vincent R, Lopez A, Sperling NM. Malleus ankylosis: a clinical, audiometric, histologic and surgical study of 123 cases. *Am J Otol.* 1999;20:717–725.
7. Kauffman RS, Schuknecht HF. Reparative granuloma following stapedectomy. A clinical entity. *Ann Oto Rhinol Laryngol.* 1967;76:1008–1017.
8. Batman C, Ozturk O, Ramadan SS. Postoperative granuloma after stapedectomy: is it destiny or avoidable? In: Arnold W, Hausler R, eds. *Otosclerosis and Stapes Surgery: Advances in Otorhinolaryngology.* Vol 65. Basel: Karger; 2007:285–295
9. Kuhweide R, Van de Steene V, Vlaminck S, Casselman JW. Reparative granuloma related to perilymphatic fistula. In: Arnold W, Hausler R, eds. *Otosclerosis and Stapes Surgery: Advances in Otorhinolaryngology.* Vol 65. Basel: Karger; 2007:296–299.
10. Gacek RR. The diagnosis and treatment of poststapedectomy granuloma. *Am J Otol.* 1970;7:420–424.
11. Harris I, Weiss L. Granulomatous complications of oval window fat grafts. *Laryngoscope.* 1962;72:870–885.
12. House HP, Patterson ME. Persistent stapedial artery: a report of 2 cases. *T Am Acad Ophthalmol Otolaryngol.* 1964;68:644–646.
13. Horn KL, Visvanathan A. Stapes surgery in the obscured oval window: management of the ptotic facial nerve and the persistent stapedial artery. *Oper Techn Otolaryngol Head Neck.* 1998;9(1):58–63.
14. Lippy WH. Special problems of otosclerosis surgery. In: Brackmann DE, Shelton CS, Arriaga M, eds. *Otologic Surgery.* Philadelphia, PA: WB Saunders; 1994:348–355.
15. Perkins R. Laser stapedotomy. In: Brackmann DE, Shelton CS, Arriaga M, eds. *Otologic Surgery.* Philadelphia, PA: WB Saunders; 1994:314–329.
16. Wiet RJ, Harvey SA, Bauer GP. Complications in stapes surgery: options for prevention and management. *Otolaryng Clin North Am.* 1993;26:471–490.
17. Proctor B, Nager GT. The facial canal: normal anatomy, variations and anomalies. *Ann Oto Rhinol Laryngol.* 1982;91(supplement 93):33–61.
18. Durcan DJ, Shea JJ, Sleeck JP. Bifurcation of the facial nerve. *Arch Otolaryngol.* 1967;86:37–49.
19. Welling DB, Glasscock ME, Gantz BJ. Avulsion of the facial nerve at stapedectomy. *Laryngoscope.* 1992;102:729–733.
20. Fergusson BJ, Gillispie CA, Kenan PD, Farmer JC. Mechanisms of cholesteatoma formation following stapedectomy. *Am J Otol.* 1986;7(6):420–424.
21. Causse JR, Causse JB. Eighteen year report on stapedectomy 1: problems of stapedial fixation. *Clin Otolaryngol.* 1980;5:49–59.

PART VII

Atlas

CHAPTER 20

The Art of Stapes Surgery

Robert K. Jackler

Christine Gralapp, Chapter Illustrator

INTRODUCTION

Many otologists would describe stapes surgery as among the most satisfying of all ear operations. The procedure is elegant, technically sophisticated, and most patients are highly appreciative for their improved hearing. It is also among the most perilous. For such a miniscule area the number of variations and anomalies the otologist might encounter are numerous and can tax even the most experienced microsurgeon. When a tympanoplasty fails it can usually be successfully redone. When stapes surgery goes wrong it can result in irremediable consequences such as deafness, vertigo, and even facial paralysis. Success in surgery is less about technical virtuosity than it is about mental preparedness, the exercise of sound judgment, and knowing one's limits. The better prepared a surgeon is the more likely to achieve success and avoid preventable complications.

One important goal in creating these illustrations was to help the novice surgeon gain competence, efficiency, and finesse with the routine aspects of stapes surgery. During training, the learning curve for stapes procedures is steeper than for most ear procedures. Stapes procedures require the surgeon to have a clear plan of the technical maneuvers that, in turn, have to occur in specific sequence. Our illustrations are intended to guide the inexperienced surgeon to learn the principles of obtaining adequate exposure by designing and raising a tympanomeatal flap of the proper size and shape as well as avoiding flap tears or disruption of the tympanic membrane. The fledgling surgeon has to master hand positions that afford high levels of stability and also master the skill of two-handed surgery. Beginning surgeons rapidly become facile with their dominant hand, but development of nondominant hand skill takes time and practice. Many of the maneuvers in stapes surgery are completed most effectively when exposure is adequate for binocular viewing. The methods of obtaining adequate exposure of the oval window and incus are central to making the procedure go smoothly. We have made an effort to show a diversity of technical options for opening the footplate (small and large fenestra; microdrill, laser, and pick) as well as illustrating some of the more commonly used stapes prostheses.

The second major goal of these illustrations was to provide stapes surgeons with the intellectual framework to be prepared for the myriad uncommon variants and technical challenges that inevitably arise from time to time. The majority of these (eg, overhanging facial nerve, narrow niche, deficient incus, thick footplate) are usually not knowable preoperatively by the surgeon. Chances are that when surgeons first encounter a stapes gusher or biscuit footplate, for example, they will be on their own never having faced these challenges before. The only way to prepare is through mental preparedness and formulation of a plan, much as an airline pilot anticipates rare emergencies. Illustrations are one means of helping surgeons recognize and deal with uncommon variants and technical challenges.

This chapter has over 160 original illustrations that were created over a several-year period (Figures 20–1 through 20–164). They are the product of an ongoing collaboration between a surgeon (Jackler) and illustrator (Gralapp), which has gone on for over 25 years and produced nearly 1,500 original illustrations. We have done our best to be comprehensive in our coverage, but it was impractical to exhaustively cover all conceivable aspects of stapes surgery. We welcome comments from readers about ways we could improve our illustrations to make them clearer and more relevant. We also welcome suggestions for additional illustrations that may be helpful in guiding safe and effective stapes surgery.

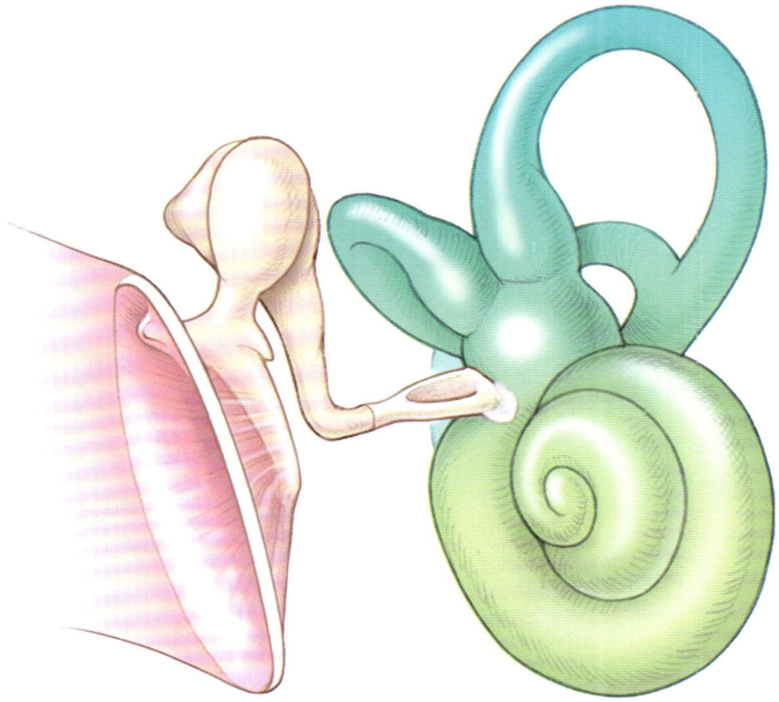

Figure 20–1. Schematic coronal view of the middle and inner ecr showing a fixed stapes due to an otosclerotic plaque at the anterior margin of the oval window.

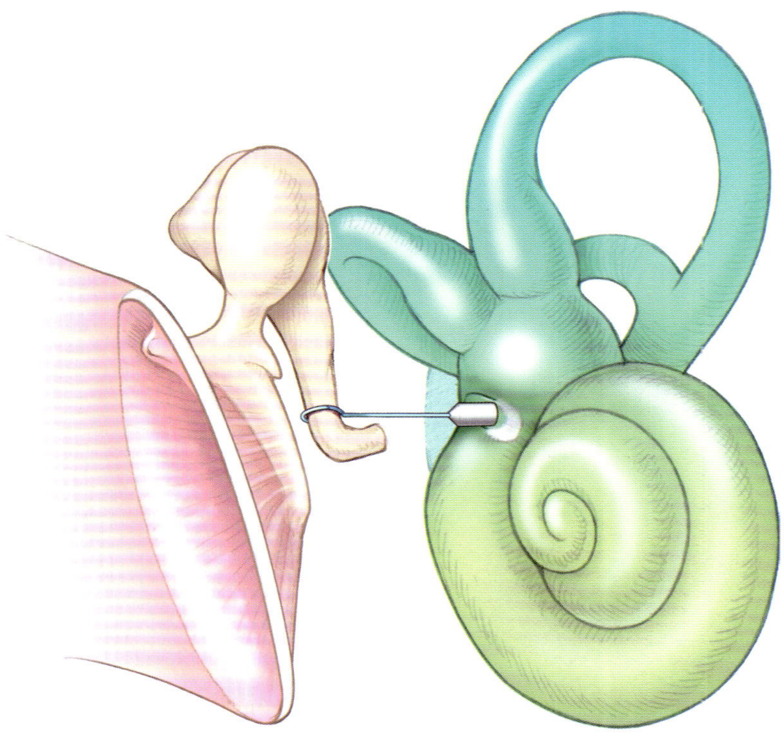

Figure 20–2. Schematic illustrating small fenestra stapedotomy with a Teflon-wire prosthesis.

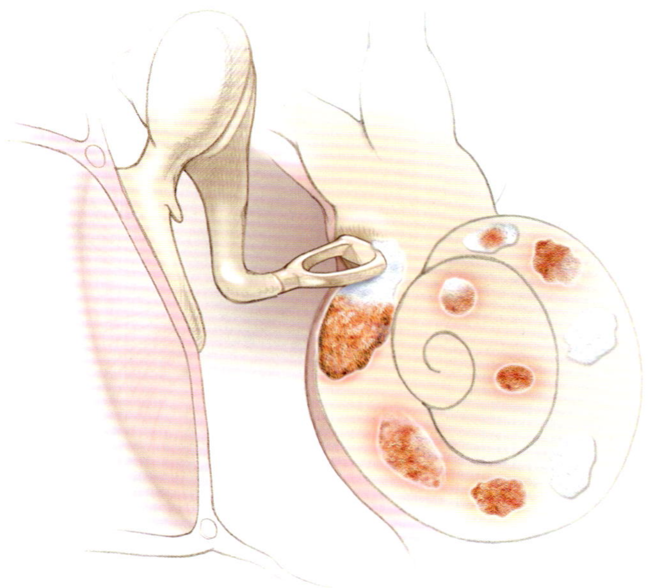

Figure 20–3. Otosclerosis is a disease of the otic capsule. In its active phase, known as otospongiosis, highly vascular lesions resorb bone surrounding the inner ear, most often in a patchy pattern. The active lesions mature into calcified otosclerotic plaques that are responsible for stapes fixation.

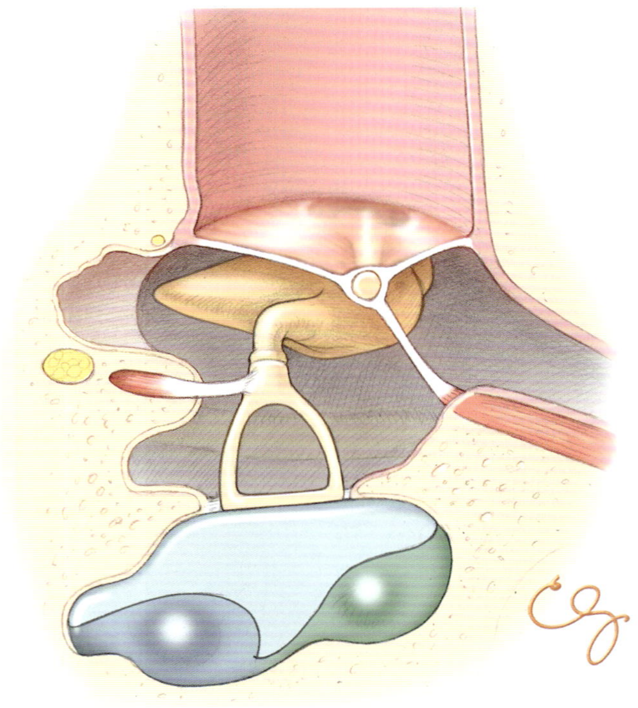

Figure 20–4. Schematic view of the middle and inner ear displayed via a perspective looking upward from the hypotympanum. This projection was chosen as a means of introducing the concepts of stapes surgery in a perspective that enables simultaneous viewing of the ear canal, middle ear, stapes, vestibule, utricle (*blue*), and saccule (*green*).

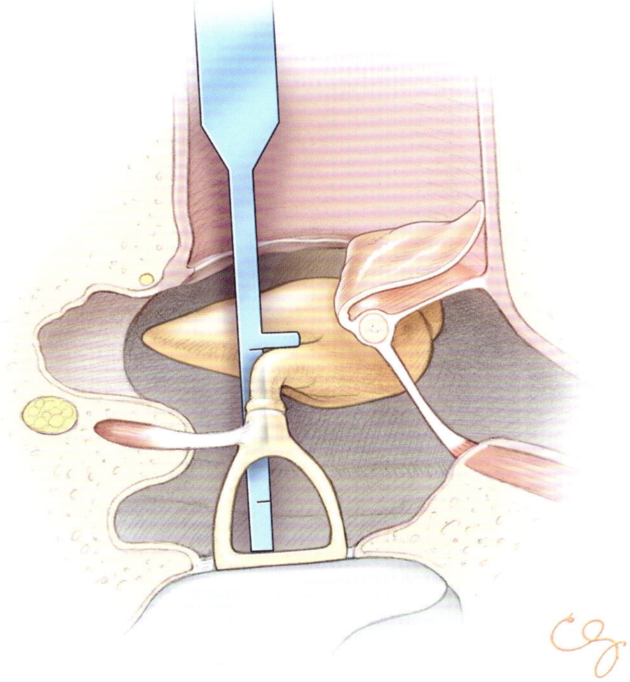

Figure 20-5. The tympanomeatal flap (canal skin and eardrum) has been raised and reflected anteriorly to expose the posterior half of the middle ear. To aid in selection of the proper length prosthesis, the distance from the lateral surface of the incus to the footplate is being measured.

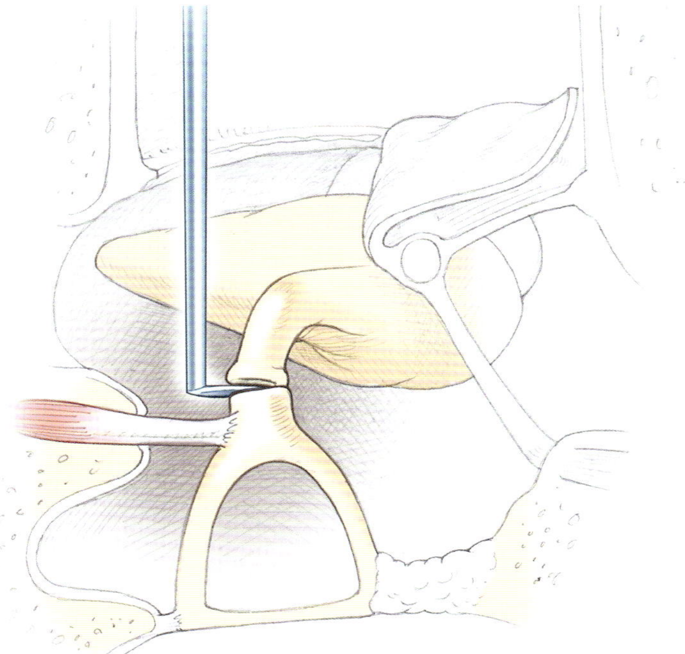

Figure 20-6. Division of the joint between the incus and stapes using an incudostapedial joint knife.

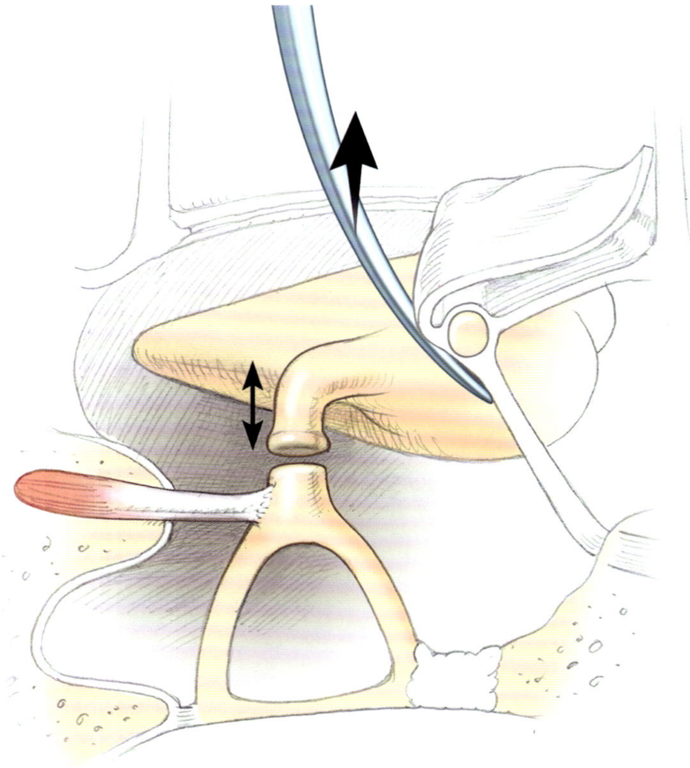

Figure 20-7. After division of the joint, mobility of the lateral ossicles (malleus and incus) is tested.

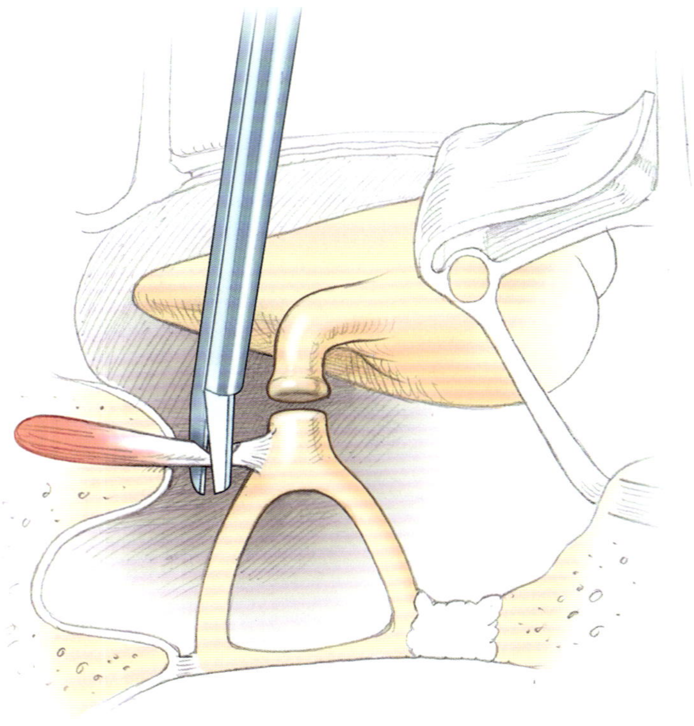

Figure 20-8. Section of the stapedius muscle with microscissors.

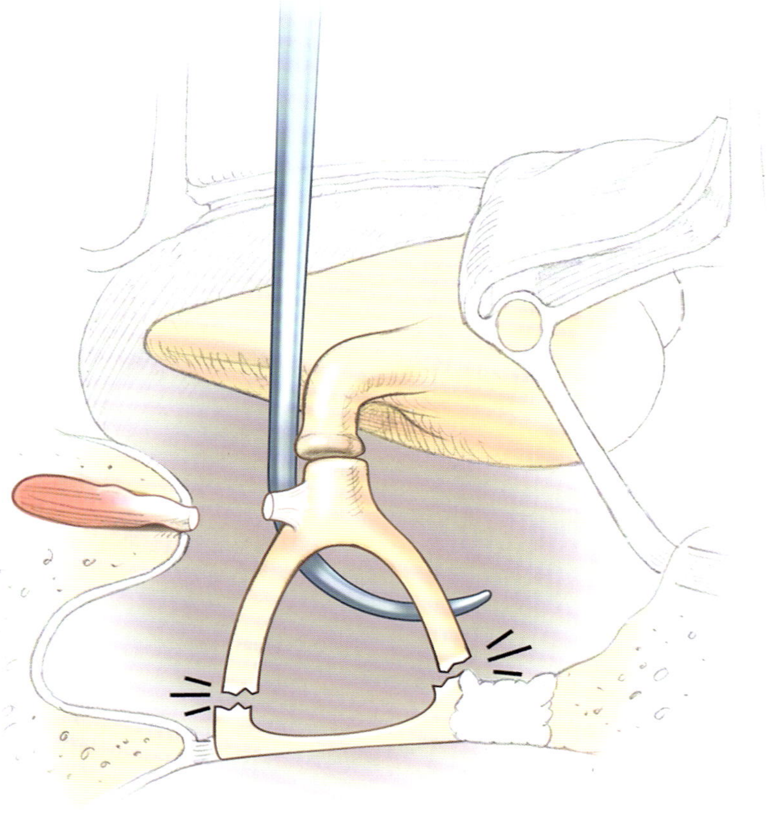

Figure 20–9. Removal of the stapes superstrructure using a curved needle.

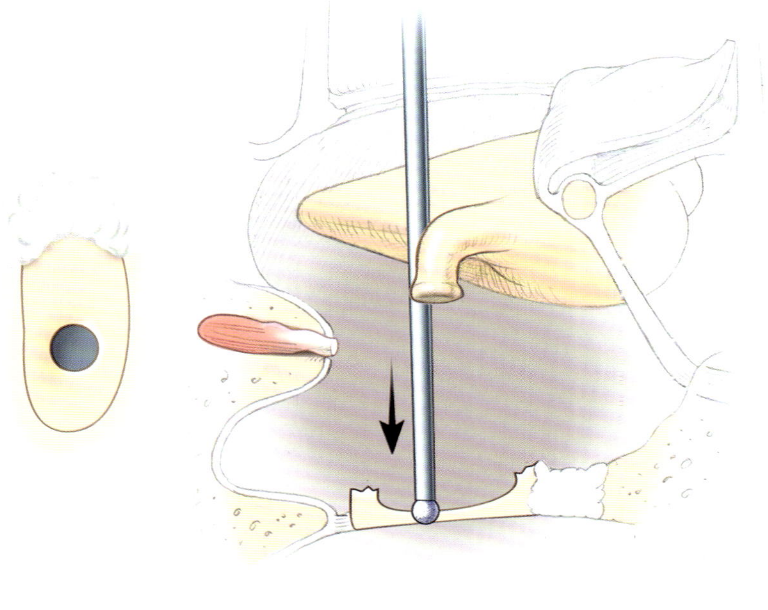

Figure 20–10. Creation of a small fenestra stapedctomy with a microdrill.

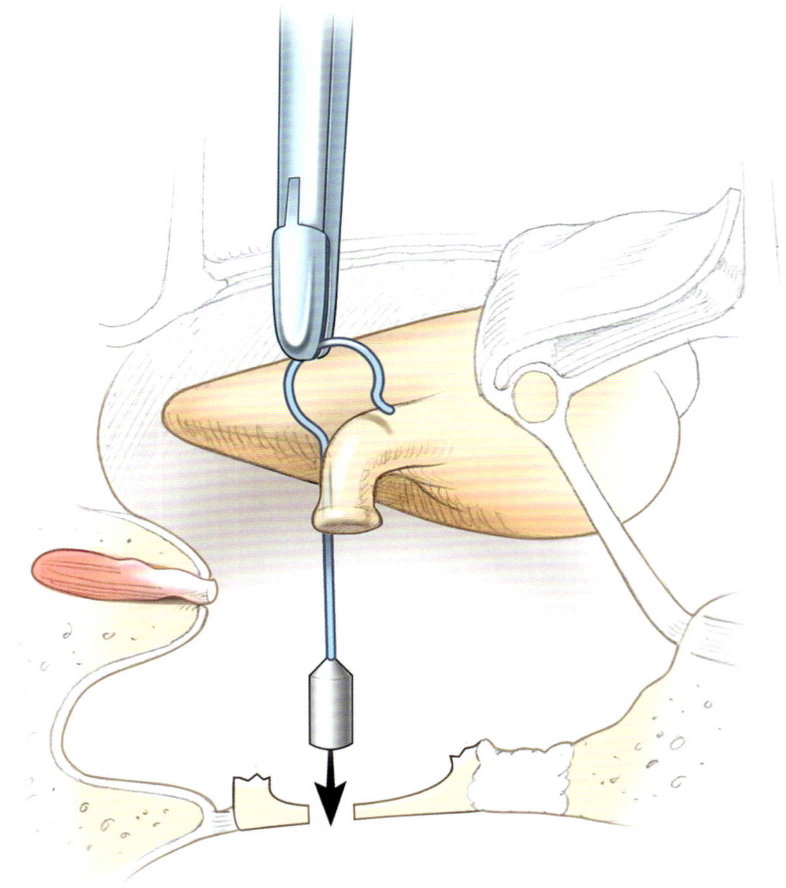

Figure 20-11. Placement of a stapedotomy piston.

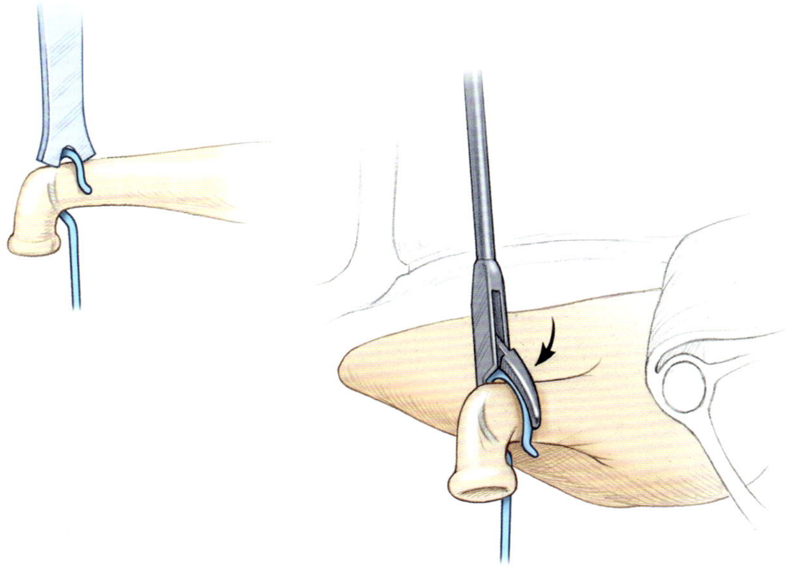

Figure 20-12. Positioning of the shepherd's crook on the incus with a notched chisel (strut guide) and closing the wire with a crimper.

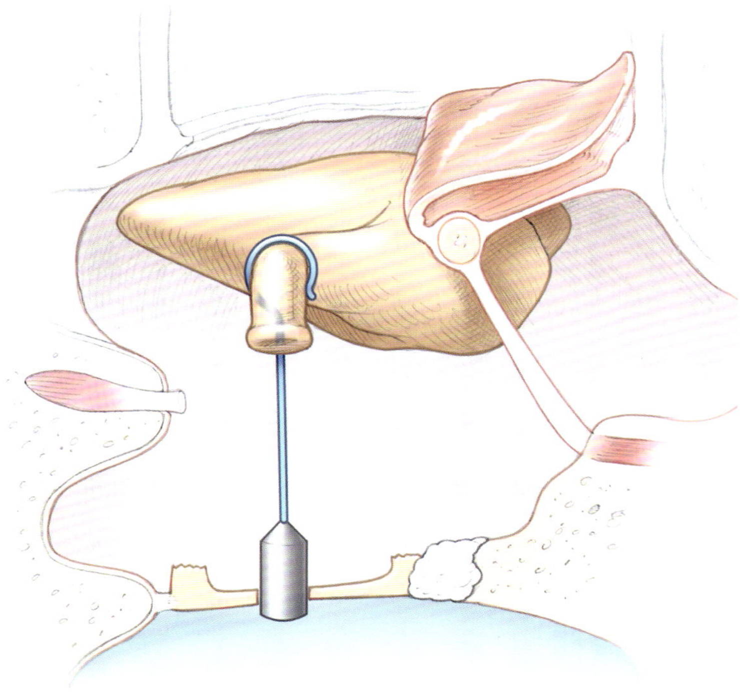

Figure 20–13. Completed placement of the stapes piston through the stapes fenestra into the vestibule.

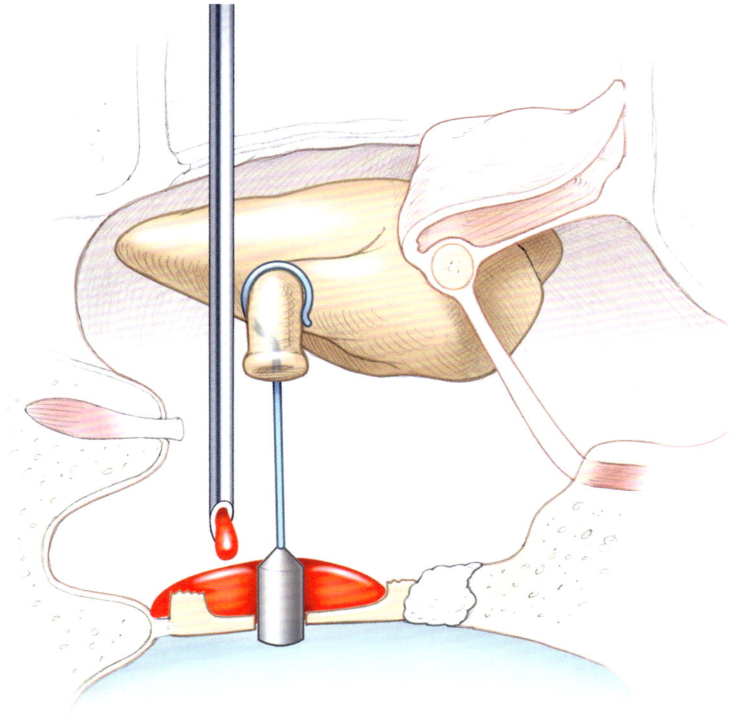

Figure 20–14. Sealing around the prosthesis with blood.

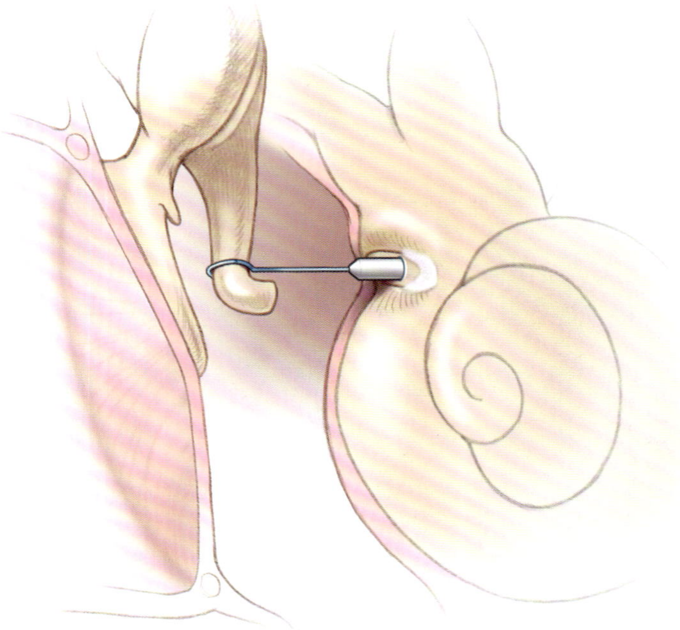

Figure 20-15. Comparison between small and large fenestra technique.

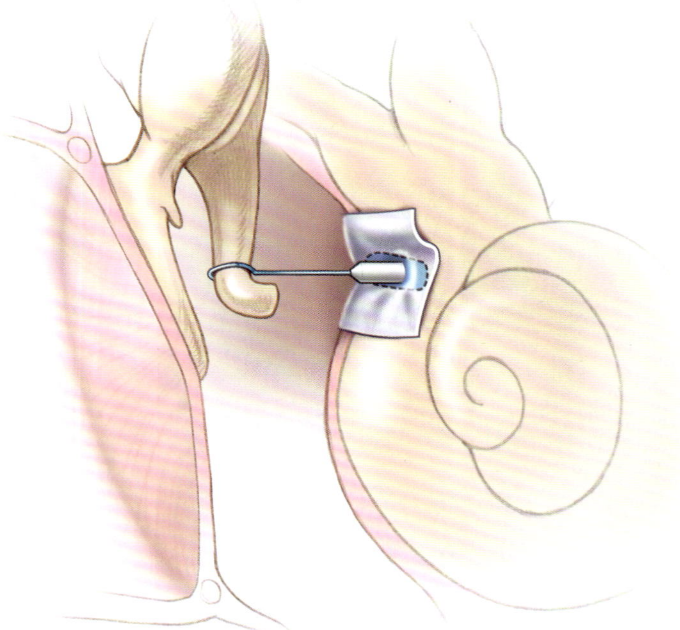

Figure 20-16. The large fenestra operation requires placement of a membrane across the oval window, most commonly tragal perichondrium, temporalis fascia, or vein harvested from the dorsum of the hand.

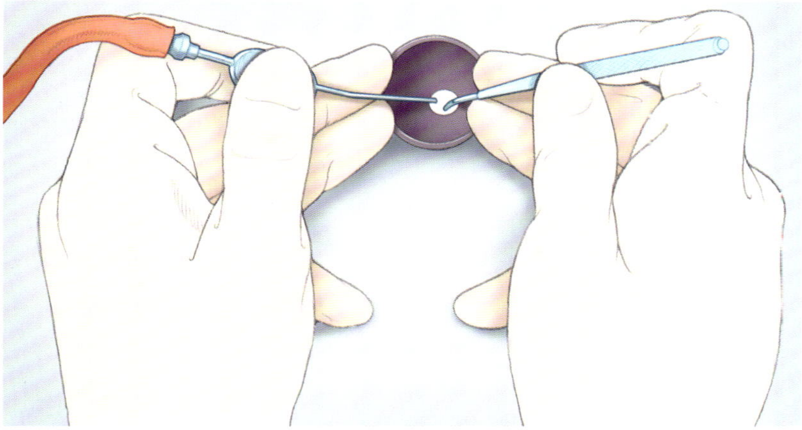

Figure 20–17. Placement of the surgeon's hands during transcanal stapes microsurgery. The third and fourth fingers of each hand stabilize the speculum. Note that the micro instrument (right hand) and suction (left hand) are held in a manner to both optimize stability and to enable binocular viewing. Some surgeons use a speculum holder to enhance stability.

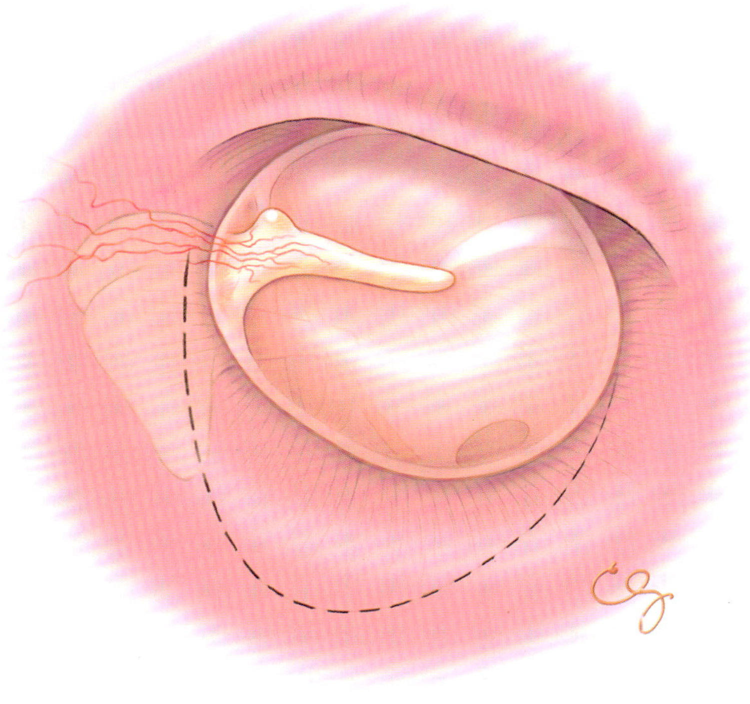

Figure 20–18. Operative view of the ear canal and ear drum as seen in a transcanal approach. Dotted line represents the canal incision of a tympanomeatal flap. The flap is longer superiorly to cover the scutectomy defect. Note that the optimal incision is not "12 to 6" but rather more like 1 PM to 7 PM on an imaginary clock face in which the malleus sits at noon. For the flap to properly fold on itself exposing the posterior superior quadrant it is best to carry the incision slightly beyond the malleus.

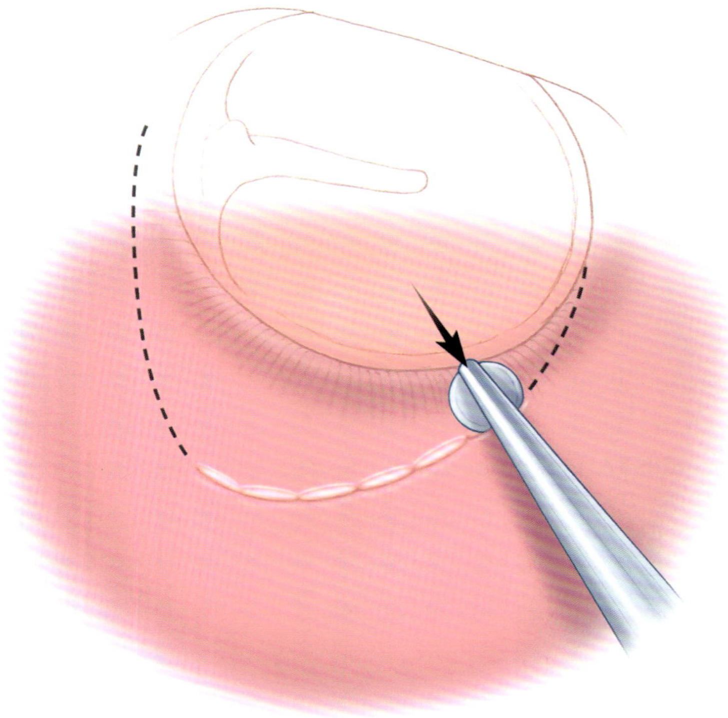

Figure 20-19. The incision line is first crushed with a round stapes knife. This maneuver squeezes closed blood vessels and thereby reduces bleeding. It also helps to minimize flap tearing during incision.

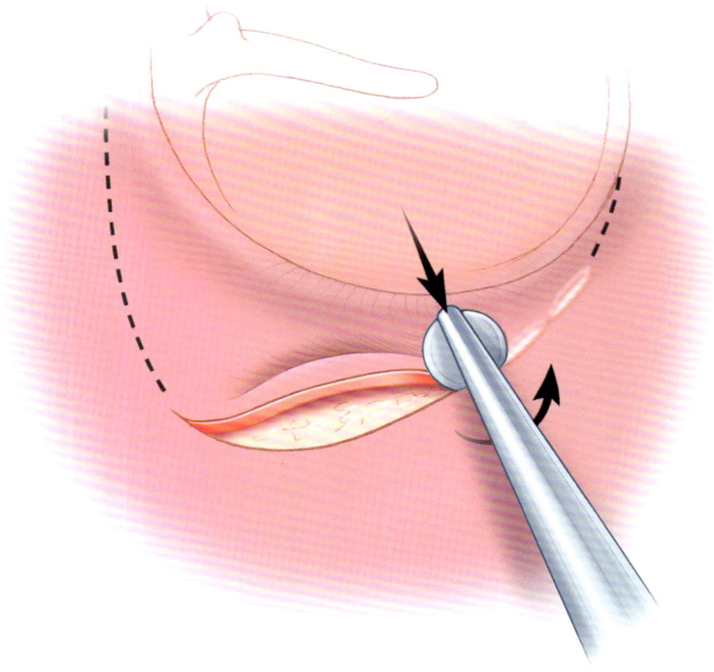

Figure 20-20. Using a twisting motion the incision is created with a stapes knife.

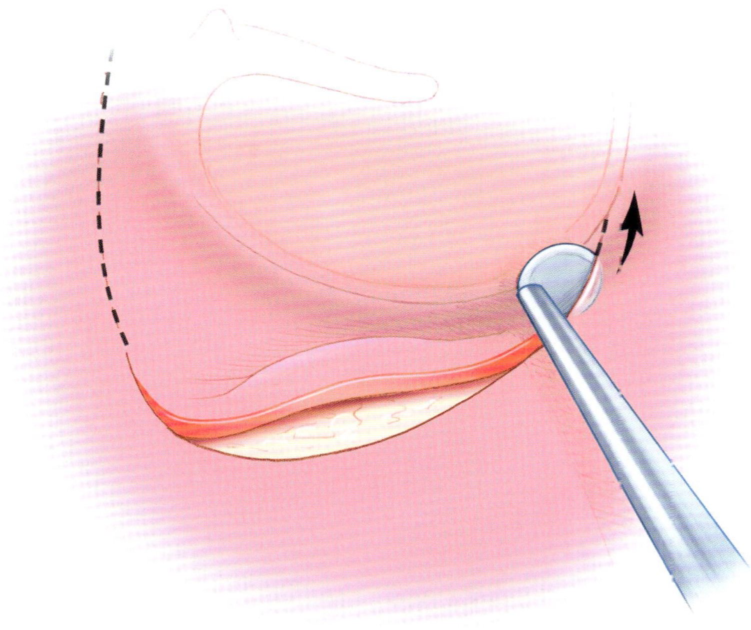

Figure 20–21. The incision if carried inferiorly. As the stapes exposure is in the superior quadrant, the inferior portion of the flap can be kept quite short.

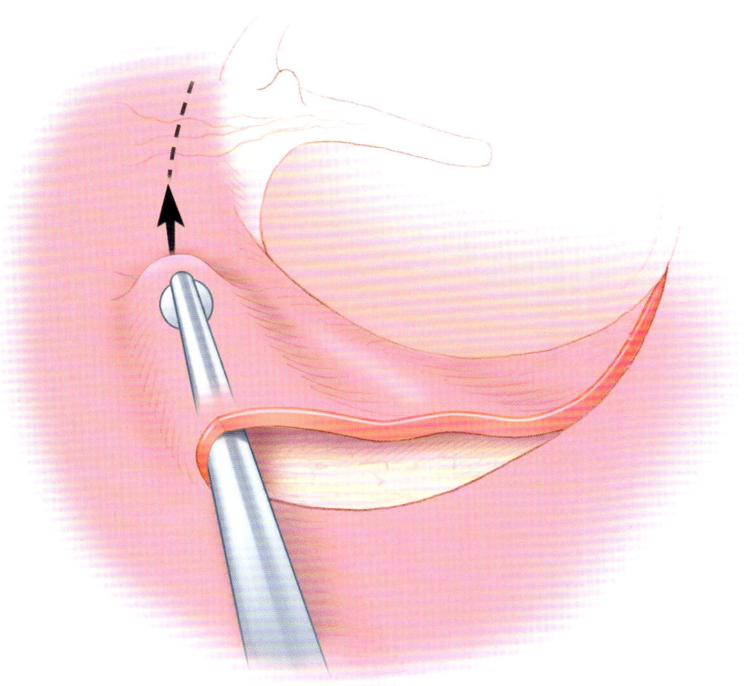

Figure 20–22. Using either a stapes knife or annulus elevator, a tunnel is created under the so-called "vascular strip," the portion of the flap most likely to bleed.

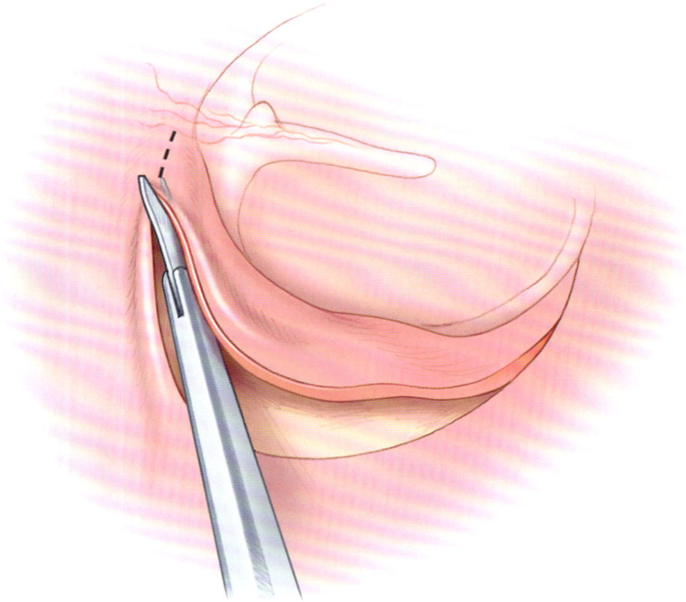

Figure 20-23. Cutting the vascular strip with scissors squeezes vessels closed and thereby reduces bleeding. It also creates a neatly designed flap without irregular edges. Some surgeons prefer to cut the entire flap with a stapes knife.

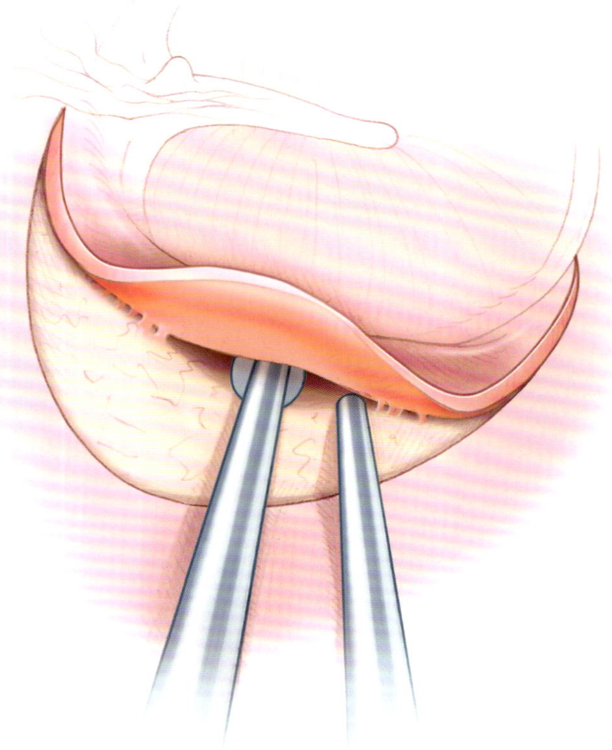

Figure 20-24. The flap is raised to the level of the tympanic annulus. Care must be taken to avoid traumatizing the flap by aspirating it with the suction. The suction is best kept about the stapes knife blade.

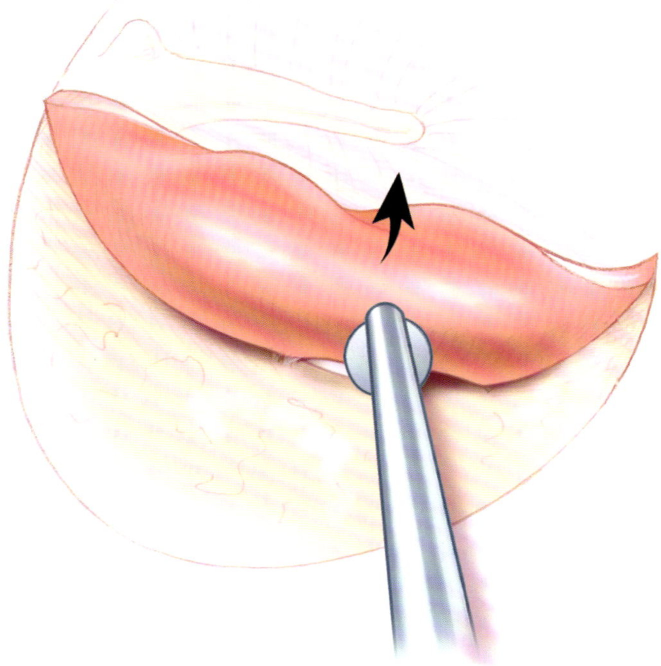

Figure 20-25. To avoid potential disturbance to the ossicles the middle ear is first entered inferiorly. The stapes knife lifts the tympanic annulus out of its bony groove. With gentle downward and inward pressure, the knife can then safely fall over the margin into the posterior tympanic space.

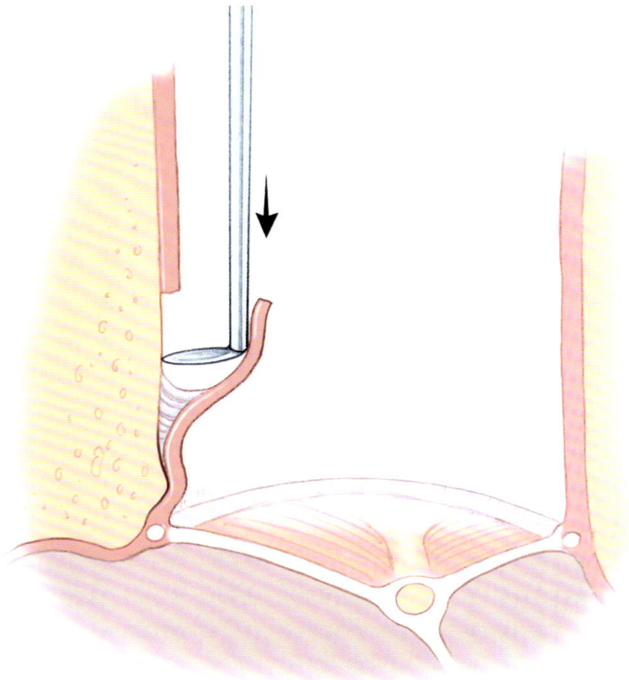

Figure 20-26. A bony prominence is often encountered slightly lateral to the tympanic membrane level.

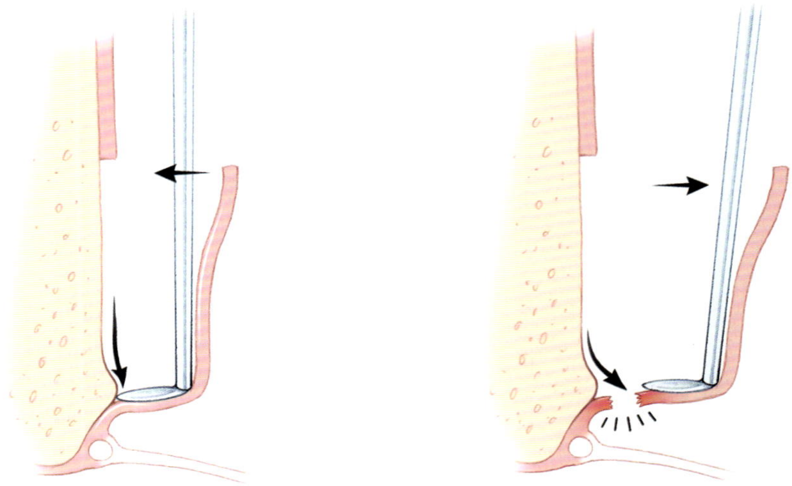

Figure 20-27. To avoid tearing of the flap or tympanic membrane it is necessary to maintain continuous pressure with the stapes knife against the bony canal. Allowing the stapes knife to disengage from the canal wall risks tearing the flap.

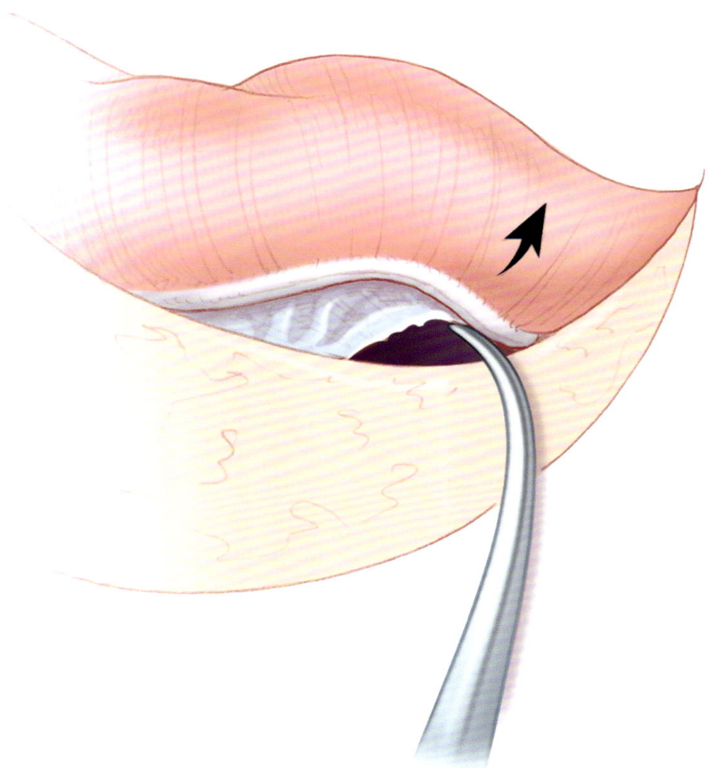

Figure 20-28. The tympanic mucosa is lysed with a curved needle. When done under local anesthesia, lidocaine is infused into the middle ear to anesthetize the tympanic mucosa. To avoid anesthetizing the labyrinth with resultant postoperative vertigo, lidocaine should be promptly suctioned from the middle ear, especially from the round window niche where it tends to accumulate.

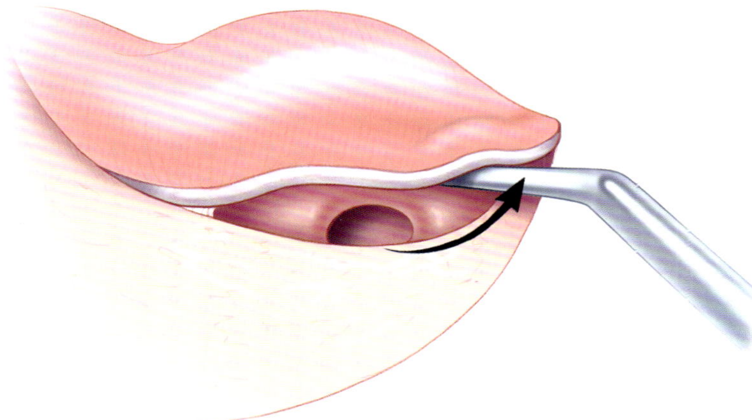

Figure 20-29. Elevation of the tympanic annulus inferiorly using an annulus elevator. To avoid tearing, it is important to maintain firm pressure against the bone. Elevation is with the side of the shaft, not the tip of the instrument. When under local anesthesia this maneuver is often incompletely anesthesized. Bleeding from the inferior edge is common after this maneuver. Application of a small cube of epinephrine-soaked Gelfoam® readily controls bleeding.

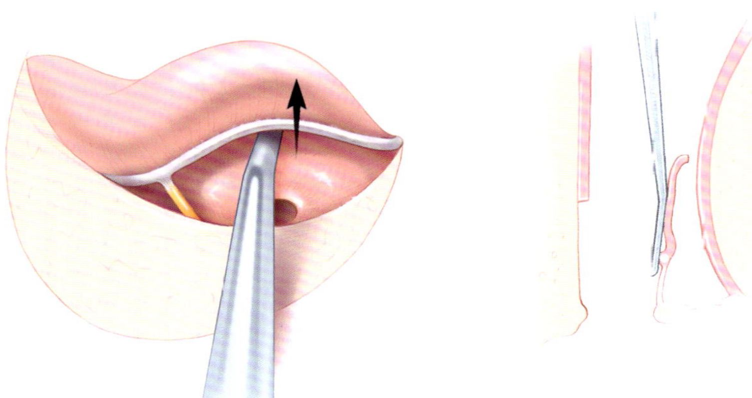

Figure 20-30. It is important to have the middle ear exposure remain adequately open throughout the surgery. Using the back of the annulus elevator the flap can be pushed against the anterior canal wall where surface tension will adhere it.

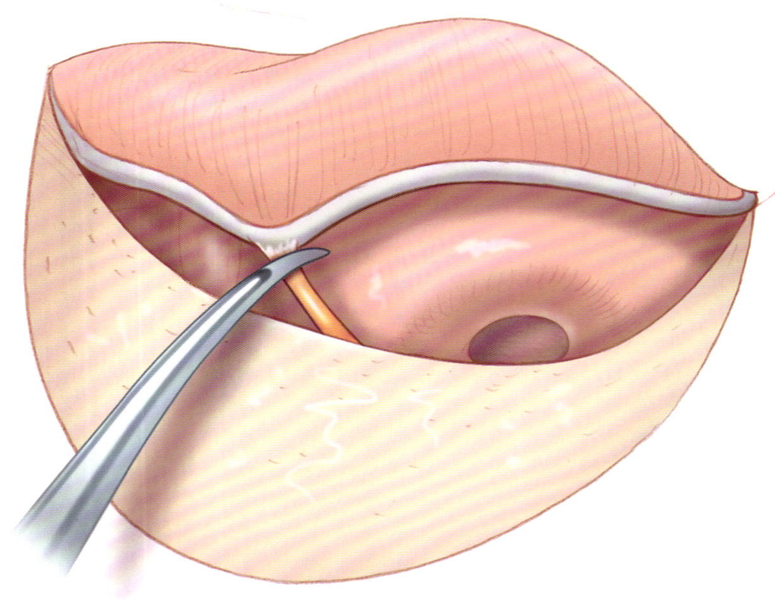

Figure 20-31. Elevation of the annulus superiorly is done with a curved needle. The chorda tympani nerve is identified and dissected free.

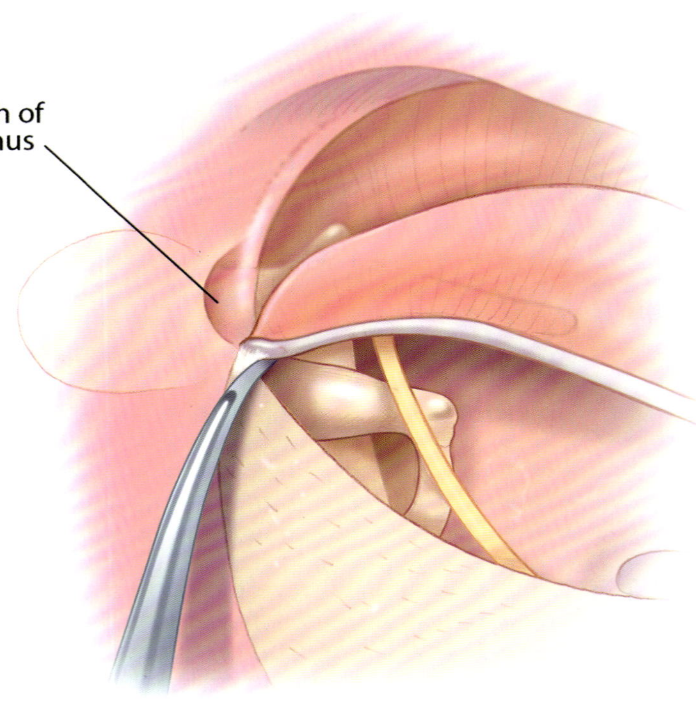

Figure 20-32. Elevation needs to be carried superiorly until the flap is free from the notch of Rivinus. This ensures that the flap will fold over the malleus handle and thus give sufficient exposure of the incus long process to enable crimping.

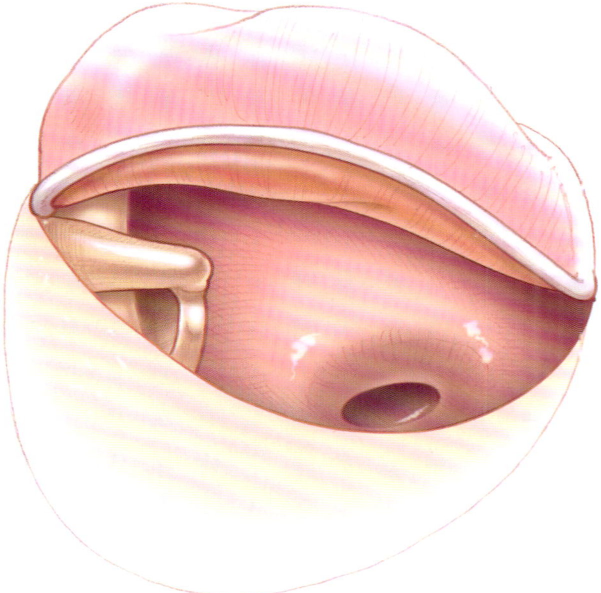

Figure 20-33. Completed flap elevation. Note that flap is folded on the umbo and that a space is available in front of the incus. If the flap does readily retain this position, further elevation superiorly or inferiorly is needed. Occasionally the flap may bulge posteriorly and compromise the exposure. This may result from a blood clot forming behind the flap, which can easily be evacuated.

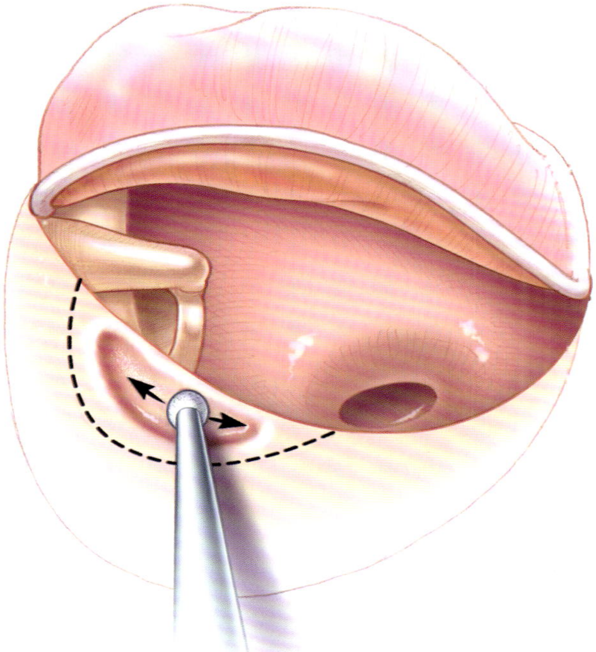

Figure 20-34. Most commonly the scutum (posterior ear canal overhang) allows at least a partial view of the stapes superstructure. It has to be removed to provide full access to the oval window. Scutum removal may be done with either a curette or microdrill or a combination of the two.

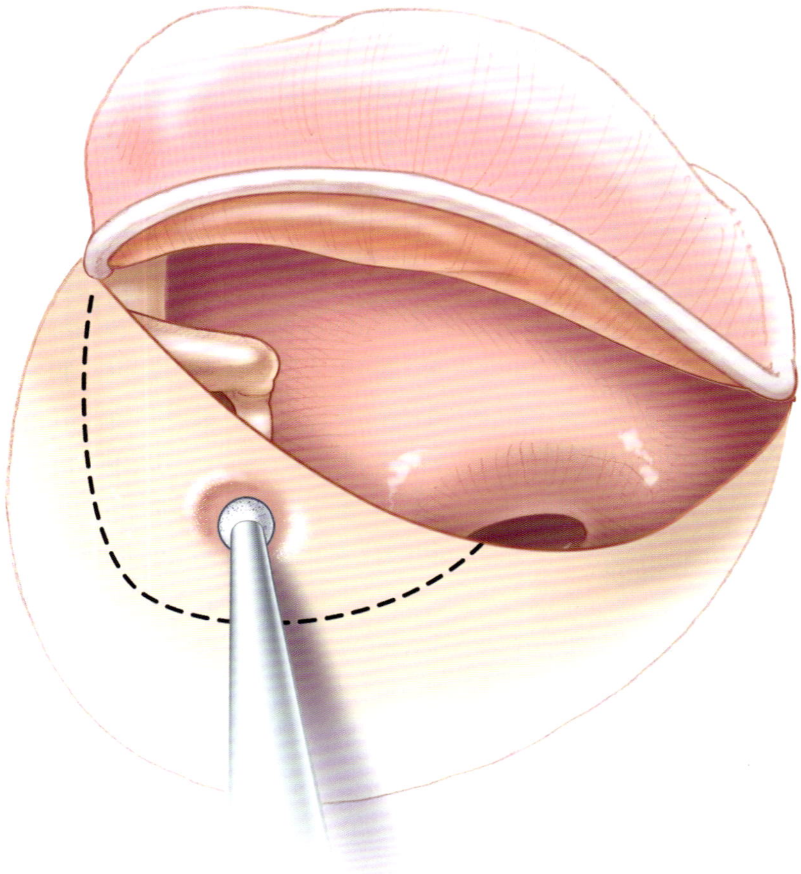

Figure 20-35. A long scutum may fully obscure the stapes and require a greater degree of bone removal. Curettage of such a thick scutum can require considerable effort.

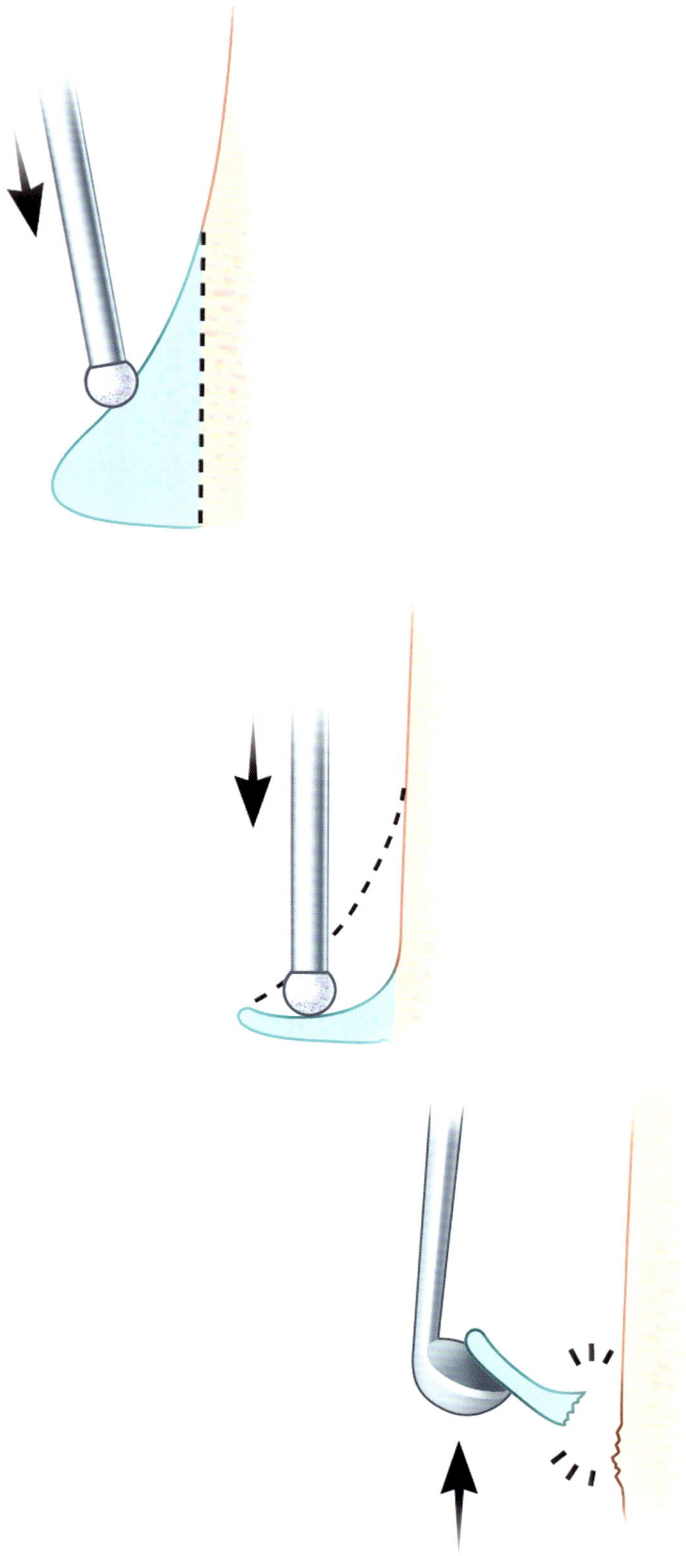

Figure 20-36. Combined technique in which the scutum is first thinned with a drill (eg, 2.3-mm diamond) and then a curette removes the last shell. A diamond burr is a bit slower, but is less likely to injure the chorda tympani, flap, or tympanic membrane.

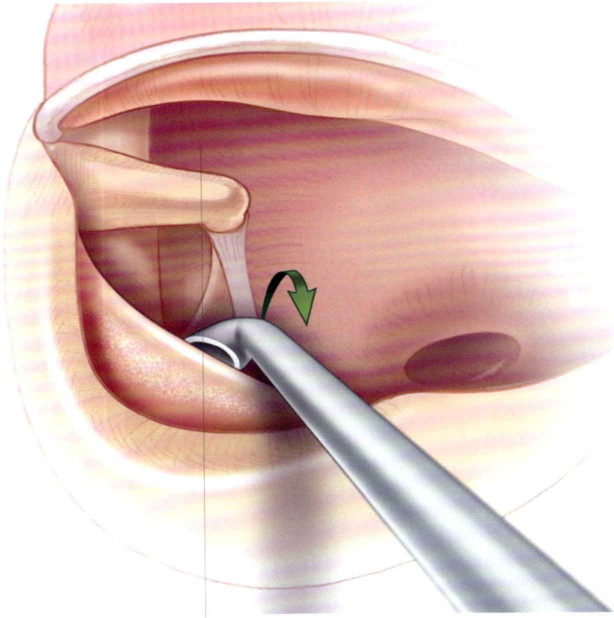

Figure 20-37. Use of a stapes curette to remove the scutum. The curette is firmly braced against the speculum to create a fulcrum effect. The motion is rotational and outward, never inward. A sudden release of inwardly directed force could lead to incus dislocation. Effective use of the curette takes practice and may be challenging for the novice. Considerable force is needed to fracture pieces of bone. When chipping away bone, it is important to avoid the curette from lurching outward where it can tear the canal skin and trigger bleeding.

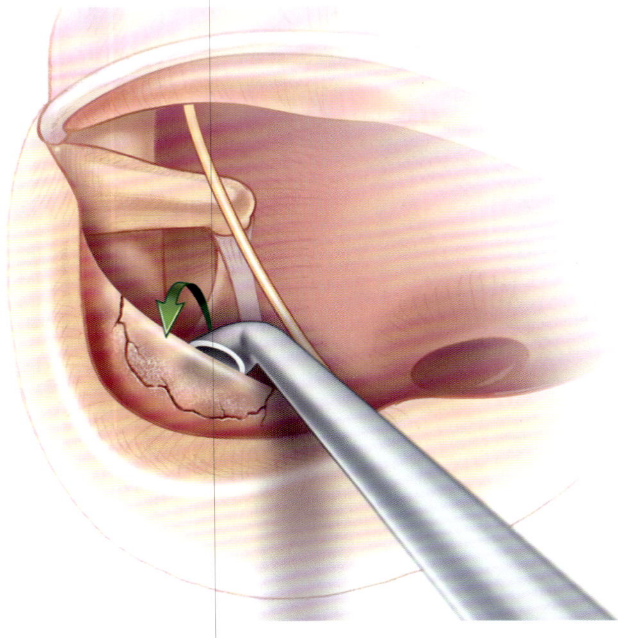

Figure 20-38. Curetting outward and away from the incus. Sometimes the scutum breaks away in a single piece. More commonly it is nibbled away in a series of small bone fragments.

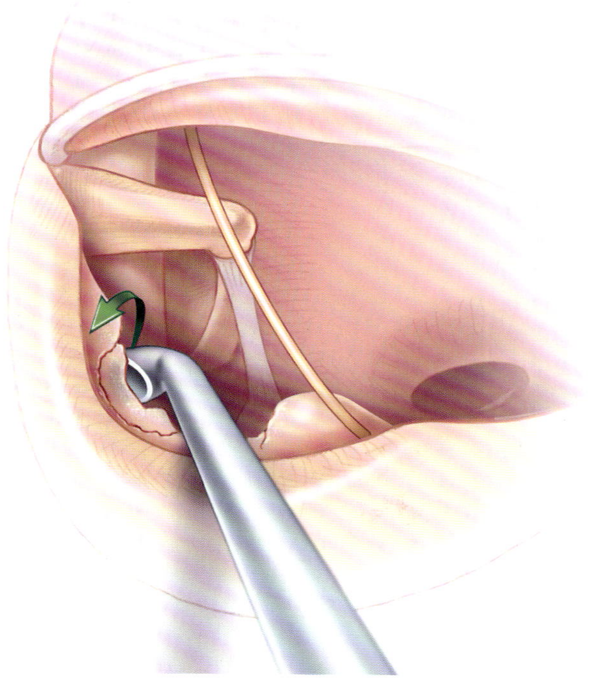

Figure 20-39. Removal of the last ridge needed for adequate exposure of the stapes. Curetting is complete when the facial nerve is in full view superiorly and the junction of the stapes tendon and pyramid are visible posteriorly.

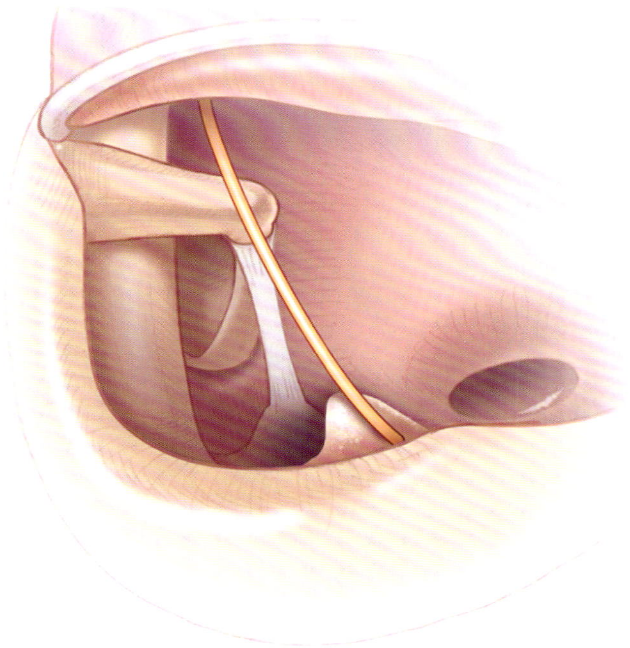

Figure 20-40. A bony prominence often exists under the entry of the chorda tympani. When the bone hinders exposure of the posterior aspect of the footplate it must be removed. This must be done carefully to reduce the risk of injury to the chorda tympani.

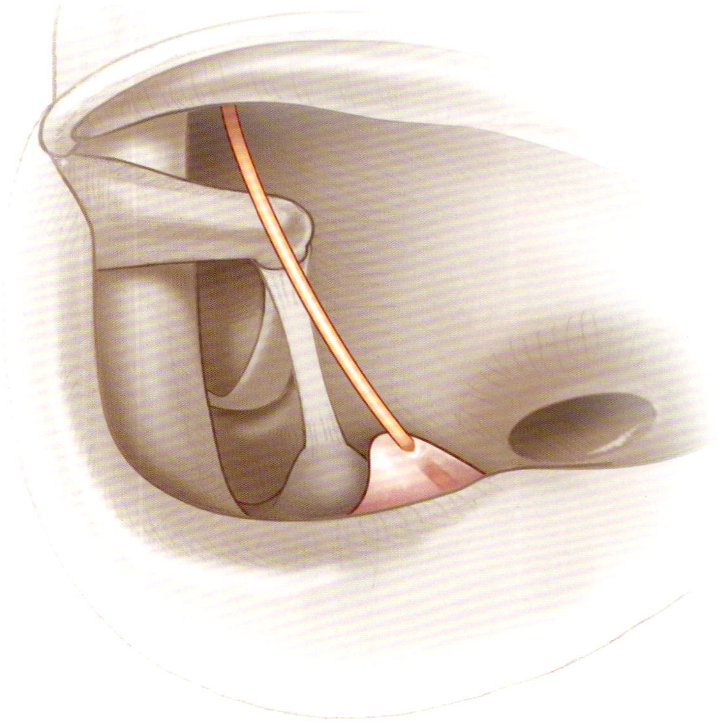

Figure 20-41. The chorda tympani sometimes actually traverses within the bone prominence.

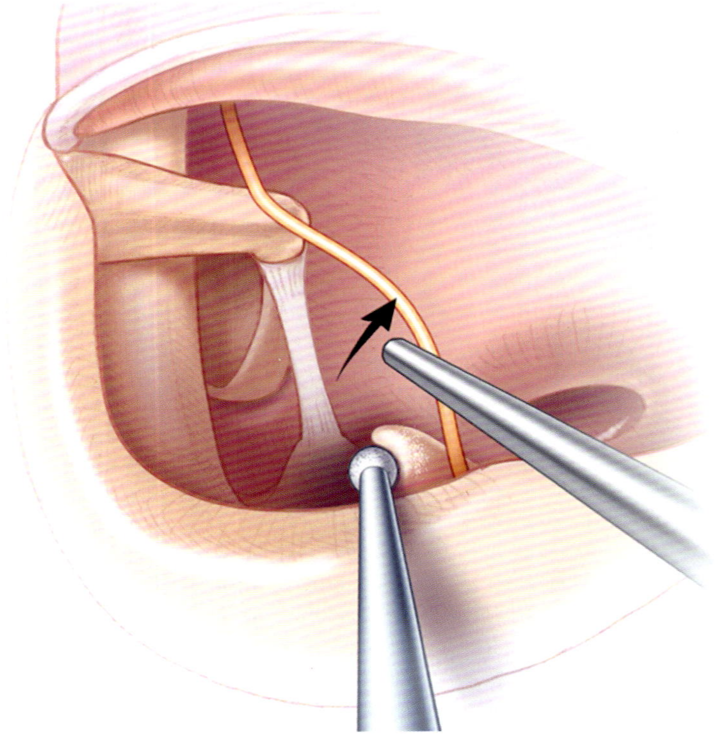

Figure 20-42. A 1-mm diamond burr is used to partially remove the prominence.

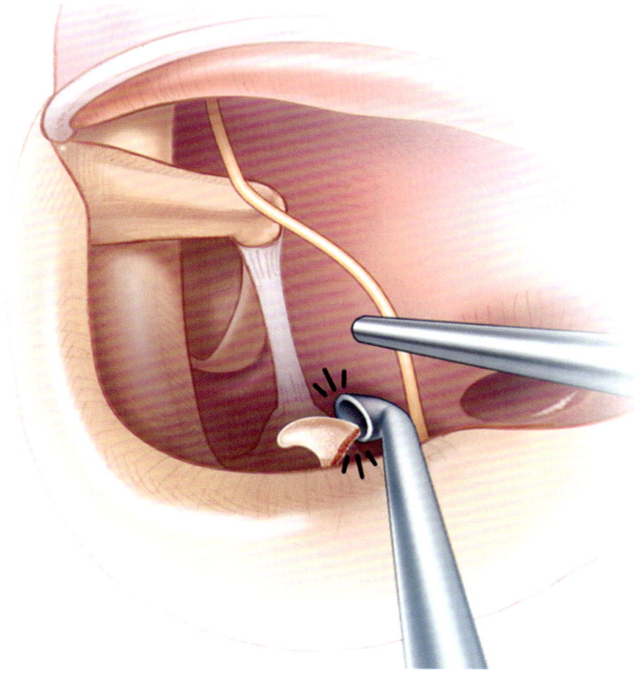

Figure 20-43. A curette is used to remove the remaining shel .

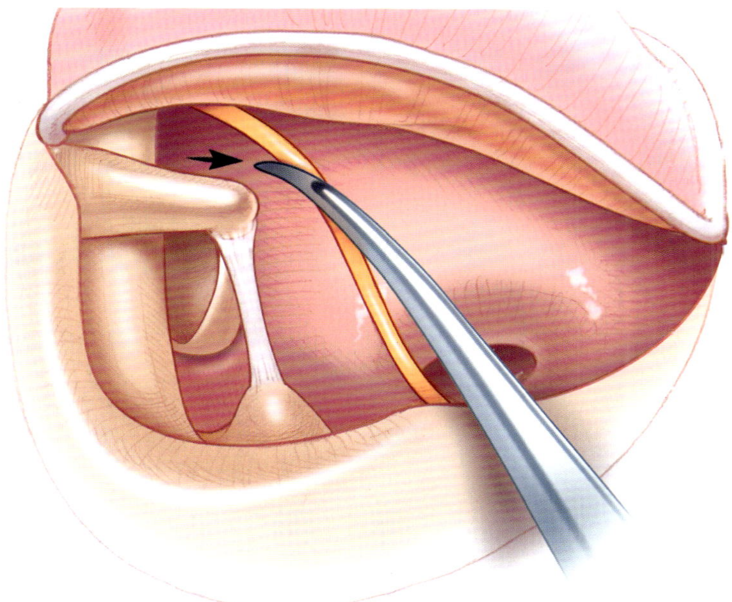

Figure 20-44. Exposure for stapes surgery is adequate when both the facial nerve and the junction of the stapes tendon with the pyramid are visible. It is important not merely to be able to see the stapes, but to have sufficient room to bring instruments into action from superior, posterior, and inferior directions. Mesenteries (often erroneously called "adhesions" when the mucosal folds are actually embryological remnants) often need to be lysed between the incus long process and the malleus. Establishing exposure anterior to the incus is essential to later placement of the prosthesis.

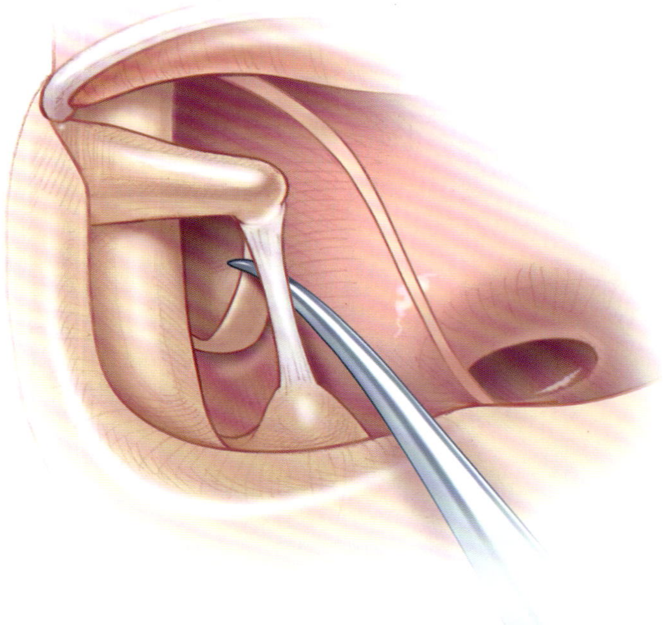

Figure 20-45. Palpation of the stapes superstructure to confirm fixation. This should be done gently as excessive force could mobilize a lightly fixed footplate.

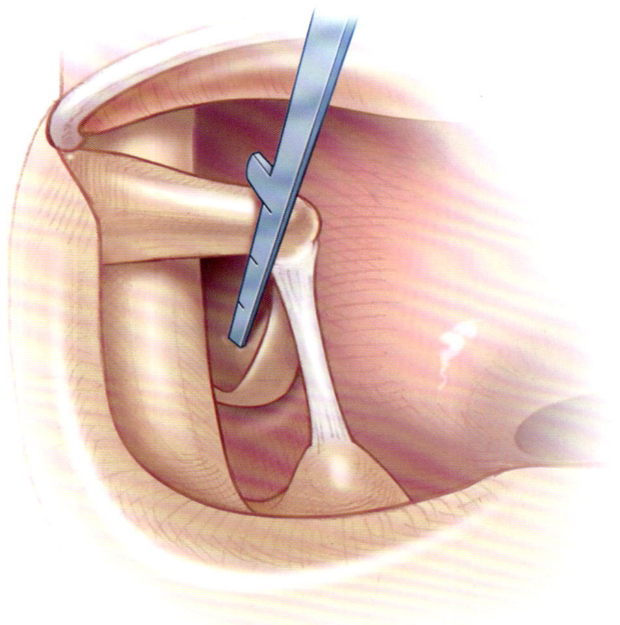

Figure 20-46. For sizing of the prosthesis, it is necessary to measure from the lateral aspect of the incus to the footplate. Note that the instrument is directly posteriorly, an angle that may require the malleable instrument to be slightly bent. To achieve the proper angle, the instrument shaft has to lean on the anterior wall of the speculum. Correct measurement is between the center and posterior third of the footplate. The measurement is 4.5 mm in the majority of cases. The maneuver must be done delicately to avoid perforation of the footplate.

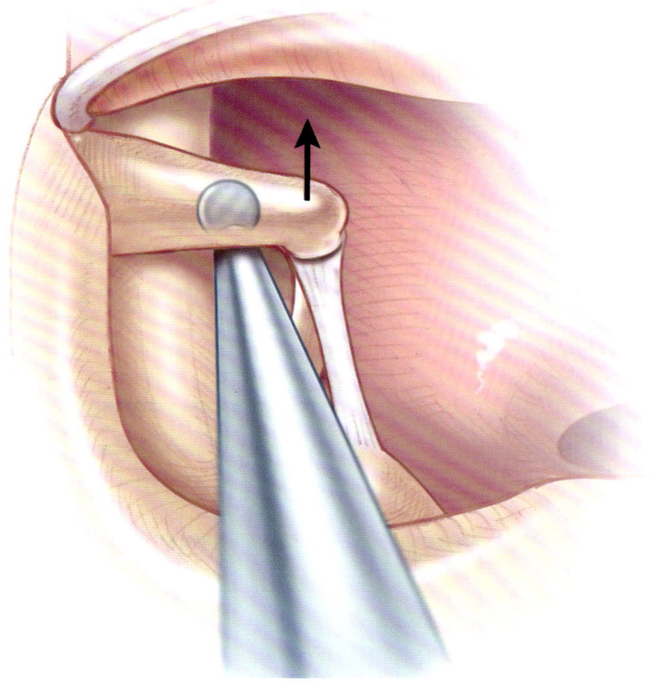

Figure 20-47. Before cutting the incudostapedial joint it is helpful to visually identify it. Slight outward pressure on the incus with the incudostapedial joint knife demonstrates the thin gray line of the joint.

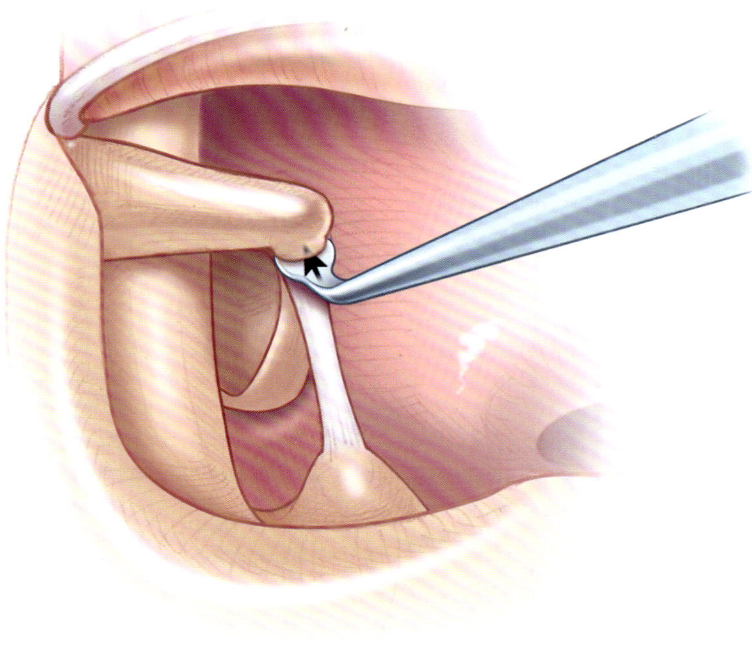

Figure 20-48. The joint is cut with a gentle "worming" motion in the anterior direction. During this maneuver gentle outward lifting of the incus is best while strictly avoiding a downward pressure on the stapes capitulum.

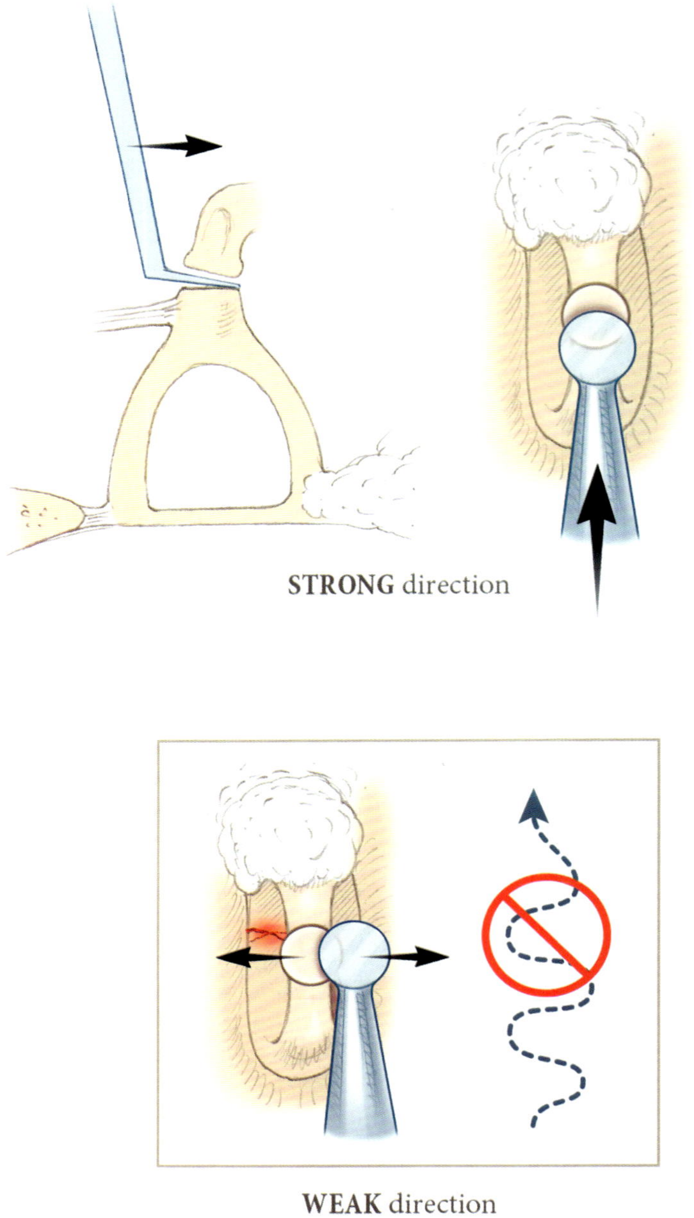

Figure 20-49. The force vector used while dividing the joint should be primarily anteriorly directed. As the footplate is fixed anteriorly but remains mobile posteriorly, side to side motion risks creating a transverse fracture in the footplate.

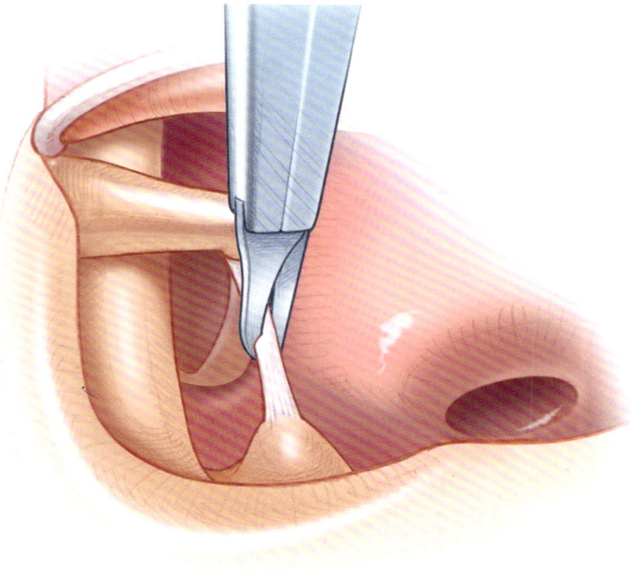

Figure 20-50. Division of the stapedial muscle tendon using microscissors (eg, Bellucci). To avoid cutting the posterior stapes crus, the trajectory of the scissors should be posteriorly directed. This is achieved by leaning the shaft of the scissors lean on the anterior side of the speculum.

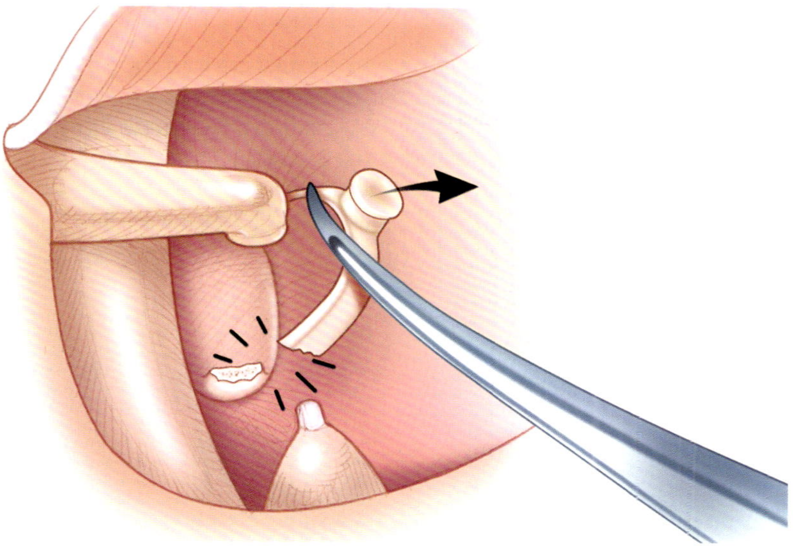

Figure 20-51. Removal of the stapes superstructure through down fracture toward the promontory. This maneuver should always be conducted away from the facial nerve. The curved needle (eg, Rosen) should contact both crura, but preferentially apply force to the anterior crus. Excessive pressure on the posterior crus will potentially lead to transverse footplate fracture. Note that this maneuver has to be done briskly. A slowly building motion may mobilize the footplate whereas a quick snapping motion will have the desired effect of fracturing the bases for both crural arches as desired. After removing the stapes superstructure, it is important to recheck that the footplate remains intact and fixed. Niche bleeding can be controlled by placing a small pledget of epinephrine-soaked Gelfoam® in the niche for a minute or two.

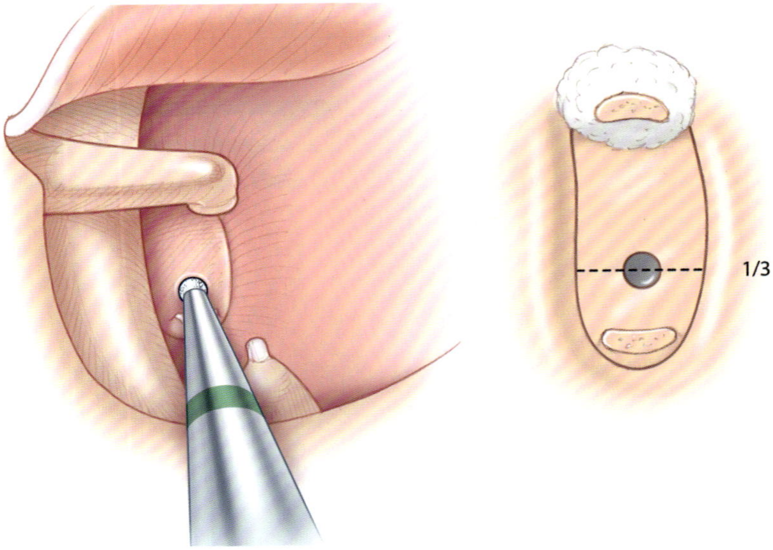

Figure 20-52. Creation of a small fenestra stapedotomy with a burr slightly larger than the intended prosthesis (eg, 0.7 mm for a 0.6-mm piston). It is best to use a diamond burr with a thin, blue footplate as a cutting burr is more likely to shatter the footplate. Optimal position of the fenestra is in the posterior central region of the footplate as the vestibule is deepest in this region. Because this procedure is delicate and potentially dangerous, a mere extra 1 mm of penetration can kill the ear, certain precautions are recommended. It is wise to remind everyone in the room to be quiet and be warned to avoid touching the patient or operating table. The surgeon's hand needs to be comfortable, well supported, and absolutely stable. The burr should be running at full speed. The drilling motion is a quick, subtle inward motion with the goal of having the burr penetrate to its meridian (ie, widest point) and not beyond. Contact with the footplate should be brief. A fenestrometer is used to ascertain the adequacy of the fenestra (see illustration in laser stapes surgery). If too small, an additional edge the shape of a crescent moon is drilled to enlarge the fenestra.

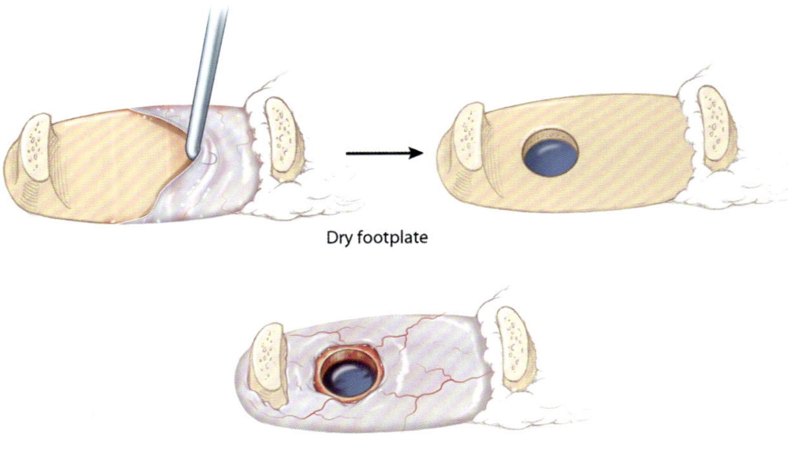

Figure 20-53. Prior to fenestration some surgeons remove the footplate mucosa. Once the bleeding has ceased, the fenestra can be created without stirring up bleeding. With the mucosa intact, oozing often occurs, which can hinder placement of the prosthesis.

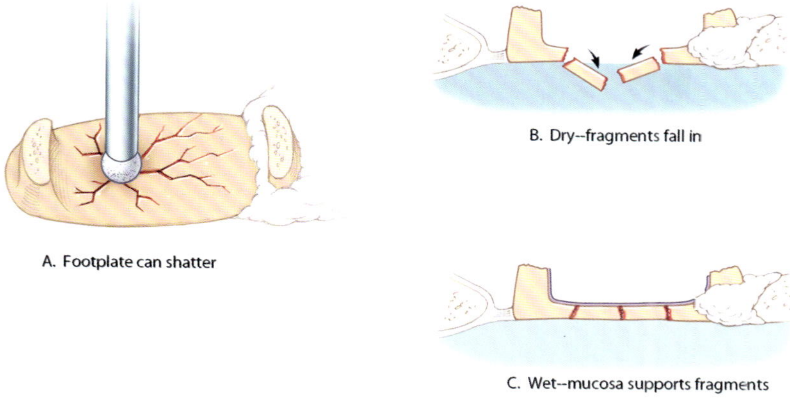

Figure 20-54. Despite the greater potential for niche bleeding, many surgeons prefer to leave the footplate mucosa intact. Should the footplate shatter during drilling, the mucosa retains the fragments at the oval window level. Without tethering mucosa, these tend to fall into the vestibule.

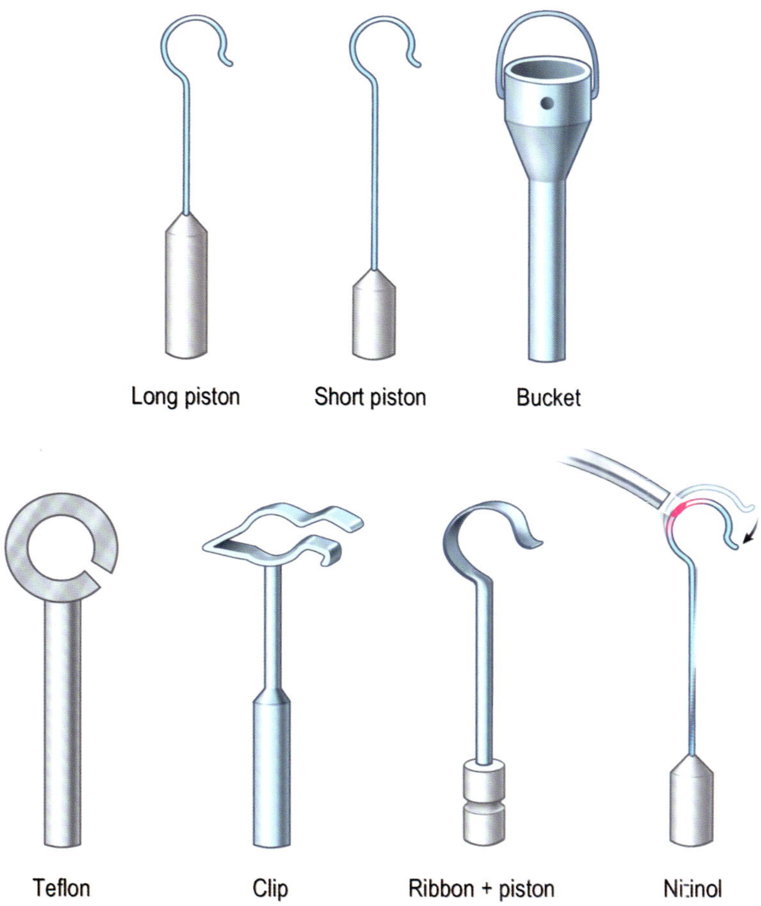

Figure 20-55. A wide variety of stapes prosthesis are available. The major types are depicted here. Most common materials used are titanium, nonmagnetic stainless steel, and Teflon. Many carry the names of their inventors.

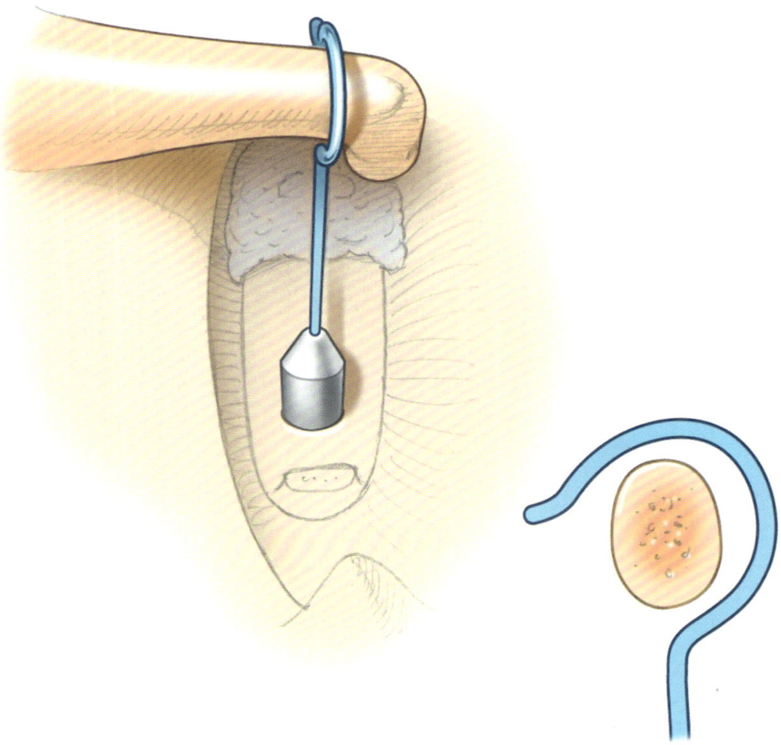

Figure 20-56. Using a smooth alligator the prosthesis is seated in position. It is important to have both the shepherd's crook engage the incus as well as the piston the fenestra. If the wire misses the incus the piston can penetrate the vestibule too deeply.

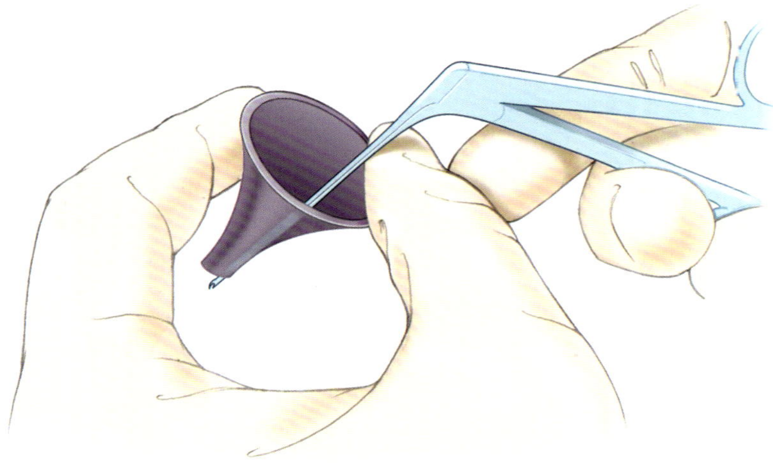

A

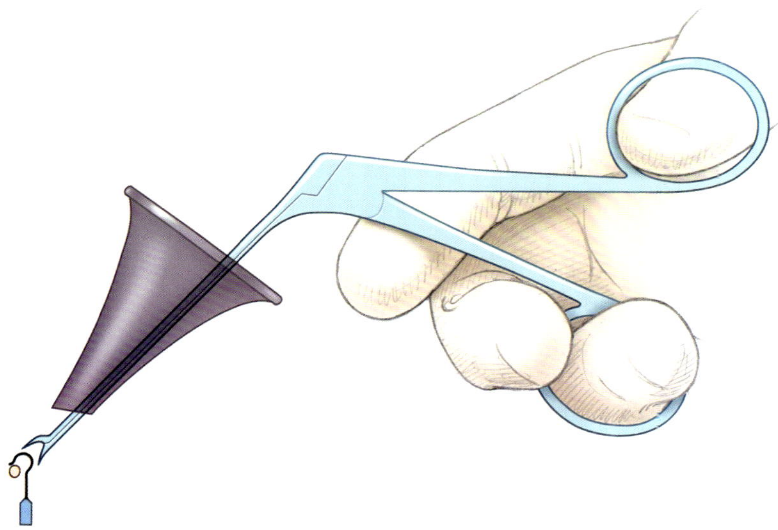

B

Figure 20-57. **A–B.** Crimping of the prosthesis on the long process of the incus is a delicate maneuver. The crimper must be stabilized on the wall of the speculum.

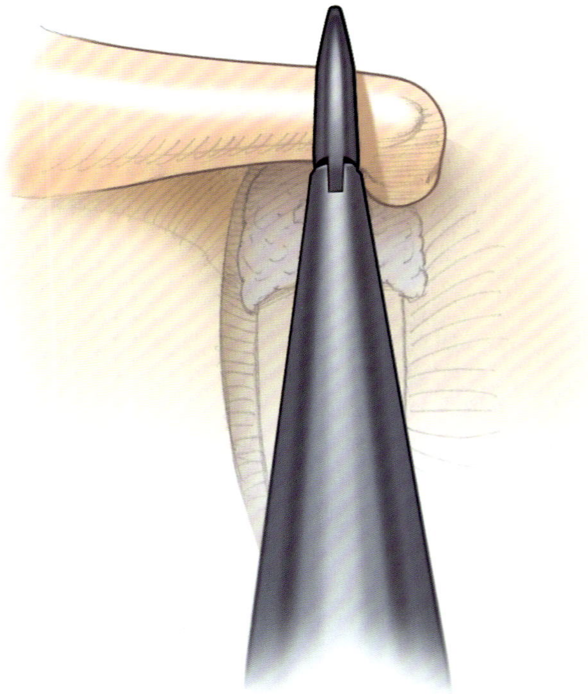

Figure 20-58. The crimper must be aligned perfectly with the wire. If misaligned, the prosthesis will not crimp but will instead twist off to one side.

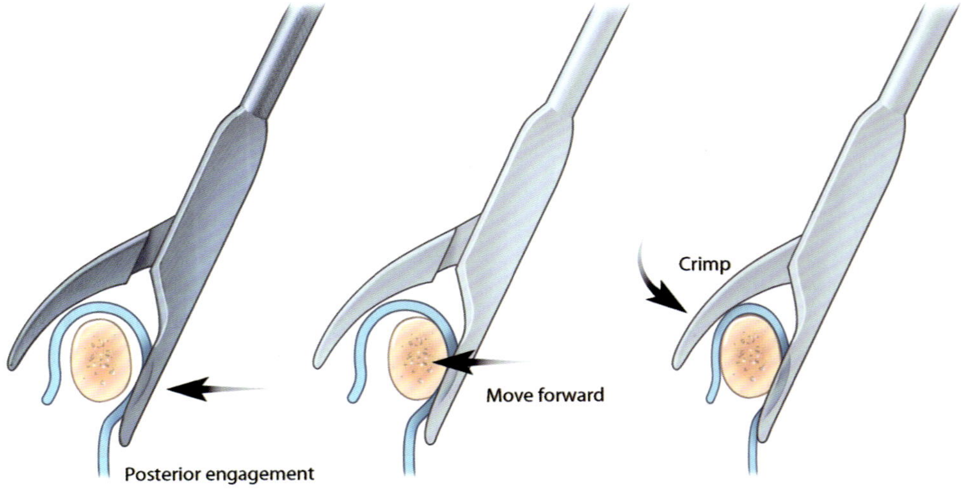

Figure 20-59. It is important to understand the crimper's action. The back tine should be held stable while the front tine actively closes onto the incus.

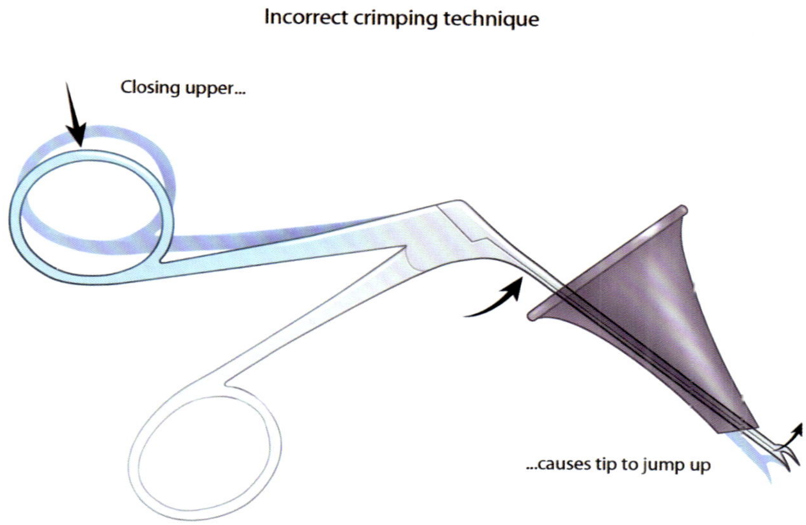

Figure 20-60. Incorrectly moving the thumb side will cause the tip of the crimper to move forward putting force on the incus.

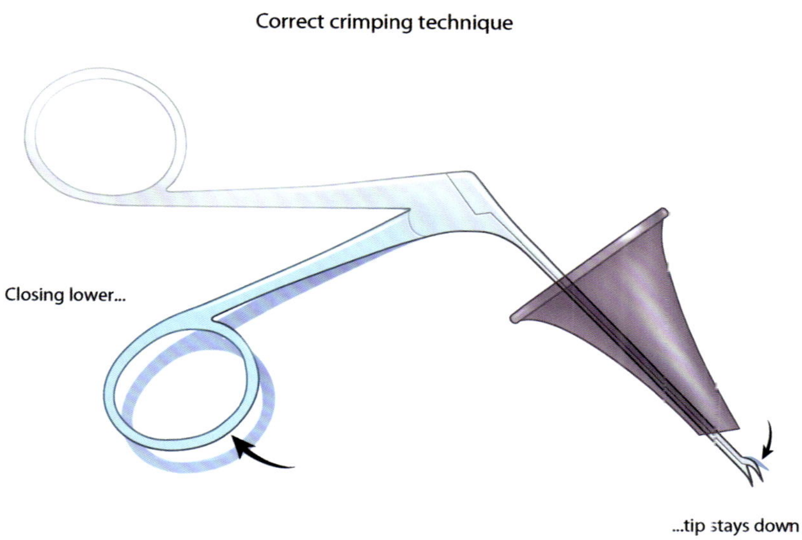

Figure 20-61. Proper crimping motion stabilizes the incus and allows the anterior tine to close the wire.

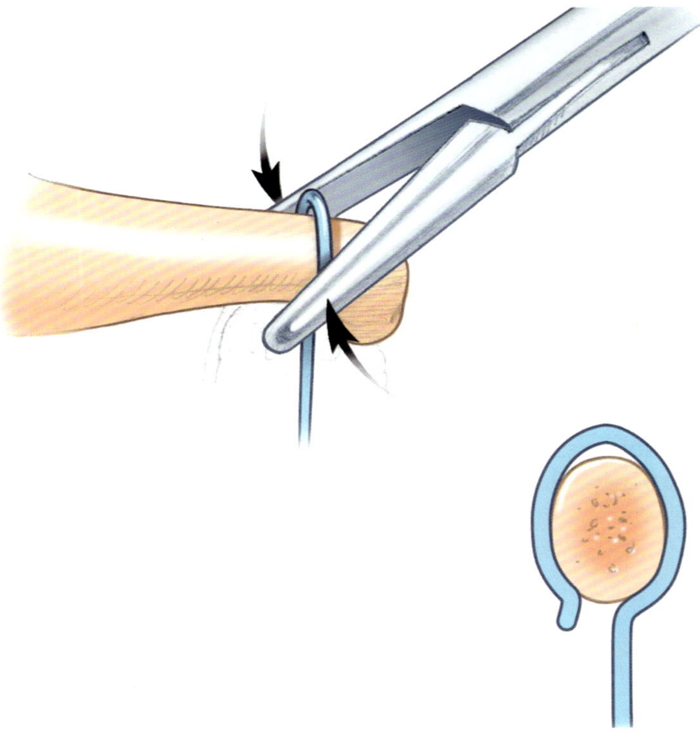

Figure 20-62. The loop closure after crimping is often too loose. To tighten, the loop is moved to the narrowest point of the incus shaft and then cinched down with a smooth alligator. The closed loop can then be slid down the incus slightly toward the lenticular process to fit snugly.

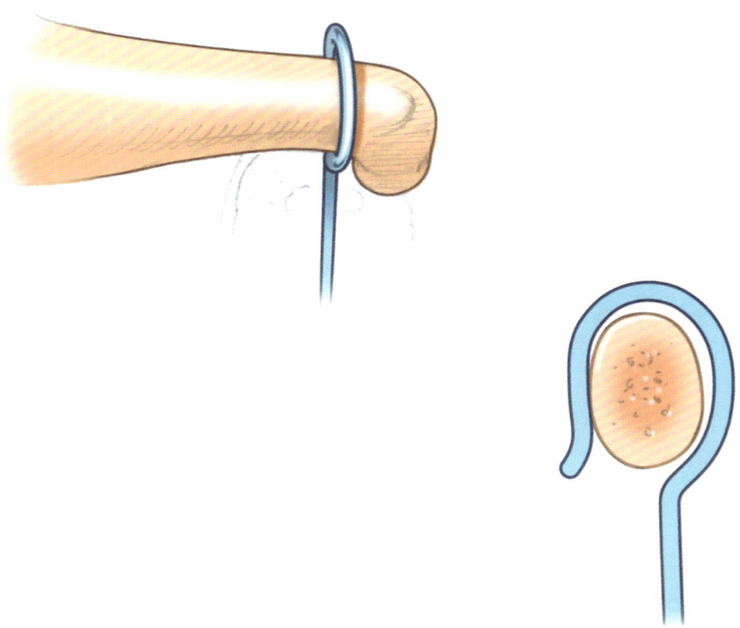

Figure 20-63. An ideal crimp is not hermetically tight around the incus as this may lead to later incus necrosis. The usual crimp may have a slight play to it.

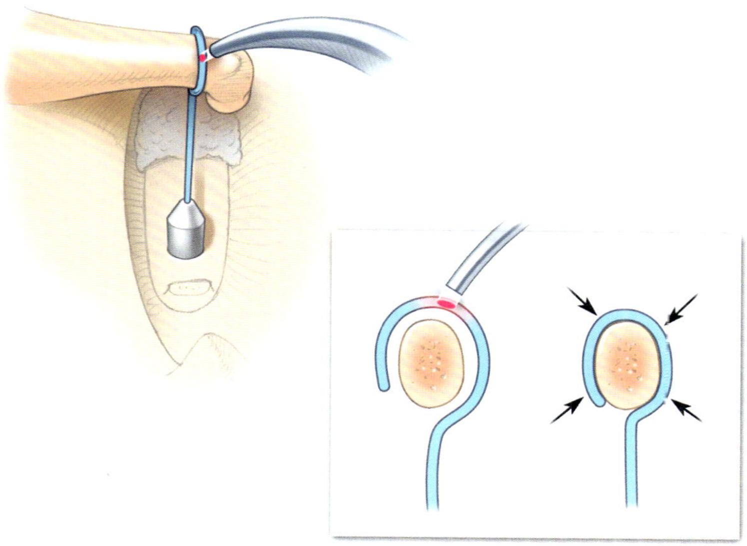

Figure 20-64. Nitinol prostheses avoid the need for mechanical crimping. The heat-activated metal crimps to the incus with the application of laser energy.

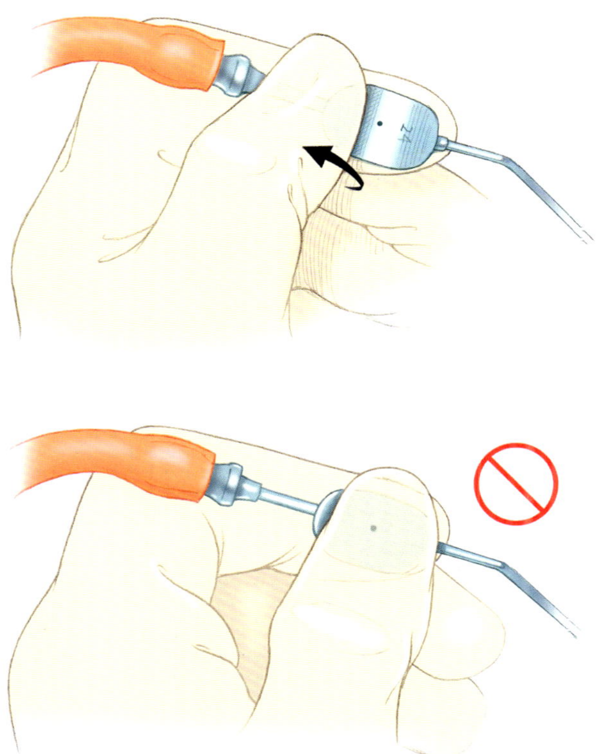

Figure 20-65. Removing blood from the vicinity of an open oval window must be done with great care. It is best to use a very small suction (eg, a #24 needle), turned down low, with the surgeon's thumb off the hole. When needed to remove tenacious clot, the thumb can briefly roll over the hole to momentarily enhance suction force. As a general rule, it is best whenever possible to remove liquid blood from the footplate before it has the opportunity to clot.

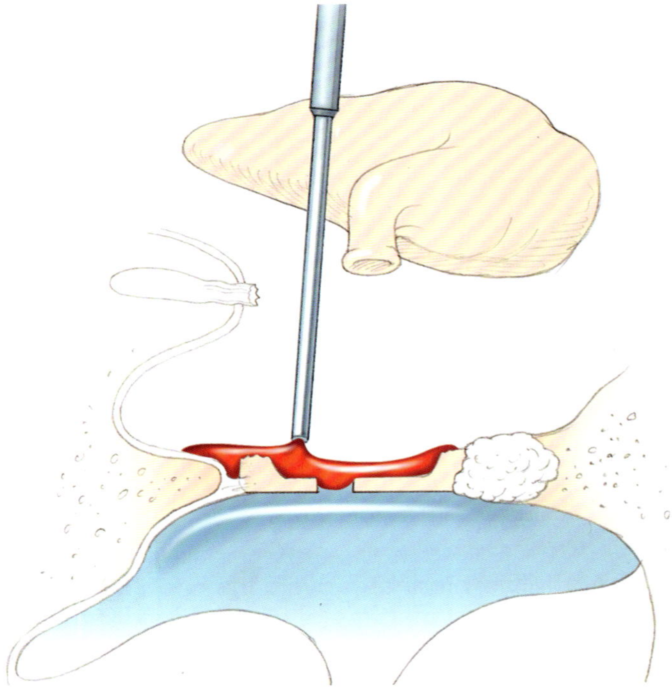

Figure 20-66. Blood is suctioned from the footplate by vacuuming anterior or posterior to the fenestra.

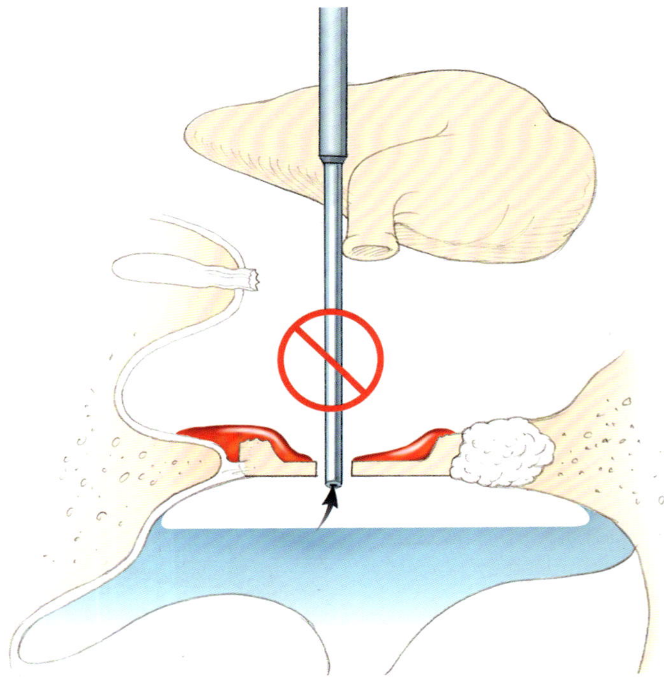

Figure 20-67. Suctioning directly over the fenestra can remove perilymph leading to a dry vestibule. This may result in sensory loss and postoperative vertigo. When air is in the vestibule some surgeons refill it with saline, but perilymph typical replenishes spontaneously via the cochlear aqueduct. Injury to the utricle or saccule, admixing endolymph with perilymph, is a much more serious injury.

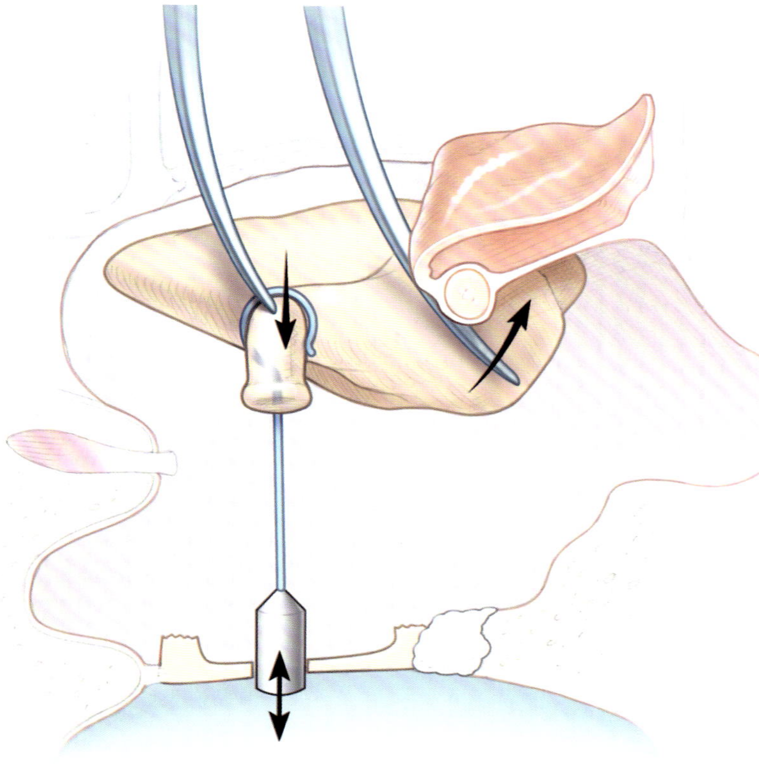

Figure 20-68. Once the prosthesis is seated and crimped, its mobility is tested both by gently moving either the incus or malleus handle. To avoid trauma to the inner ear, this maneuver is done only once or twice. The author does not use the round window reflex as it is unnecessary and risks traumatizing the inner ear.

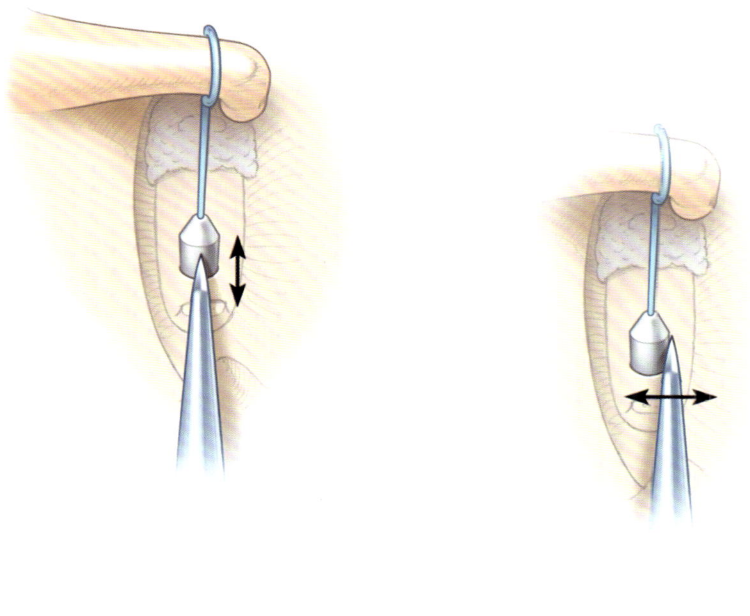

Figure 20-69. A needle or hook tests the adequacy of the piston's depth of insertion.

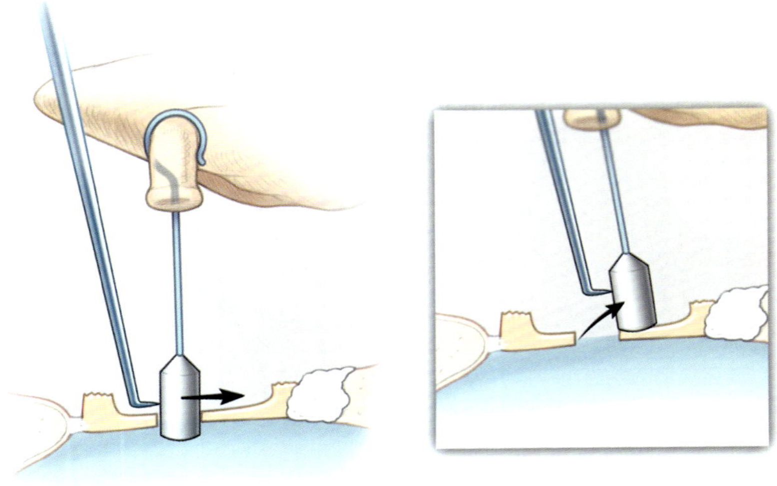

Figure 20-70. Although a well-placed prosthesis will retain under gentle pressure (*left*), a shallowly placed prosthesis will pop out when subjected to stress (*right*). If this occurs, the prosthesis is replaced with one 0.25 mm longer.

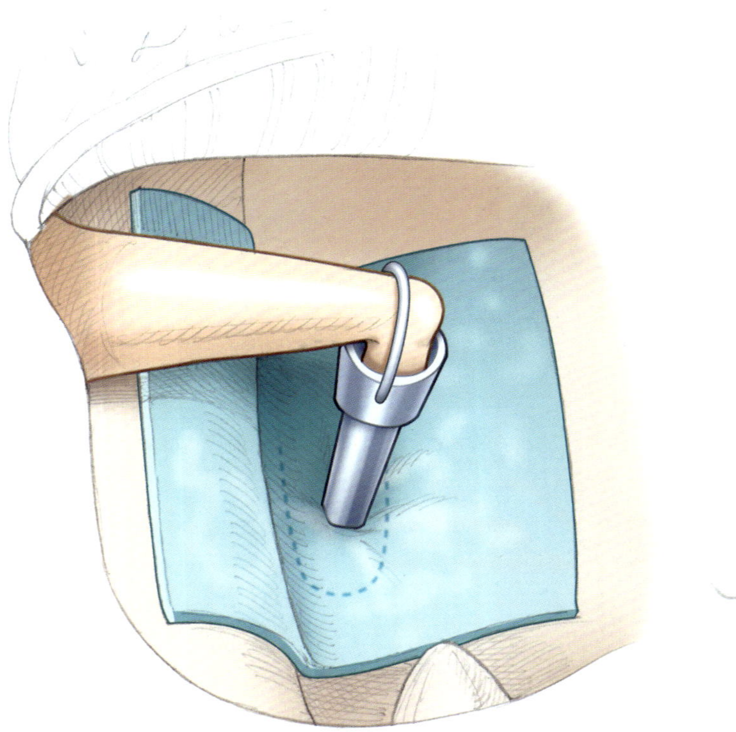

Figure 20-71. A bucket handle prosthesis requires no crimping, the loop is simply pulled over the incus. A tissue membrane is shown sealing a large fenestra.

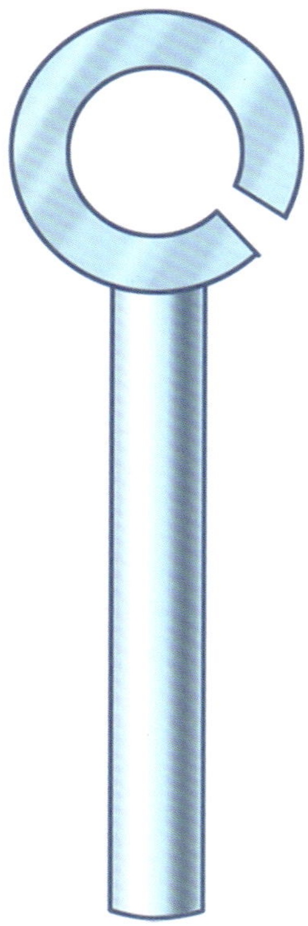

Figure 20-72. A Teflon prosthesis of the Causse type.

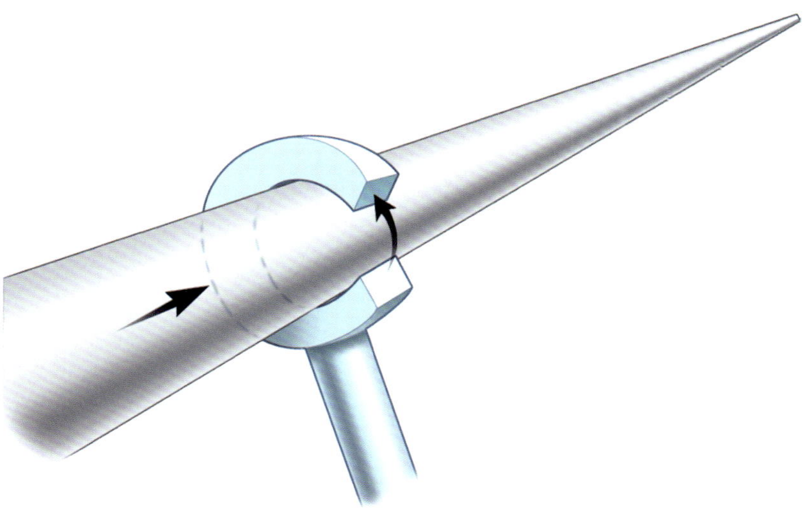

Figure 20-73. The loop is dilated to accommodate the incus long process.

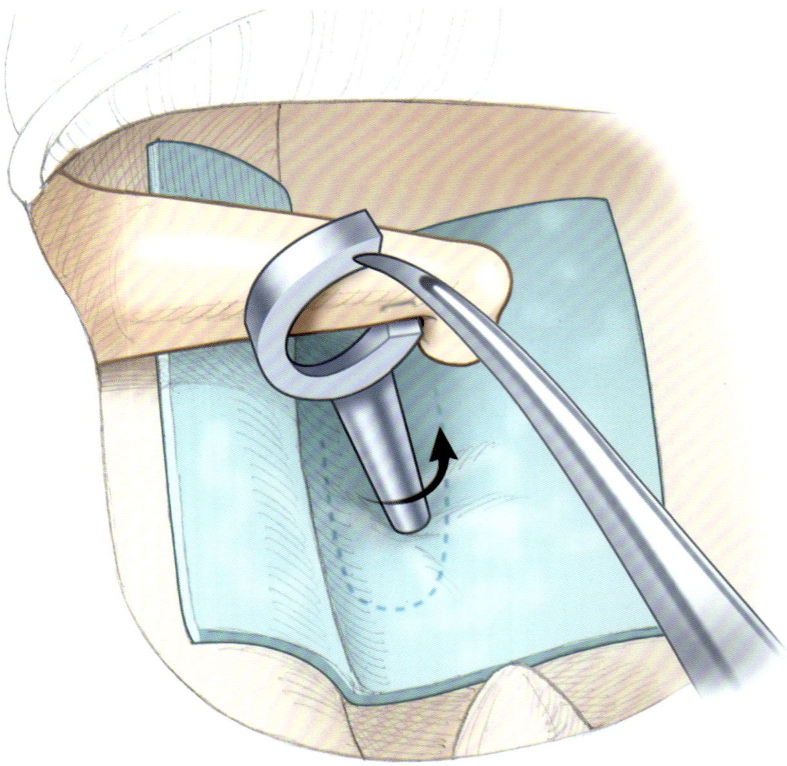

Figure 20-74. The prosthesis is rotated to engage the incus.

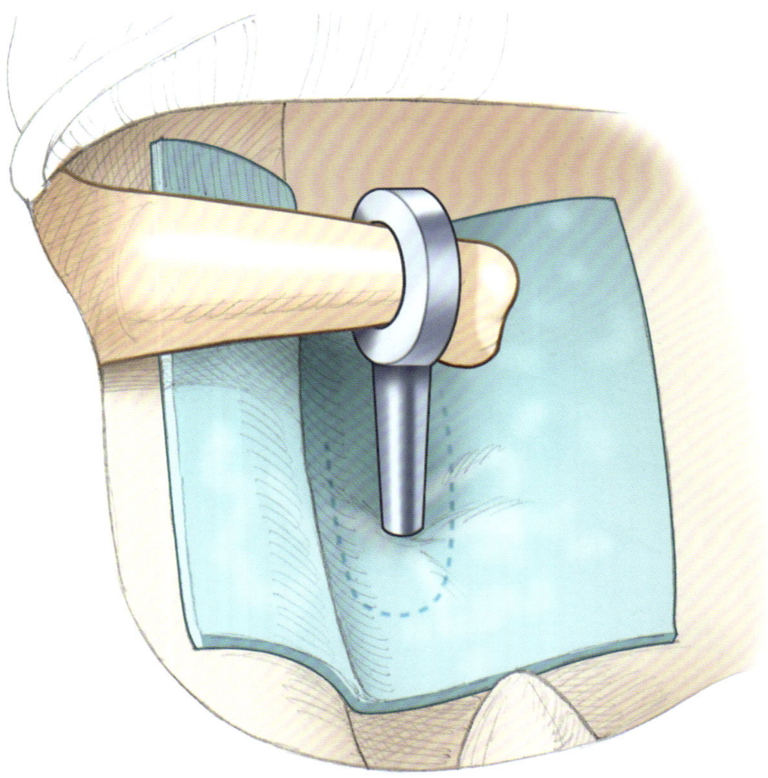

Figure 20-75. The Teflon loop prosthesis is seated into the fenestra.

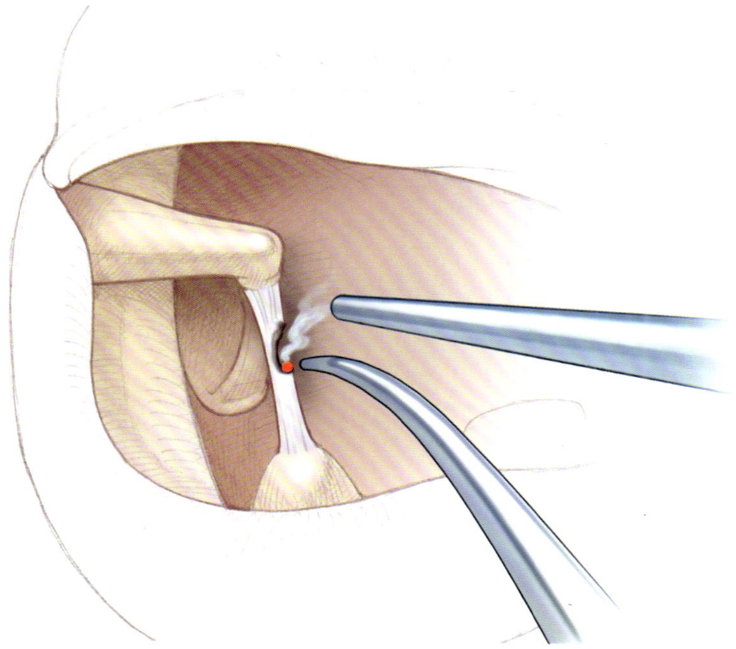

Figure 20-76. In laser stapes technique, the stapedial tendon is divided with the laser. The illustration depicts a hand-held laser fiber delivery system, which is favored in most centers over micromanipulator systems. One advantage of the hand-held laser fiber is its divergent beam, which dissipates laser energy away from the tip thus reducing the risk of overshoot injury. The fiber can also be brought in from various angles, whereas a micromanipulator beam is restricted to line of sight.

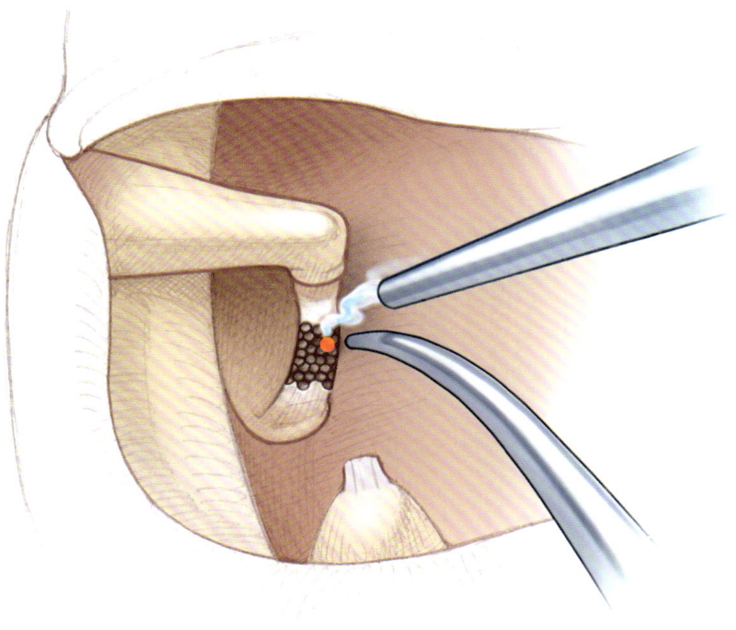

Figure 20-77. Charring of the posterior crus with multiple, overlapping laser bursts.

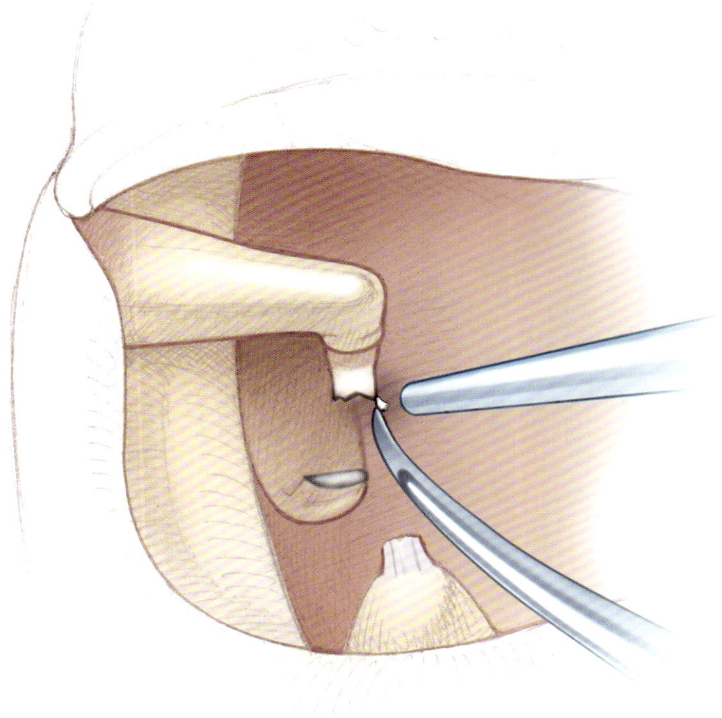

Figure 20-78. The charred posterior crus is chipped away.

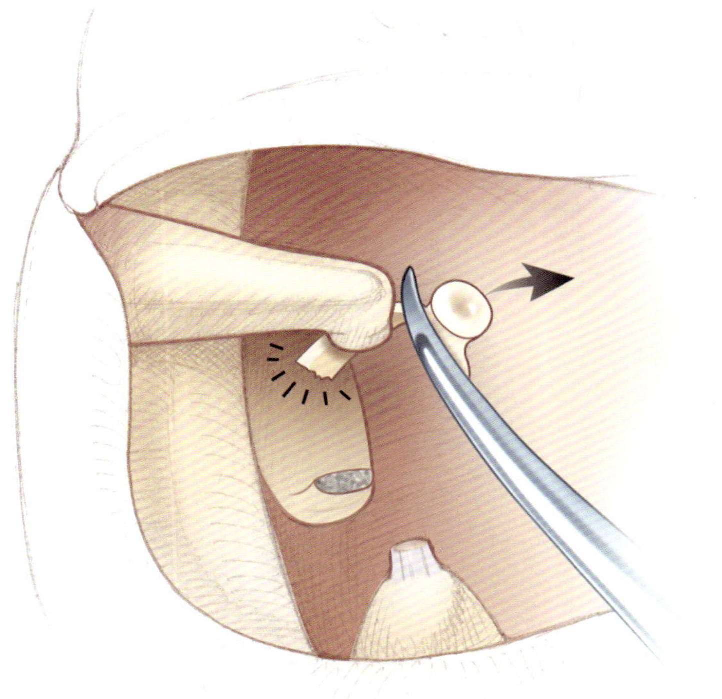

Figure 20-79. In most cases, it is difficult to target the anterior crus with the laser so it is snapped off mechanically.

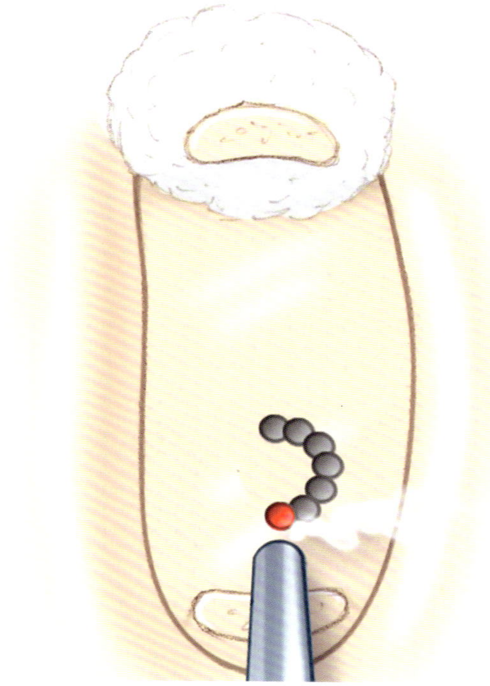

Figure 20-80. Small fenestra stapedotomy with a laser is usually created with a series of overlapping rosettes. As the unpigmented footplate may act like a laser mirror, the process may require initiation by allowing a drop of blood to form on the footplate. To catalyze energy absorption, each successive laser shot overlaps the char from the last one slightly.

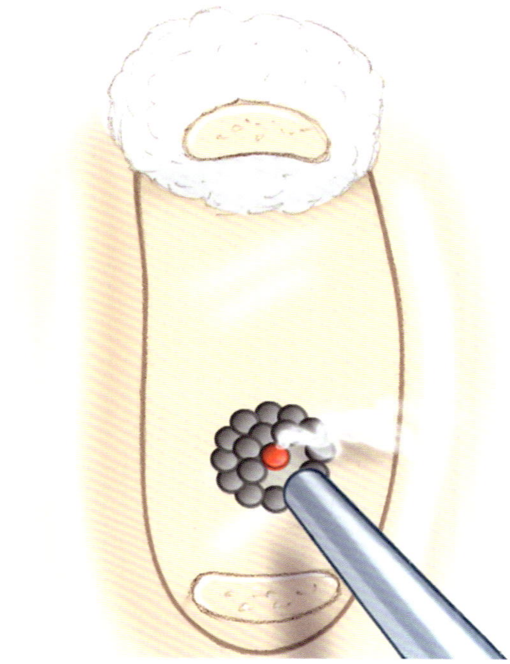

Figure 20-81. The rosette is completed by charring the entire area to be removed.

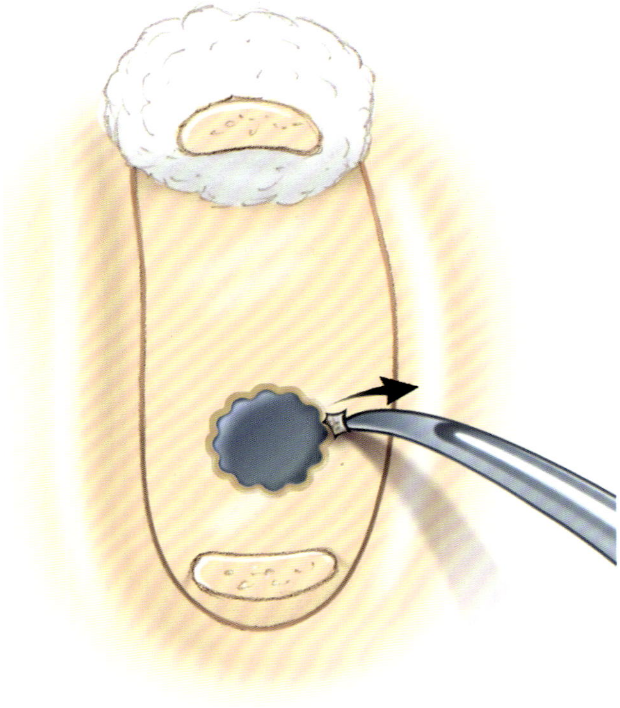

Figure 20-82. The char overlying the fenestra is then picked away. Other surgeons simply push the piston through the char.

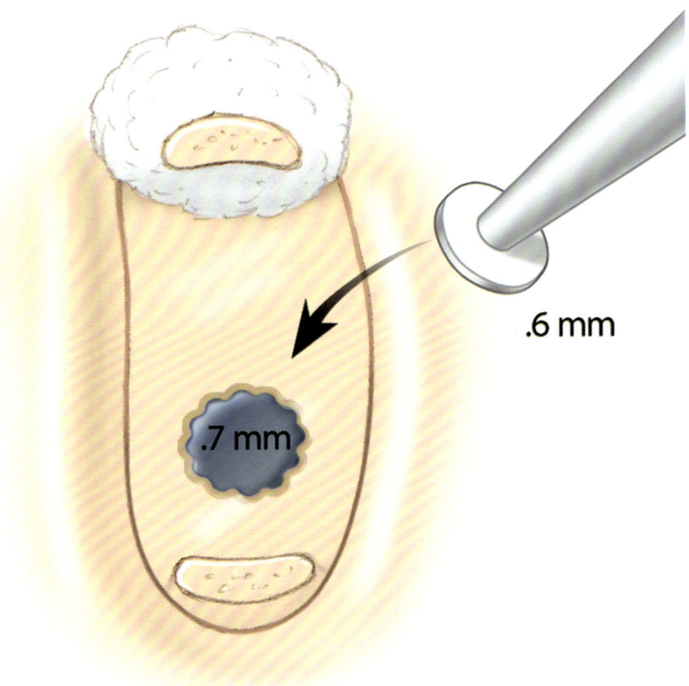

Figure 20-83. A fenestrometer (eg, 0.6 mm) can be used to evaluate the adequacy of the fenestra. The ideal fenestra is 0.1 mm in diameter wider than the piston.

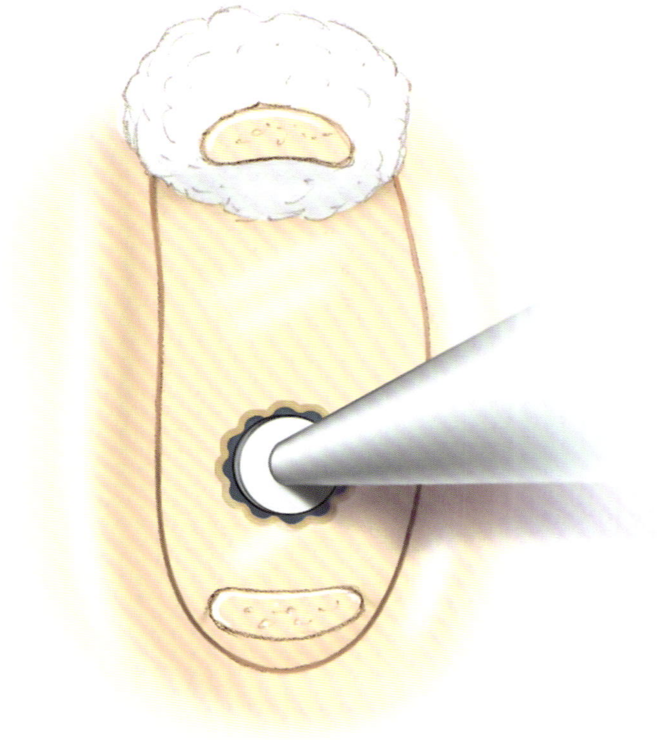

Figure 20-84. The fenestrometer is for visual reference only; it is best kept superficial to the fenestra.

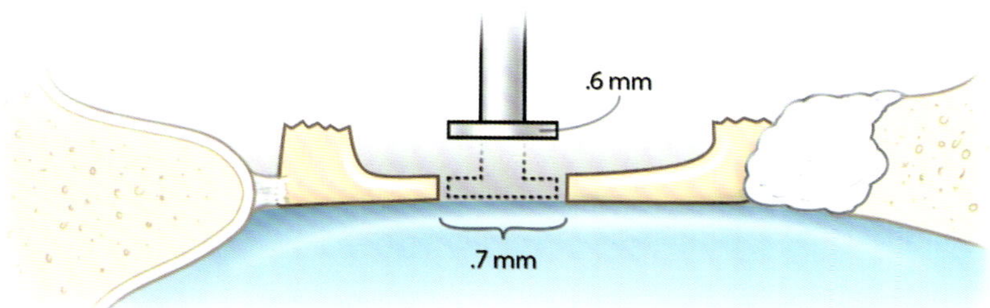

Figure 20-85. Placing the fenestrometer within the fenestra risks damage to the footplate.

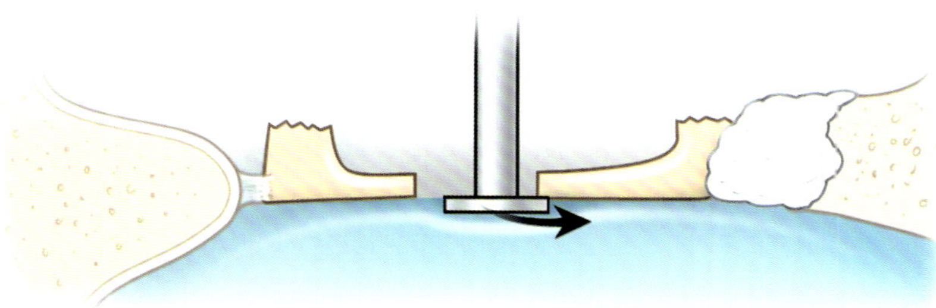

Figure 20-86. Once beneath the plane of the fenestra, it is difficult to remove without chipping away additional bone from the fenestra margins.

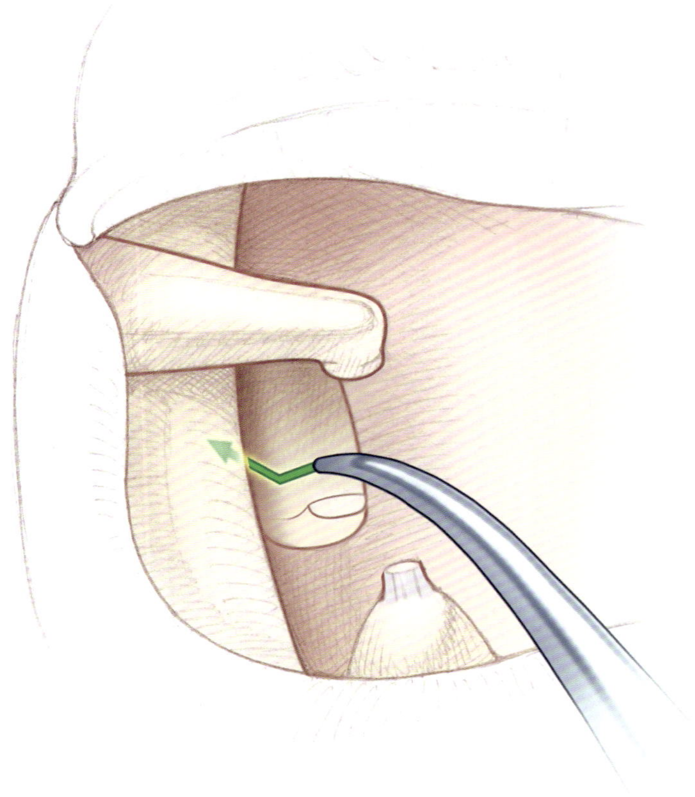

Figure 20-87. The footplate can act like a mirror reflecting laser energy, which becomes deposited elsewhere in the middle ear.

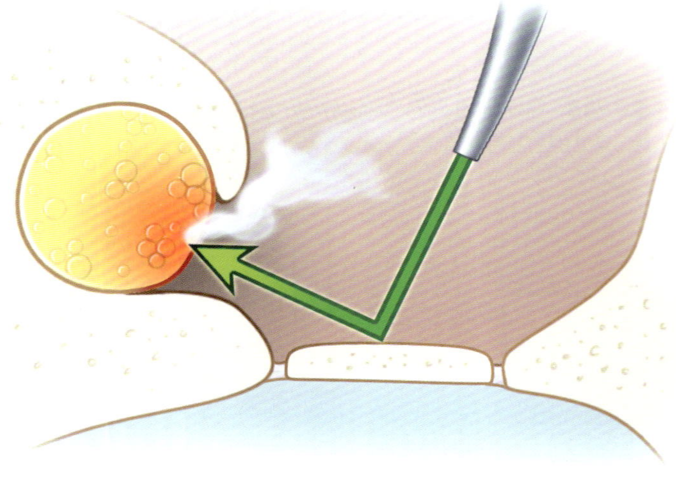

Figure 20-88. Facial nerve injury has occurred when the surgeon inadvertently heated the adjacent facial nerve, which is often dehiscent on its undersurface facing the footplate.

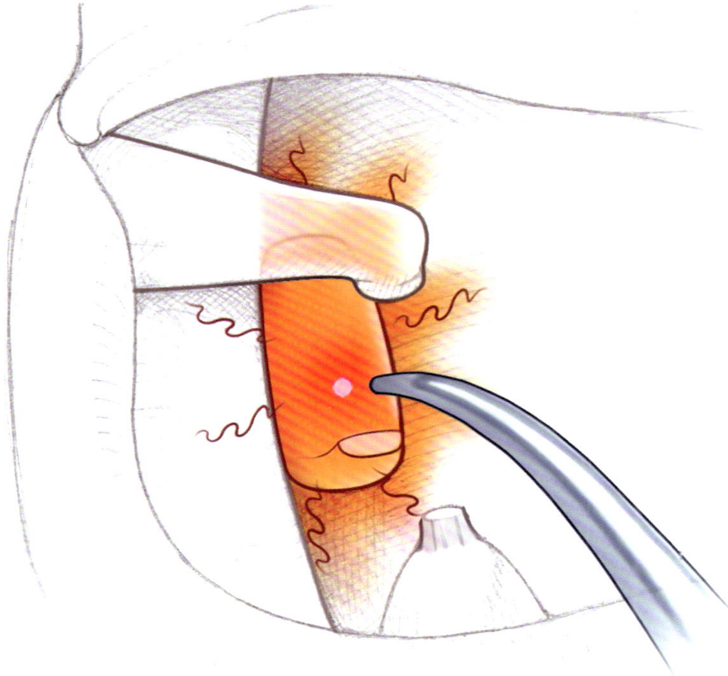

Figure 20-89. Both repeated laser impulses that fail to char the footplate (ie, a large fraction of the energy is reflected) and excessive laser power may contribute to the risk of facial nerve or inner ear thermal injury.

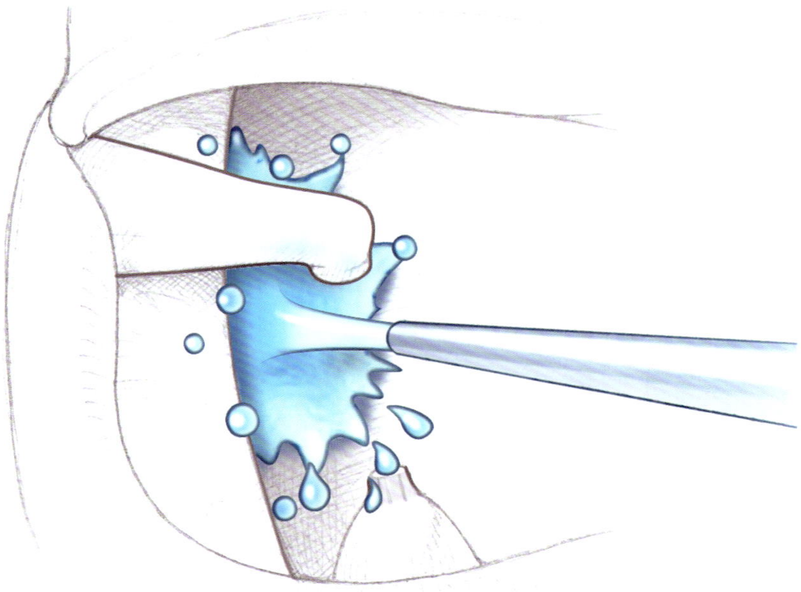

Figure 20-90. When delivering laser pulses to the footplate it is wise to periodically flush with cool saline as a means of mitigating unwanted heat buildup.

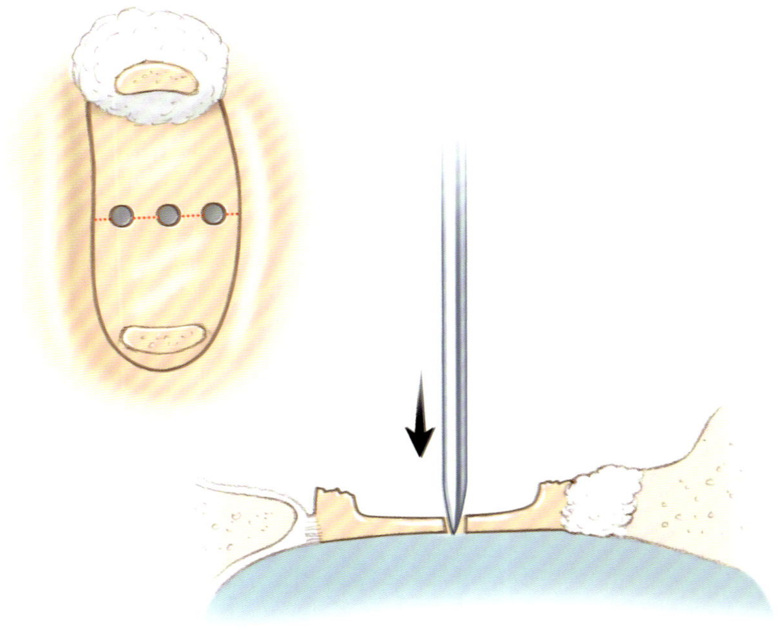

Figure 20-91. In traditional large fenestra technique, one-half or more of the footplate is removed. A sharp straight needle is used to create a series of footplate perforations across the meridian of the footplate. Some surgeons keep a sharpening stone on their set to remove any barbs from the needle before this maneuver. A dull needle might crack the footplate.

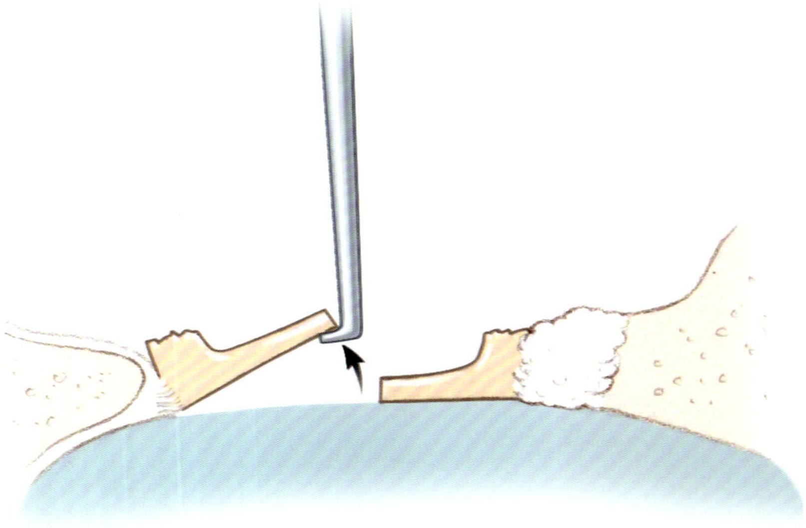

Figure 20-92. A hoop is used to extract the posterior half of the footplate.

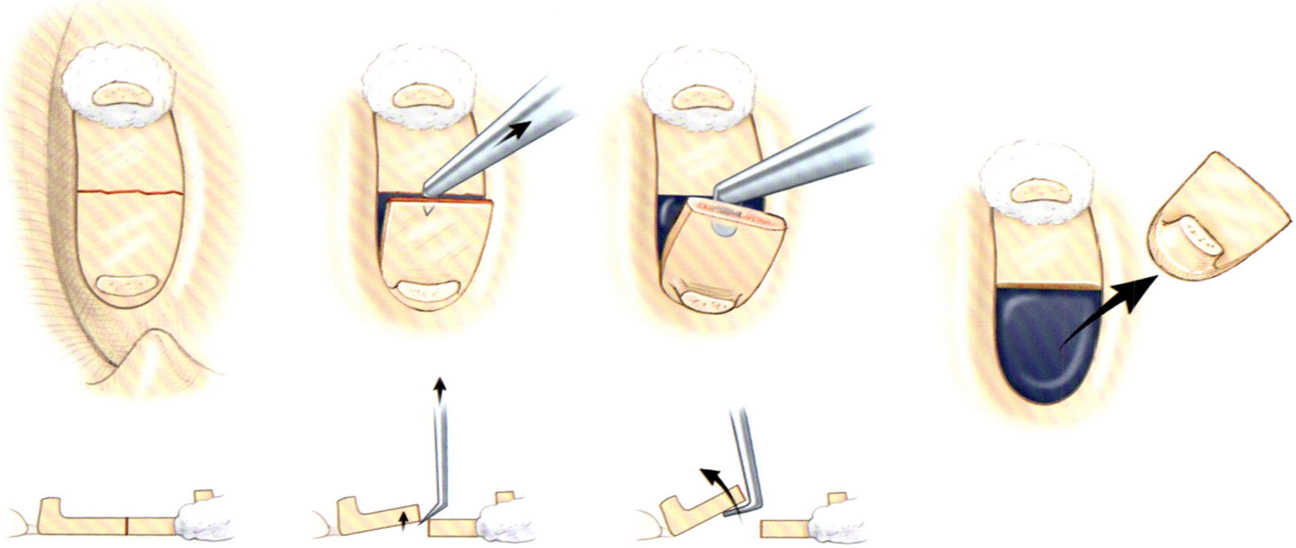

Figure 20-93. When the footplate crack is thin and nondisplaced, an obtuse (45-degree) hook is needed as a crack opener. This is a most useful tool to have on a stapes set. Once the posterior half has been elevated, a broad 90-degree hook (eg, Hough hoe) can be used. When access is adequate, it is better to use a broad-surfaced hook rather than a pointed one, as the latter can chip fragments of bone rather than lift the segment whole.

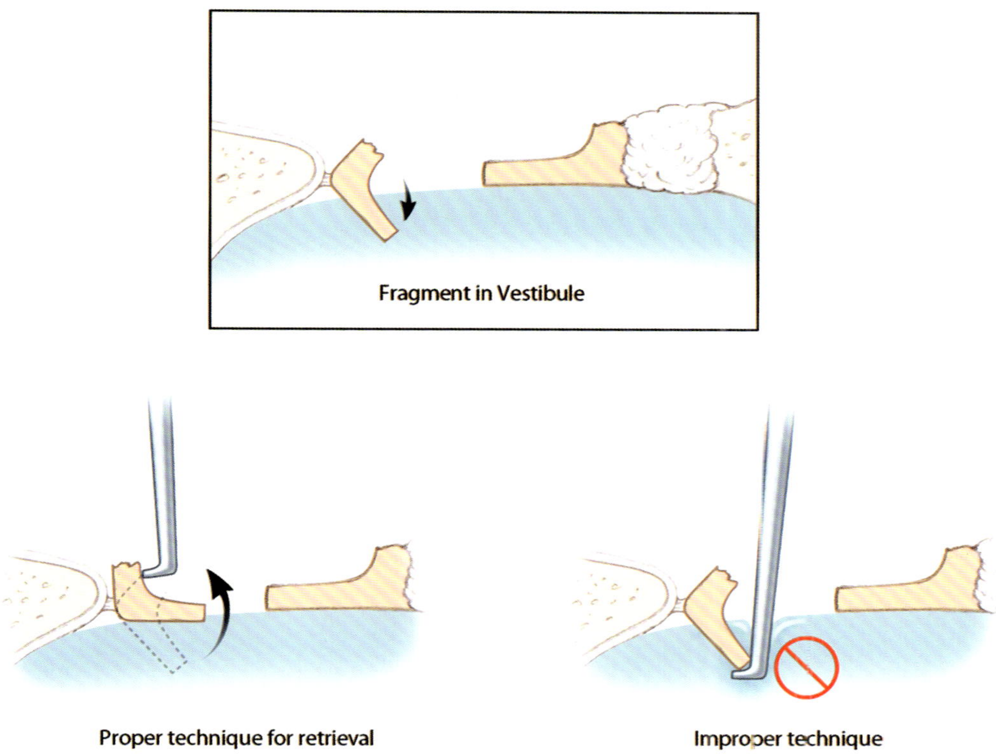

Figure 20-94. When a footplate fragment begins to fall into the oval window, it is a central axiom of stapes surgery not to reach into the vestibule. Often the fragment can be retrieved by engaging the crural base remnant with a hook.

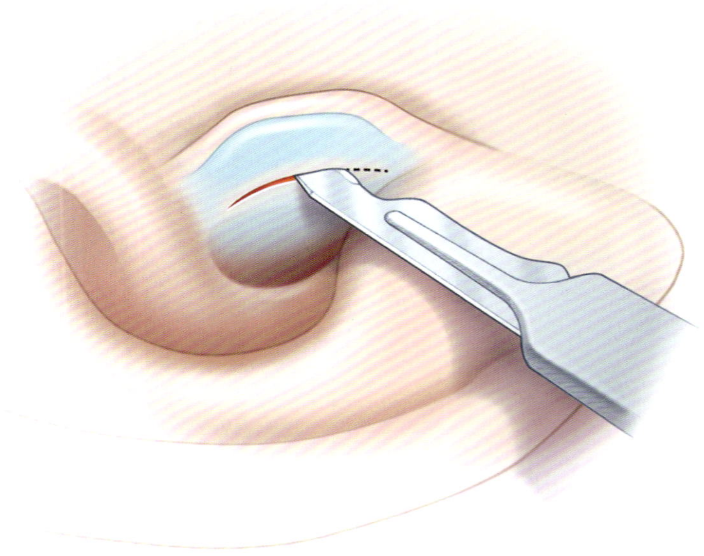

Figure 20-95. Larger fenestra stapedotomy requires a tissue seal. Options include vein from the back of the hand, temporalis fascia, or tragal perichondrium. As the tragus is readily available in the operative field, many surgeons prefer to obtain perichondrial grafts. To avoid a visible scar, the incision is placed on the dorsal surface of the tragus.

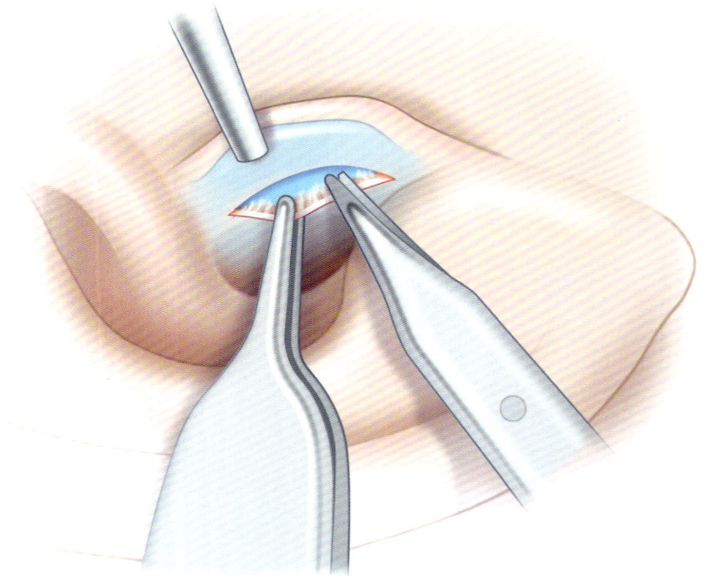

Figure 20-96. Scissors dissected the subcutaneous tissue from the perichondrium.

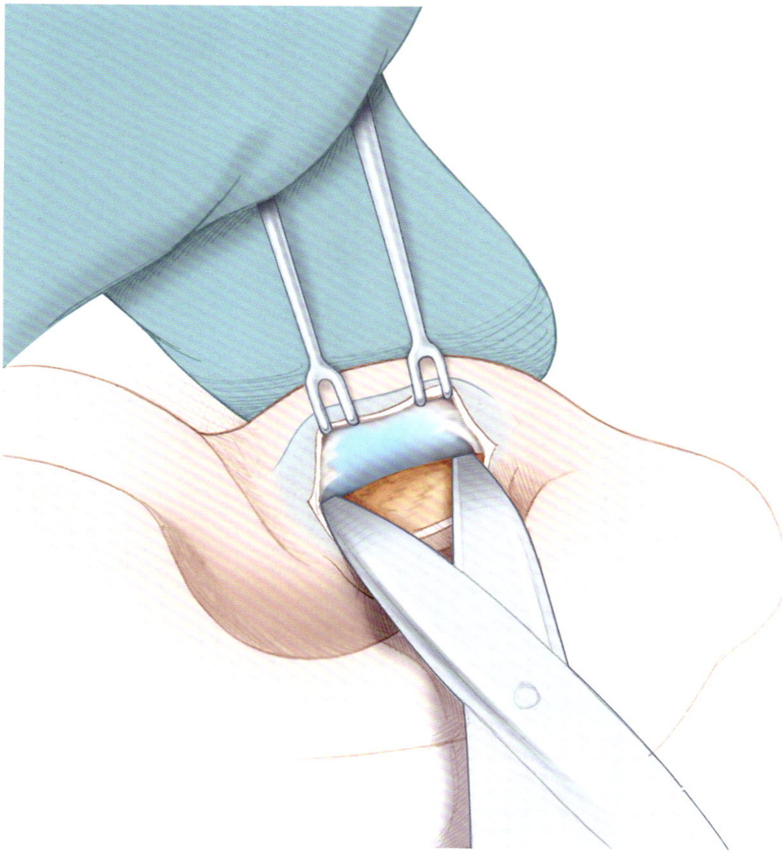

Figure 20-97. The tragal cartilage is widely exposed by scissor dissection.

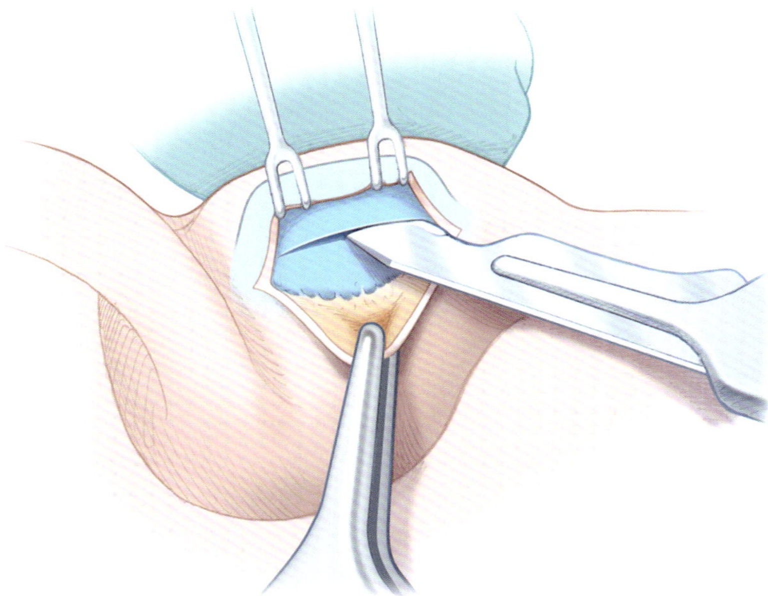

Figure 20-98. Fifteen blade incises the perichondrium and partial depth into the cartilage.

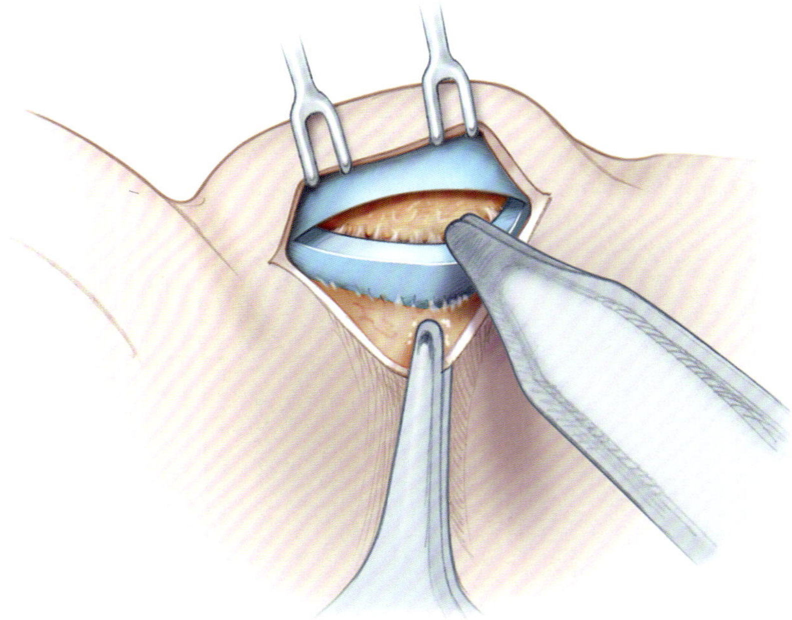

Figure 20-99. Scissors complete the division of the cartilage.

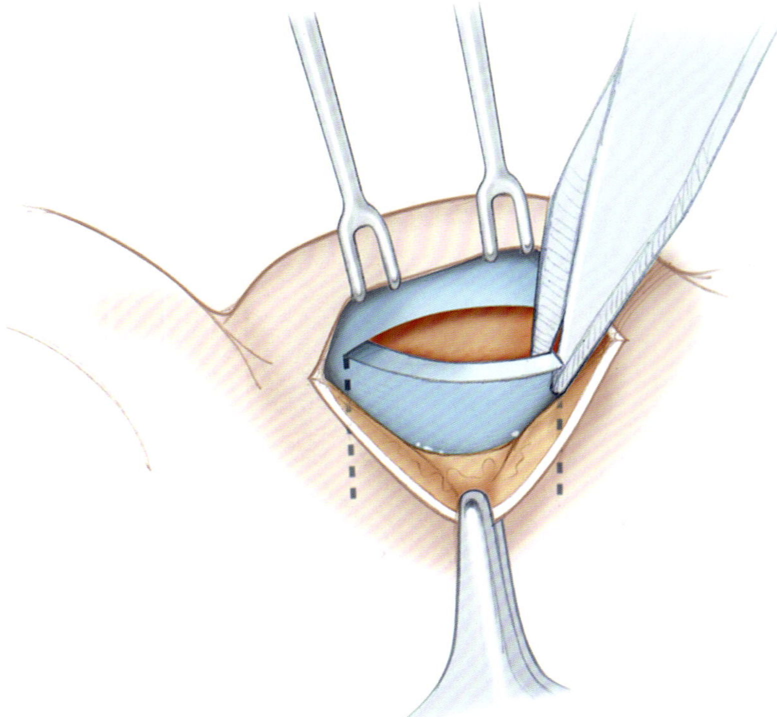

Figure 20-100. Vertical cuts are made in the cartilage.

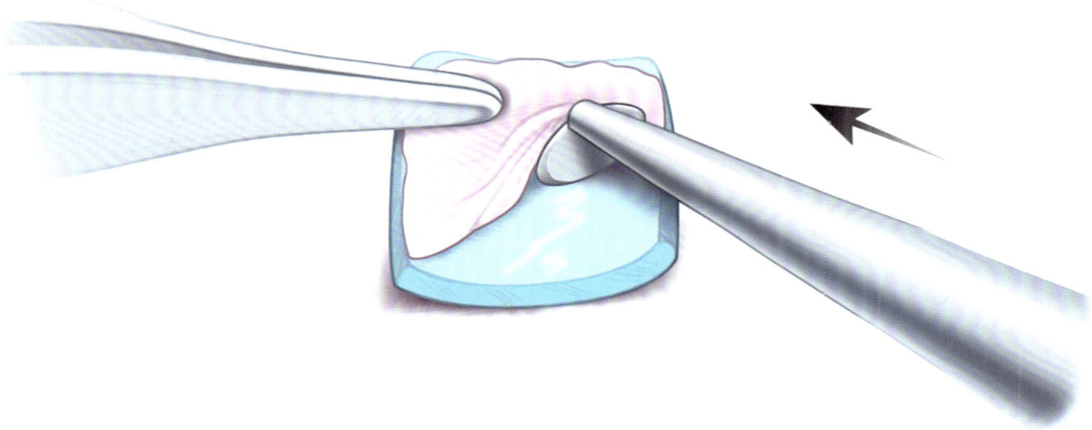

Figure 20-101. Perchondrium is dissected from the tragal cartilage.

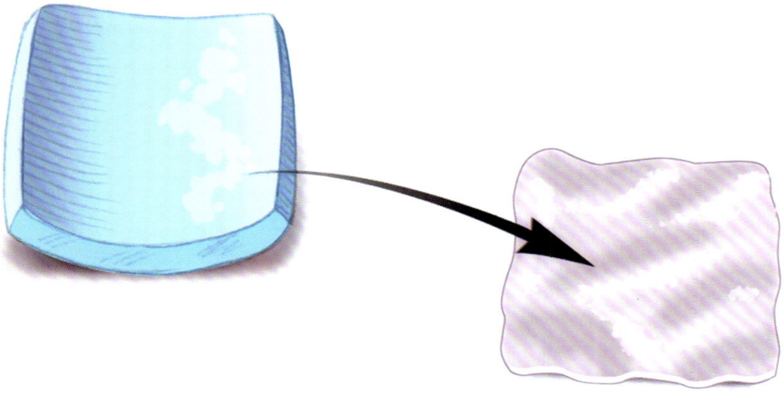

Figure 20-102. The cartilage can then be replaced and the wound closed loosely with two absorbable sutures.

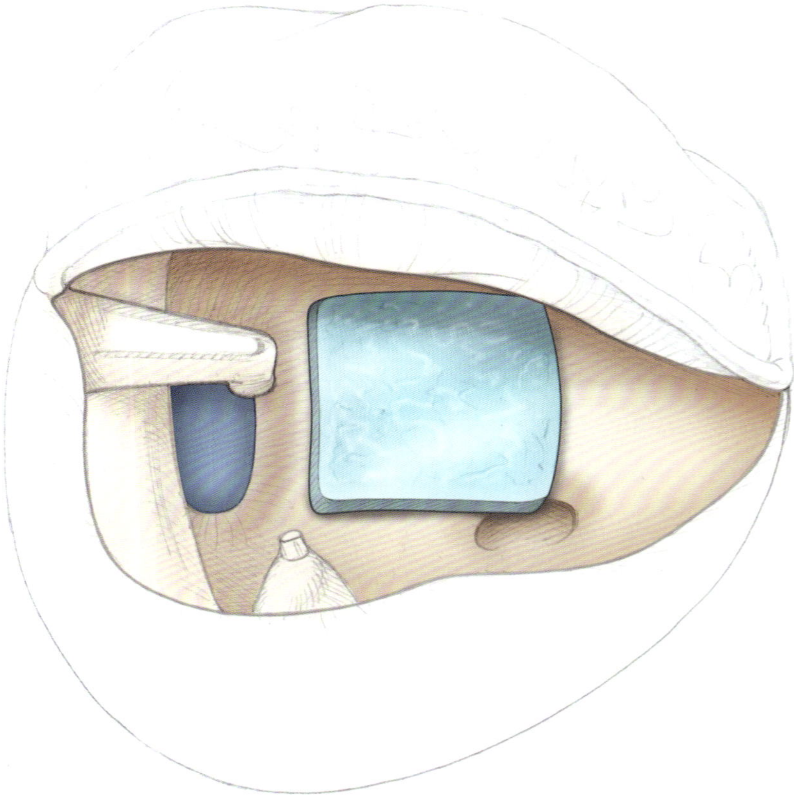

Figure 20-103. The perichondrial graft is first placed on the promontory.

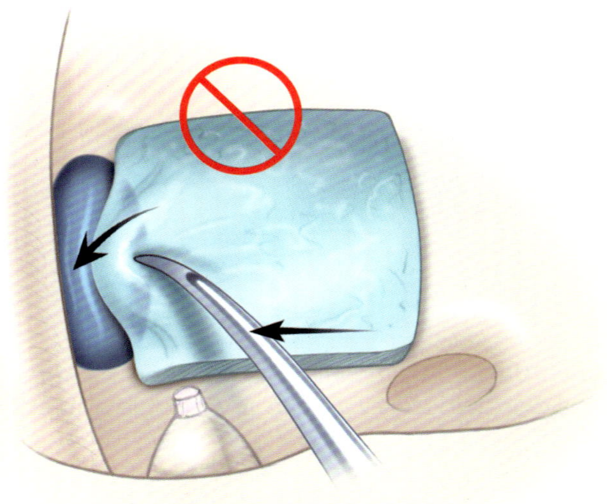

Figure 20-104. If the graft is simply pulled toward the oval window the lead edge tends to turn in toward the vestibule.

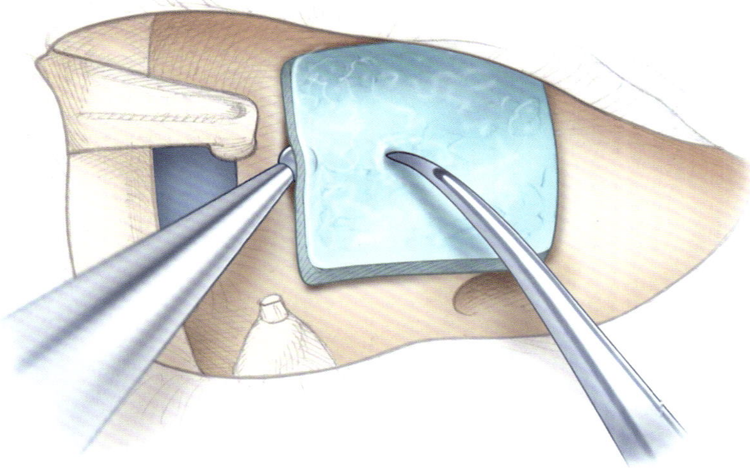

Figure 20-105. The graft must be lifted up over the facial nerve. This can be accomplished with a two-handed maneuver in which a joint knife serves as elevator while the needle propels. Lifting the graft with a 24-gauge needle is an alternate technique.

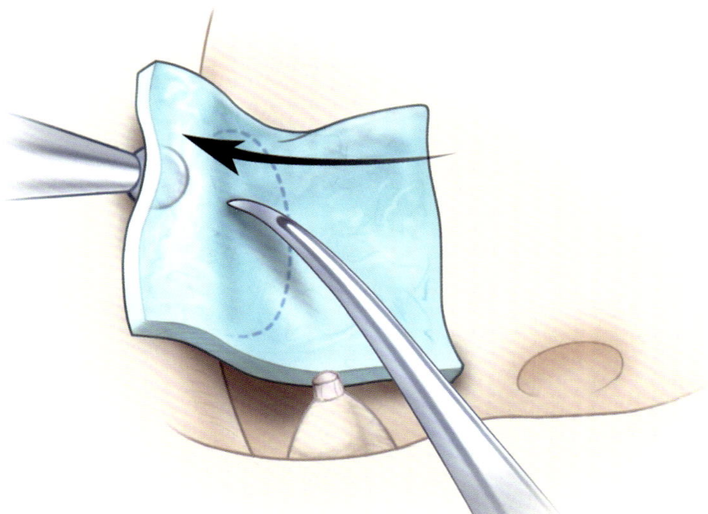

Figure 20-106. It is far preferable to use a generous size graft than risk an uncovered corner of the oval window. Getting the graft well up on the prominent ridge created by the facial nerve is important as the inadequate lead edge will fall off when the prosthesis is inserted.

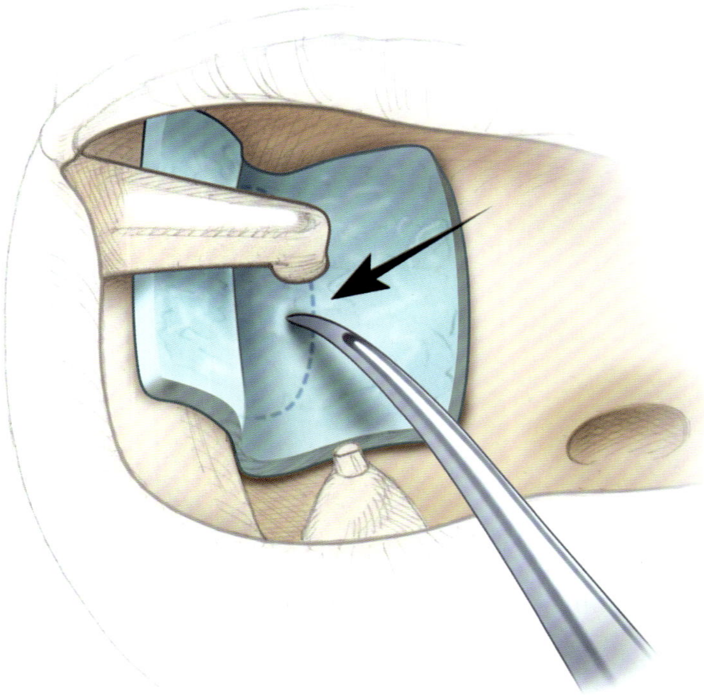

Figure 20-107. Using the extra length on the promontory the graft is seated deep into the oval window niche.

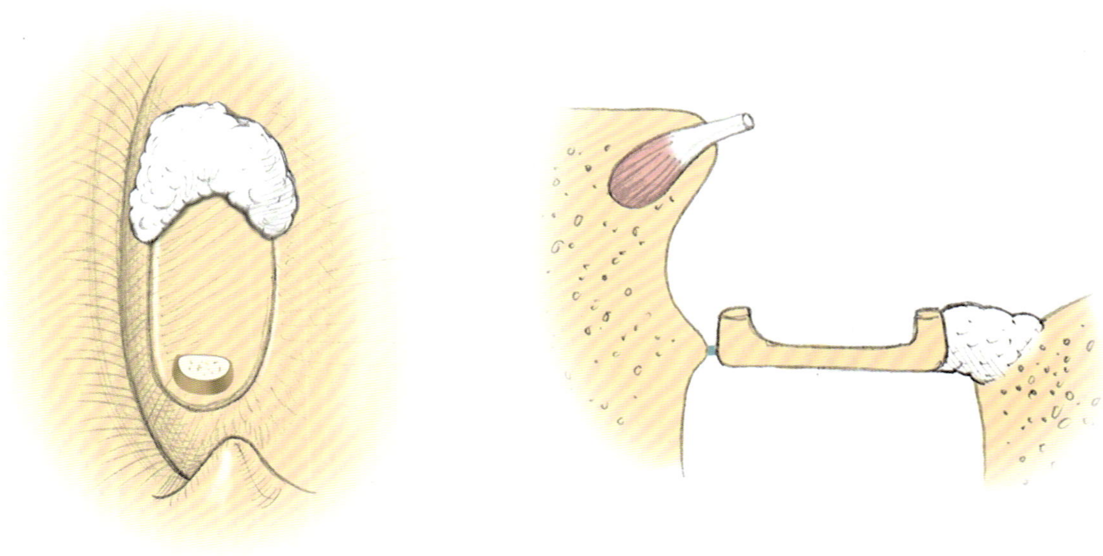

Figure 20-108. Anterior fixation of the footplate is most commonly encountered.

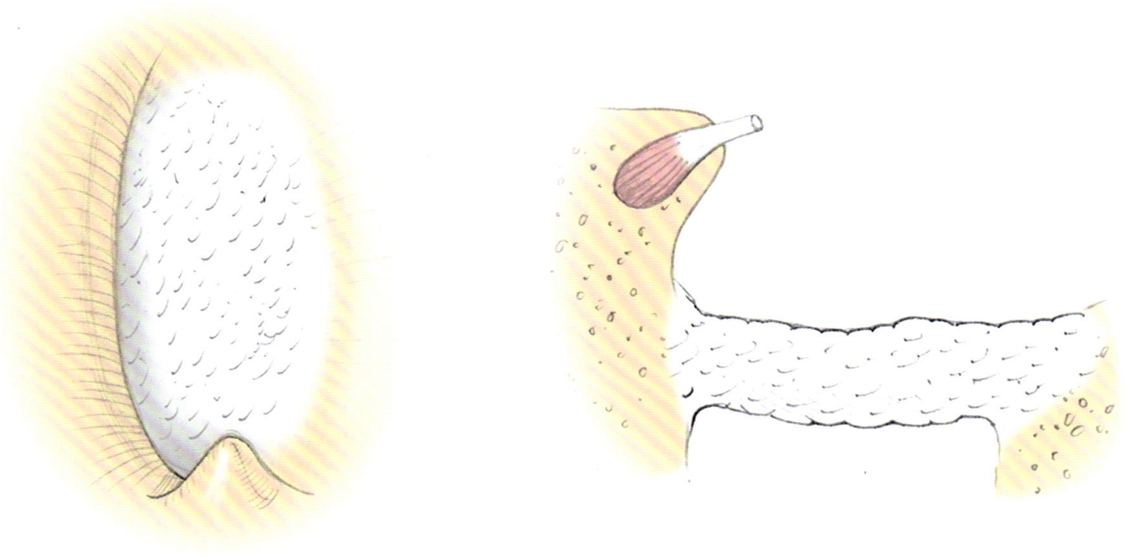

Figure 20-109. An obliterative footplate is thick and tightly fixed. The footplate appears chalky white and blood tends to accumulate in its center.

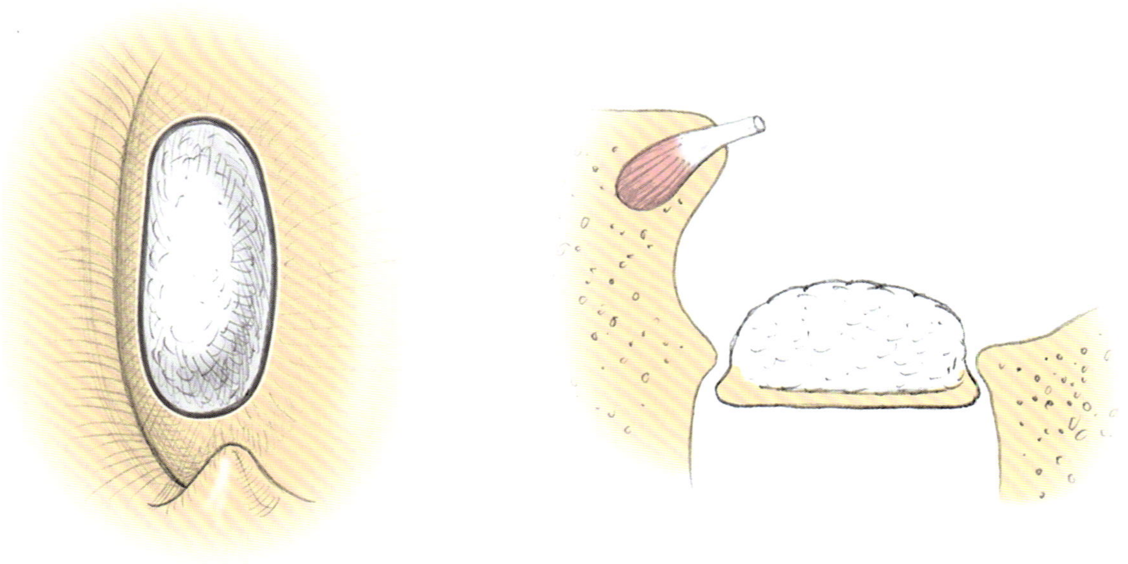

Figure 20-110. A biscuit footplate is thick and white, but is lightly fixed. Blood poo's peripherally around the annual ligament. A flange may be present on the vestibule side, which makes its extraction difficult.

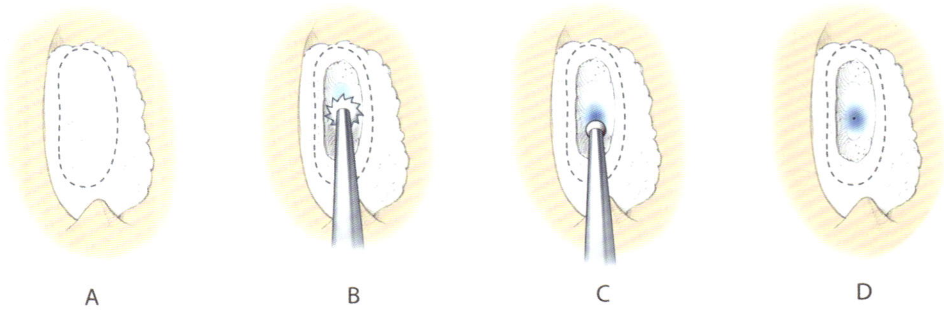

Figure 20–111. A–D. Managing obliterative otosclerosis is straightforward. Using a cutting burr (eg, 0.8 mm) the footplate is thinning until a blue region has been created. A routine small fenestra opening may then be formed with a diamond burr through the thin area.

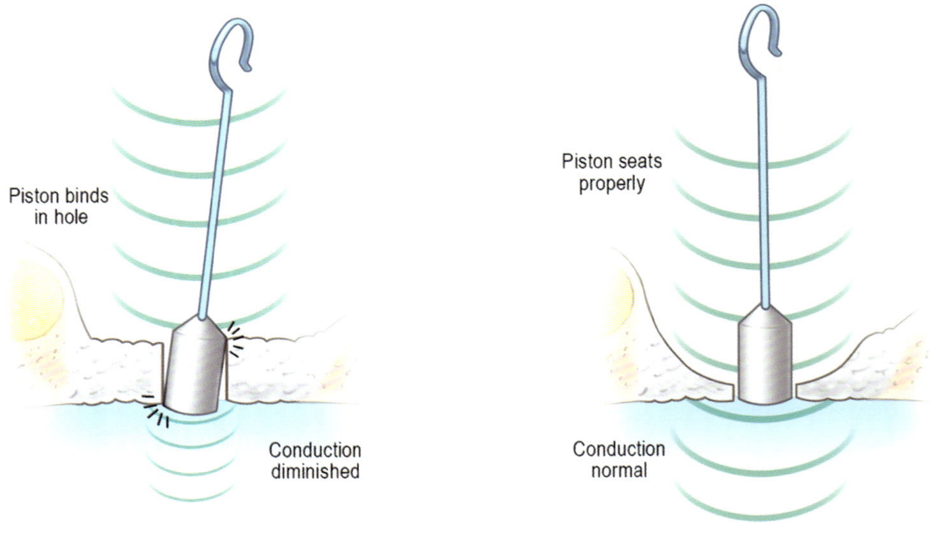

Figure 20–112. In reducing the thickness of the footplate in obliterative otosclerosis, it is important to create an adequate thin area. If the opening is too narrow (*left*) the prosthesis will rub if it is even slightly off line with the opening.

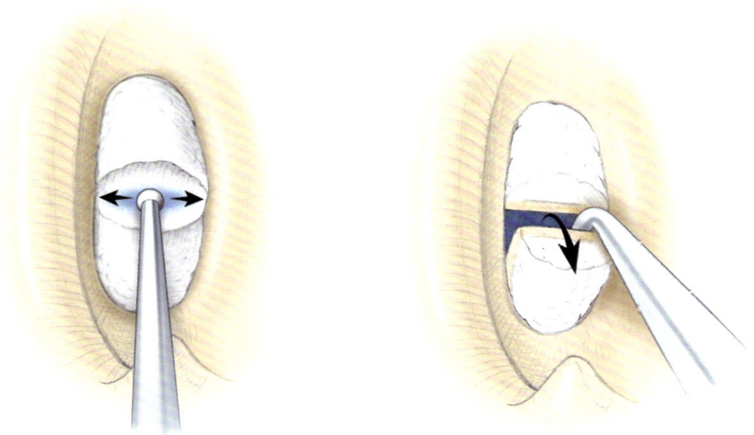

Figure 20-113. Dealing with a biscuit footplate is one of the great challenges in stapes surgery. The problem is that when drilling starts, it tends to become mobile. Drilling on a mobile footplate is forbidden due to risk of sensory loss. Once mobilized, manipulation tends to depress the biscuit footplate into the vestibule. Under favorable circumstances, the thick footplate can be bisected and the posterior half delivered.

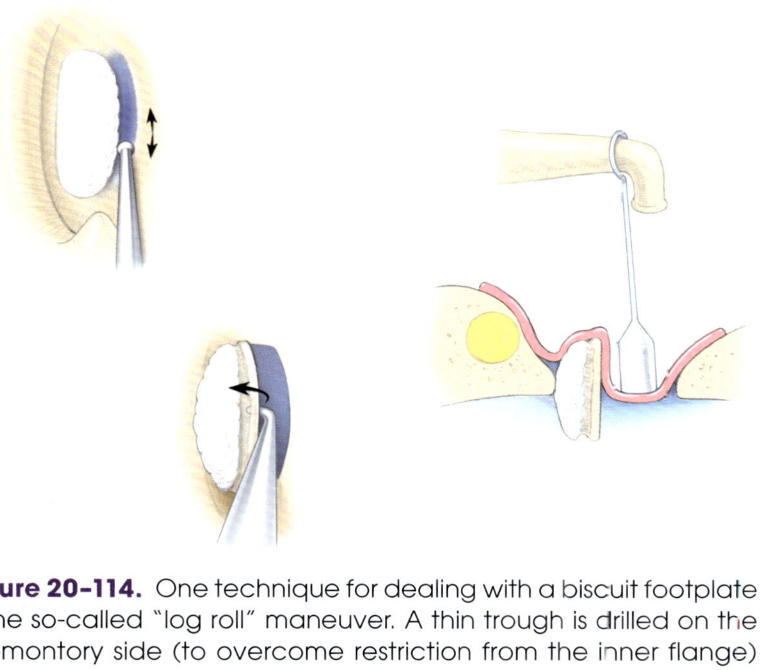

Figure 20-114. One technique for dealing with a biscuit footplate is the so-called "log roll" maneuver. A thin trough is drilled on the promontory side (to overcome restriction from the inner flange) and the footplate is rolled up on its side.

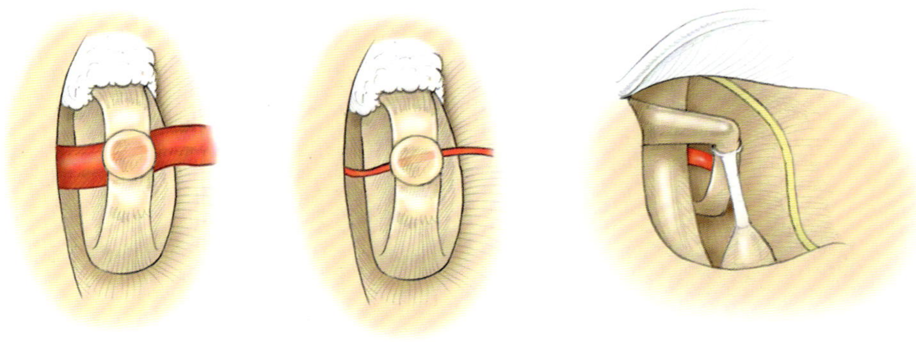

A. B. C.

Figure 20-115. A–C. If the surgeon encounters a large persistent stapedial artery, it is best to stop the procedure and recommend amplification. A vestigial stapedial artery remnant is quite common and should not deter completion of the procedure.

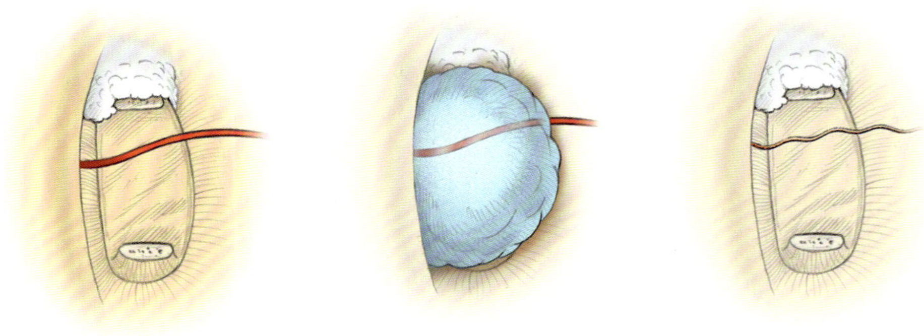

A. B. C.

Figure 20-116. A–C. Placing an epinephrine-(1:1000) soaked Gelfoam® pledget can help to shrink the stapes artery remnant. The fenestra can usually be placed posterior to the vestigial artery without disturbing it.

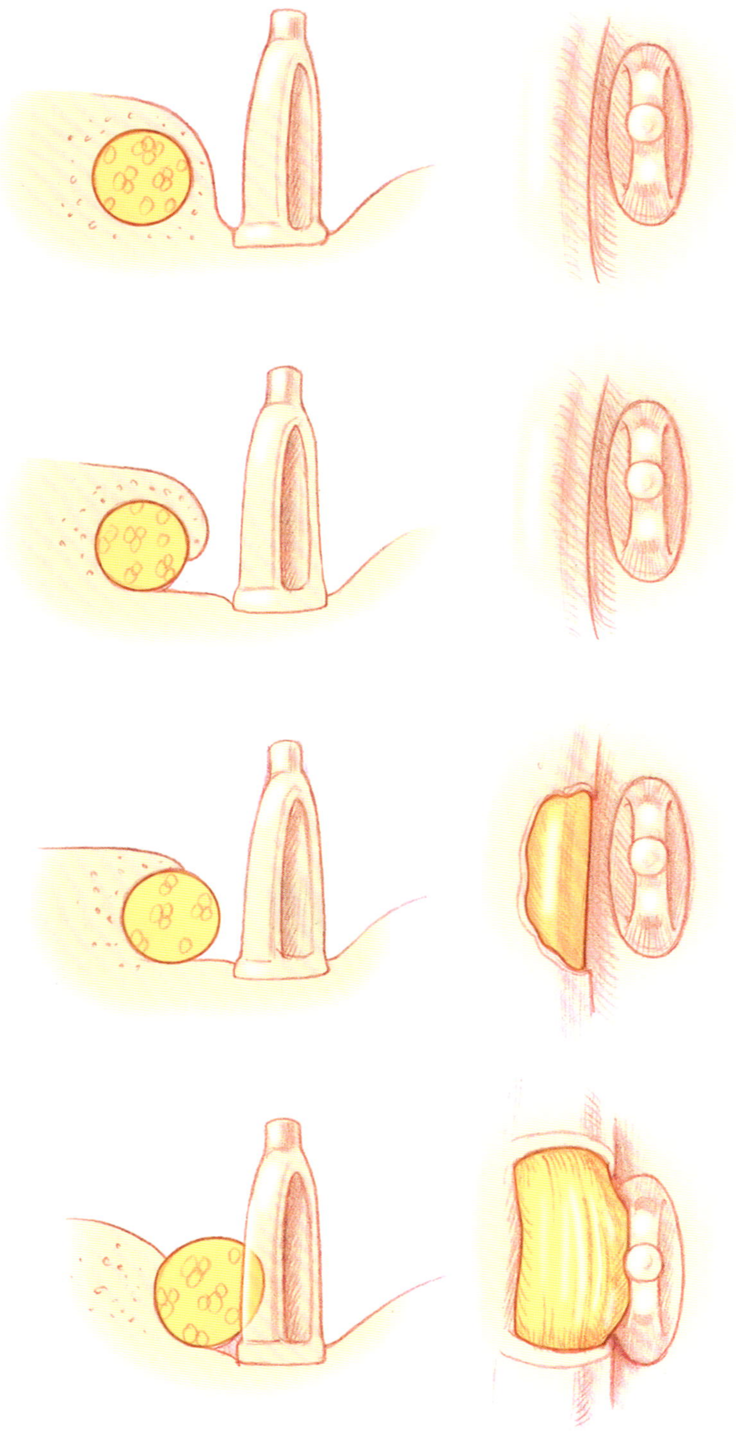

Figure 20-117. The facial nerve is situated immediately superior to the oval window. It is often dehiscent on its lower surface, out of the surgeon's line of sight. Occasionally, it lies fully dehiscent (ie, lacking any bony covering). Rarely the facial nerve may prolapse from its canal and even impinge on the stapes arch. In such cases surgeon must determine if the conductive hearing loss is due to stapes fixation or merely from the facial nerve leaning on the crura.

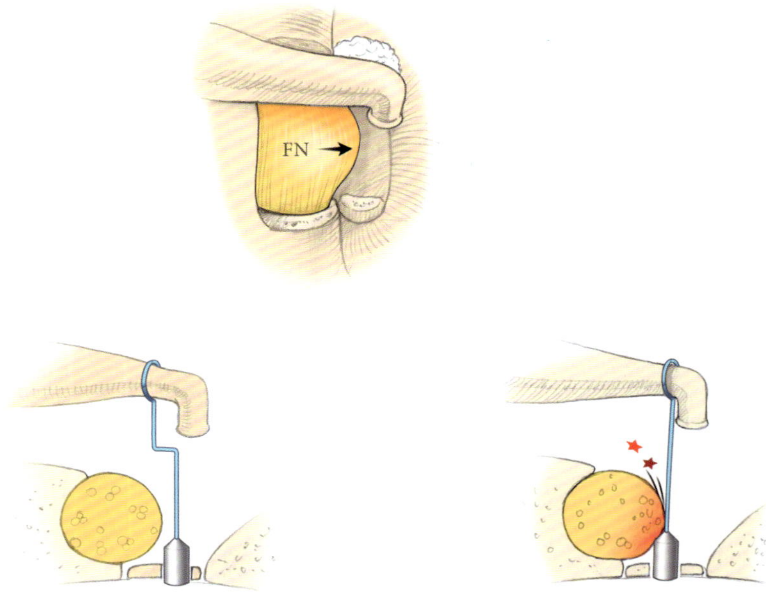

Figure 20-118. Although a severely protruding facial nerve renders stapes surgery impossible, minor degrees of prolapse can be accommodated by routing the wire around the nerve using the double-bend technique.

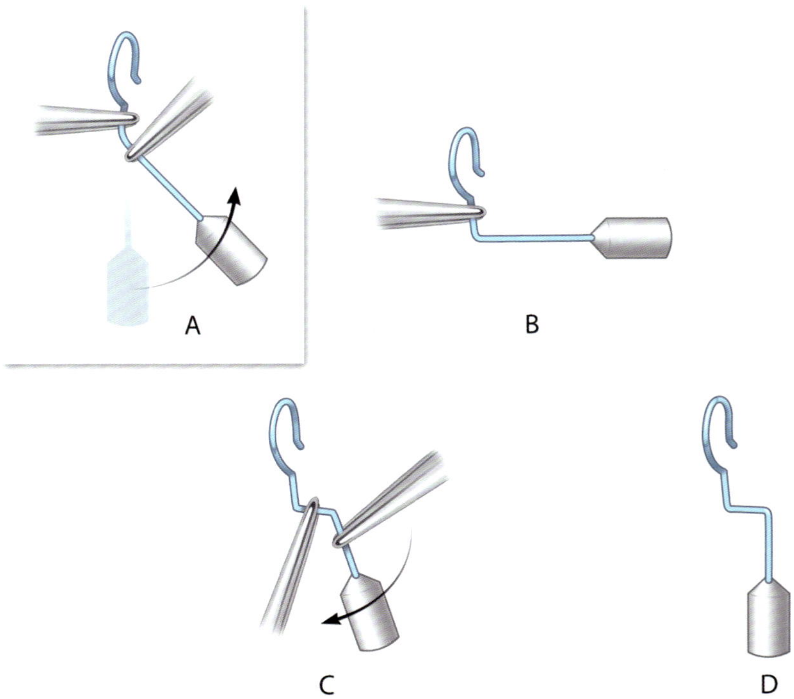

Figure 20-119. A–D. To route the wire around a dehiscent facial nerve the double-bend technique may be used. This requires adding 1 mm to the length of the wire. Using two smooth alligators, two bends are created as depicted.

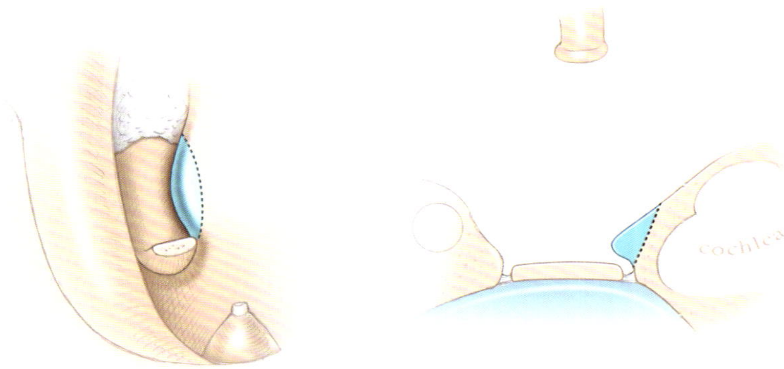

Figure 20-120. An oval window may be narrowed by a promontory scroll that limits access for footplate fenestration.

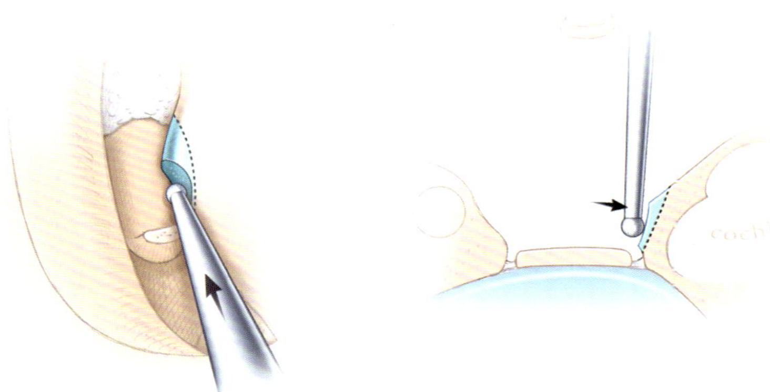

Figure 20-121. Using a diamond burr, the promontory scroll can be removed slightly inferior to the level of the annular ligament with no fear of entering the cochlea.

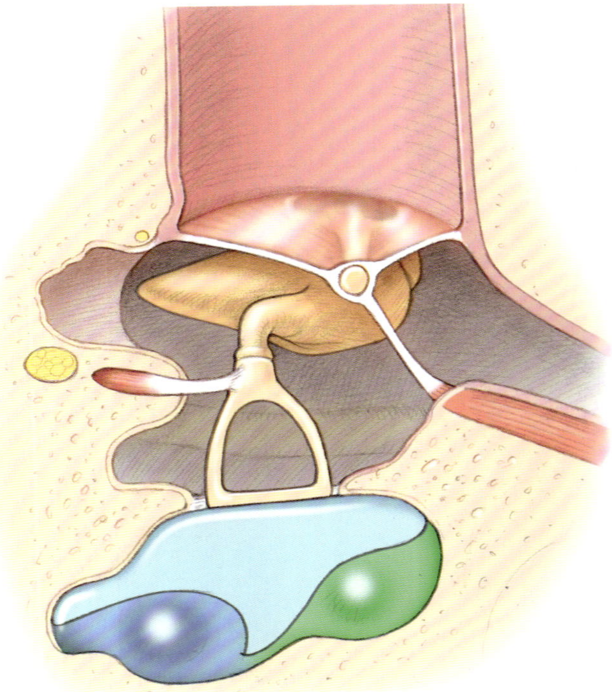

Figure 20-122. The normal relationship of the utricle (*blue*) and saccule (*green*) to the footplate. The distance from footplate to the utricle is approximately 2 mm whereas the space to the saccule is about 1.25 mm.

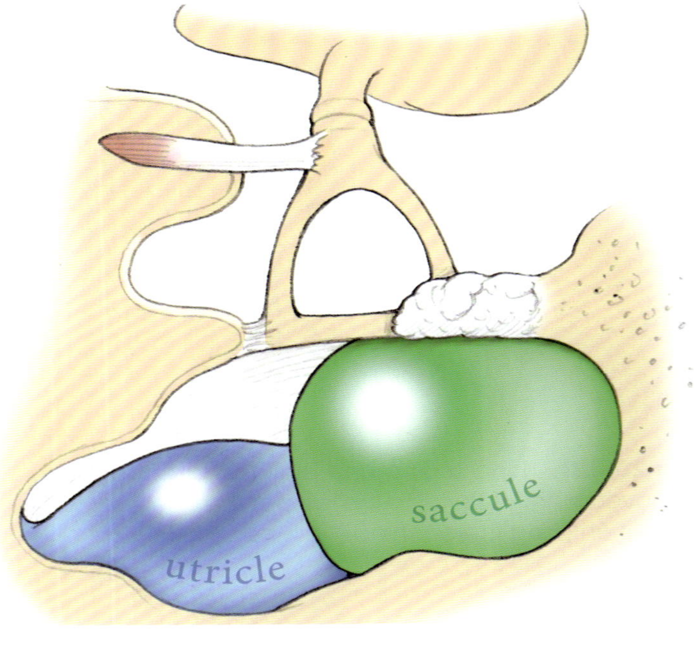

Figure 20-123. In endolymphatic hydrops (eg, Ménière's disease), the saccule may swell against the undersurface of the footplate. For this reason, hydropic symptoms contraindicate stapes surgery. Hydrops and otosclerosis may co-exist, as depicted here, perhaps due to otosclerotic involvement of the vestibular aqueduct.

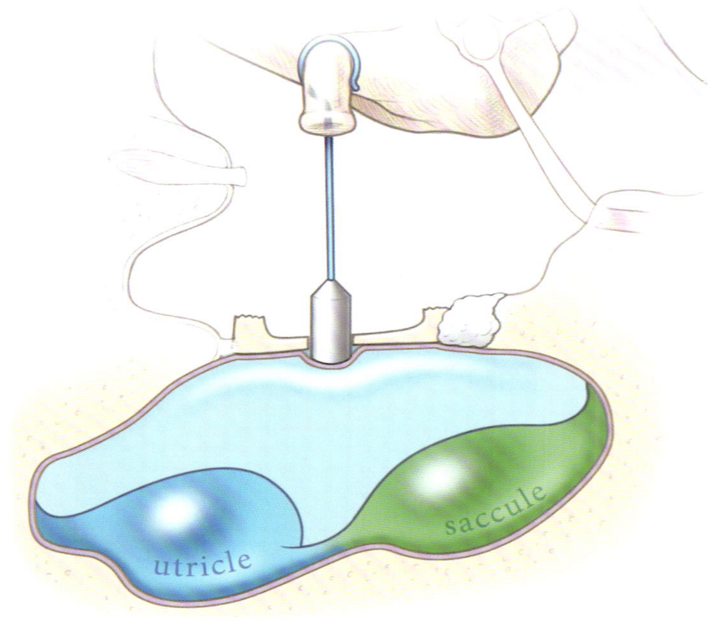

Figure 20-124. The normal position of a stapes piston in the vestibule. The piston should be only approximately 0.5 mm into the vestibule. Over time, the endosteal membrane re-forms underneath the piston. Once this membrane has re-formed, the piston does not directly contact perilymph. Once this membrane has re-formed, the piston does not come in direct contact with perilymph. It can be thought of as residing in a diverticulum of the middle ear.

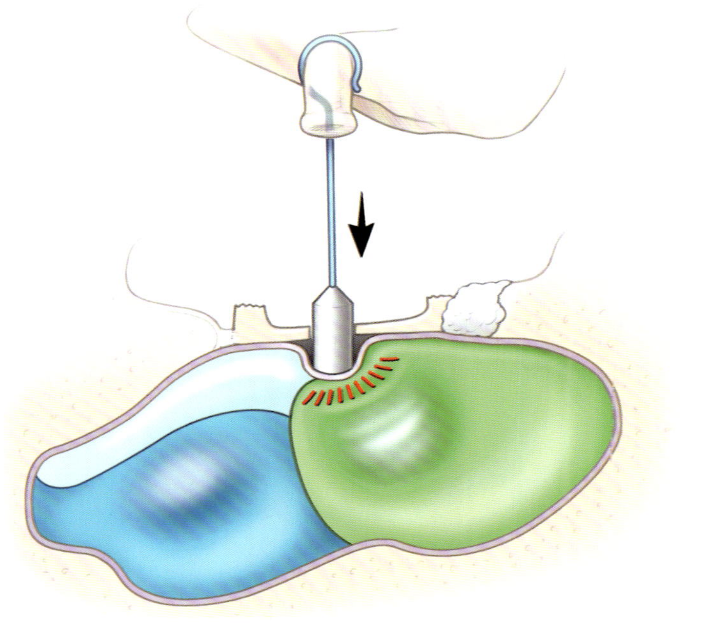

Figure 20-125. Stapes surgery is contraindicated in hydrops due to risk of the piston traumatizing the otolithic organs. Among other complications, this can lead to Tullio's phenomenon (vertigo with loud noise).

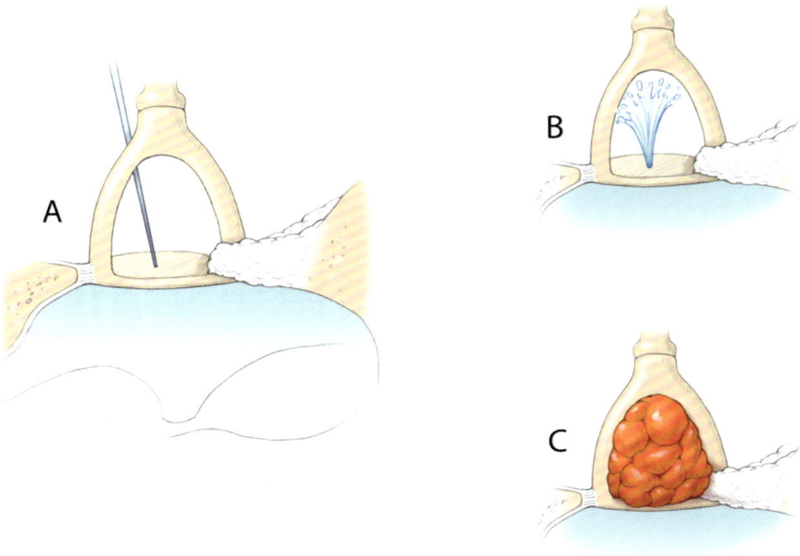

Figure 20-126. In rare instances, the inner ear may have CSF pressure within it. This may occur in certain inner ear malformations (eg, large vestibular aqueduct) as well as the X-lined gusher syndrome. In congenital conductive hearing loss a CT scan should be obtained to rule out inner ear malformation. Stapes surgery is contraindicated in inner ear malformation as the audiogram may reflect a pseudoconductive hearing loss and the risk of hearing loss is high. **A.** In conductive loss existing since early in life (whether in a child or adult) creation of a control hole may help to detect a gusher. **B–C.** Should a gusher occur, a soft tissue plug can be placed beneath the stapes arch.

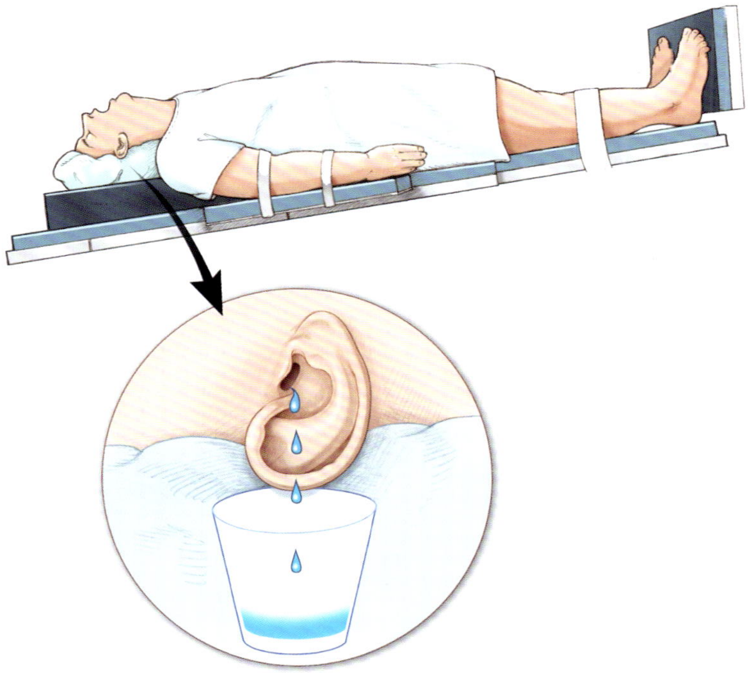

Figure 20-127. In true stapes gusher, brisk CSF flow prohibits orderly microdissection. Rather than packing the oval window in panicked fashion with poor visualization, it is better to drop the head into Trendelenberg and allow the CSF to escape.

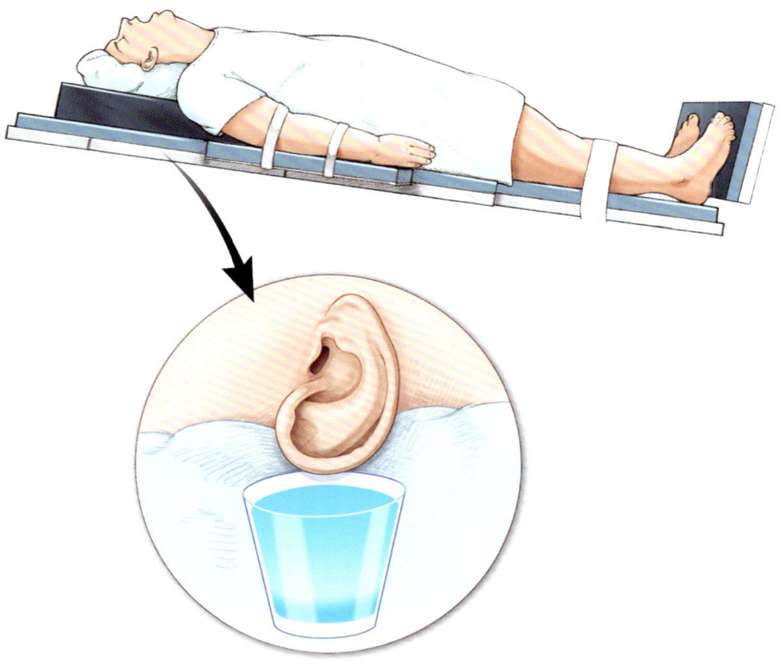

Figure 20-128. When the drainage has ceased, the head is elevated into reverse Trendelenberg. The surgeon can then complete the soft tissue closure of the oval window in a dry field. A lumbar subarachnoid drain may be placed.

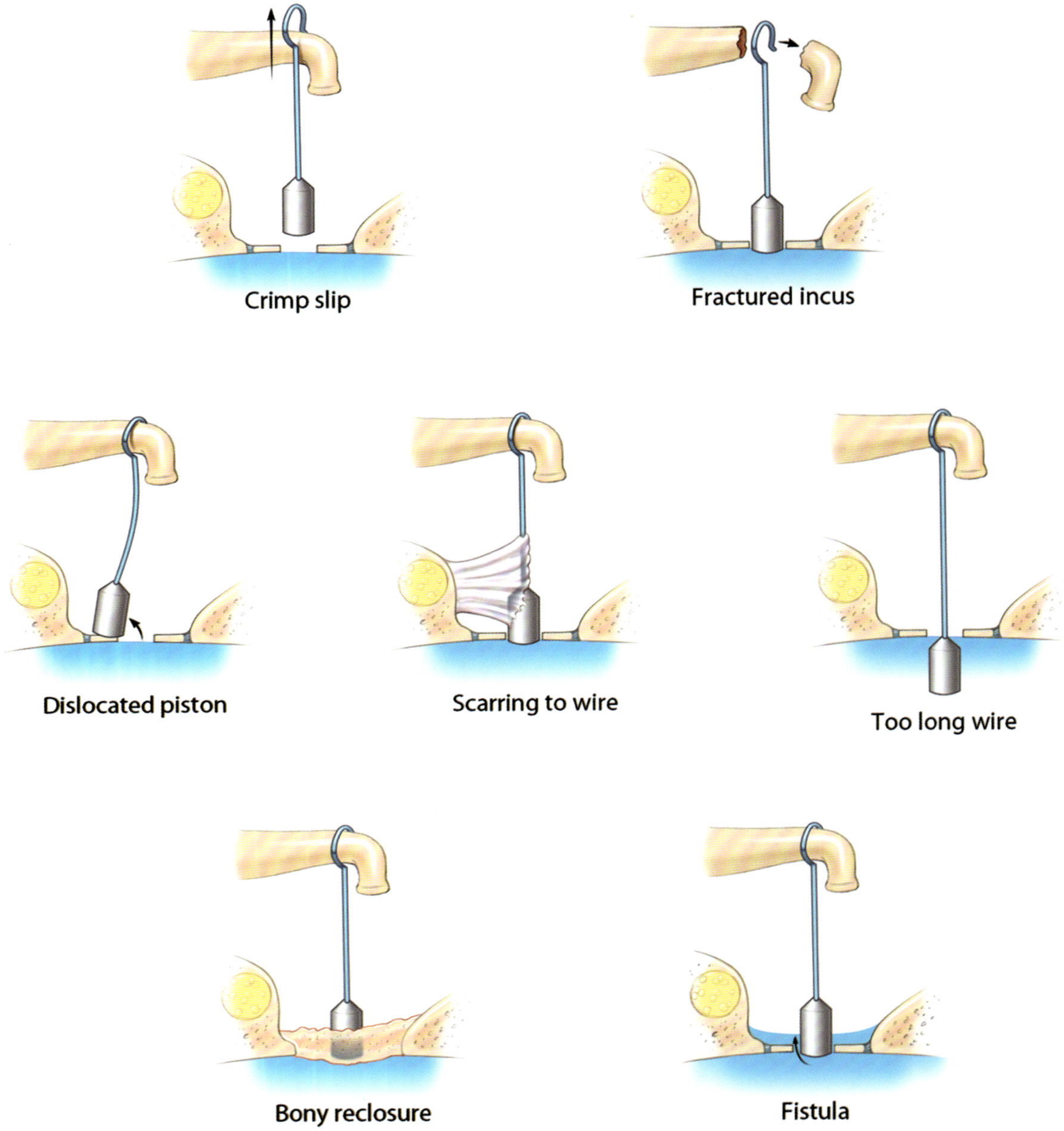

Figure 20-129. The seven most common findings encountered during revision stapes surgery.

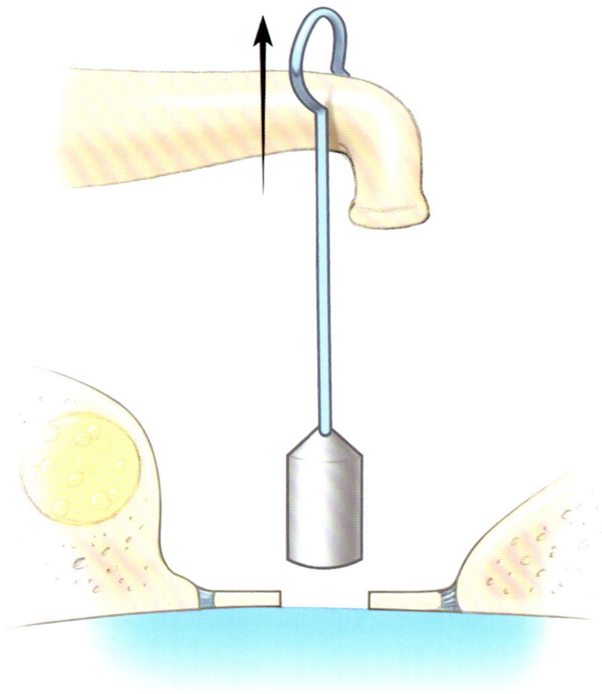

Figure 20–130. Displacement of the prosthesis due to loosening of the crimp from the incus. A fully slipped crimp will cause major conductive hearing loss whereas loose crimp may be associated with variable conductive hearing loss that comes and goes as middle ear pressure varies.

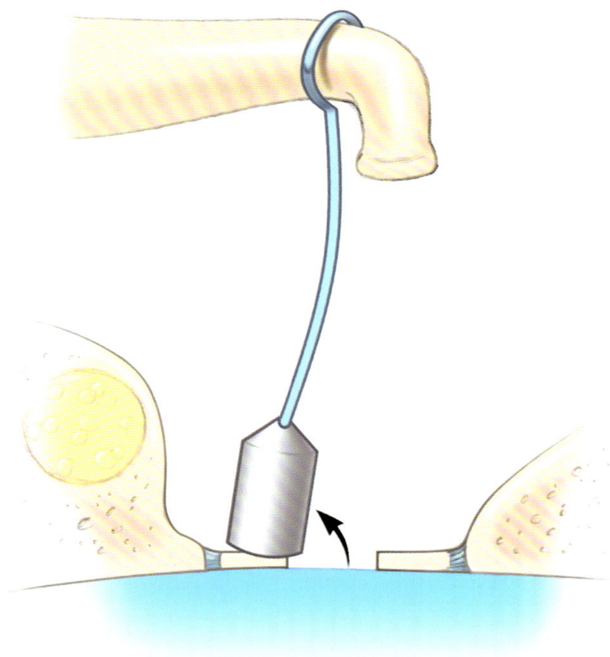

Figure 20–131. Dislodgement of the prosthesis from the oval window fenestra. Too short of a prosthesis can contribute to this complication. Sometimes it occurs during vigorous autoinflation.

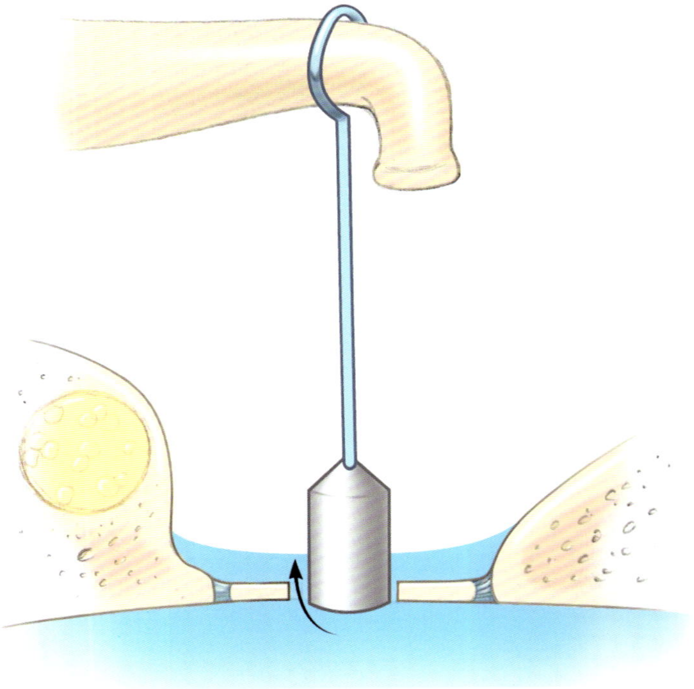

Figure 20-132. Perilymphatic fistula may be associated with sensory loss and/or vestibular symptoms.

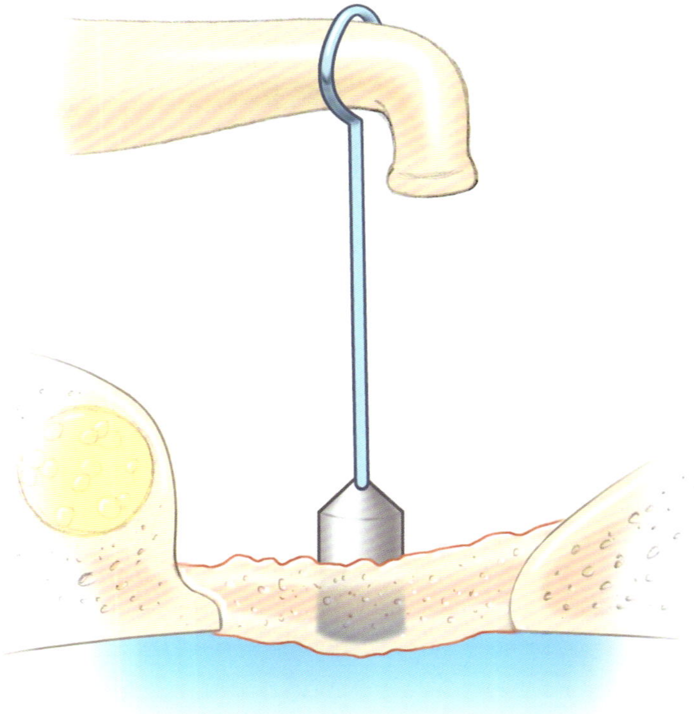

Figure 20-133. Bony reclosure of the oval window. Because repeat drill-out of recurrent obliterative otosclerosis carries a heighted risk of sensory loss, consideration should be given to amplification.

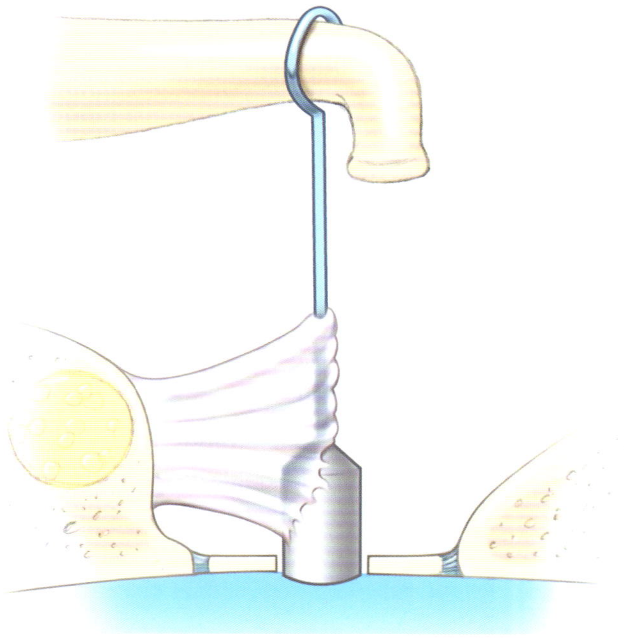

Figure 20-134. Scarring between the margins of the ova window (especially the facial nerve canal) and the prosthesis can reduce its mobility. Laser removal of the scar bands may be effective, but scarring tends to recur.

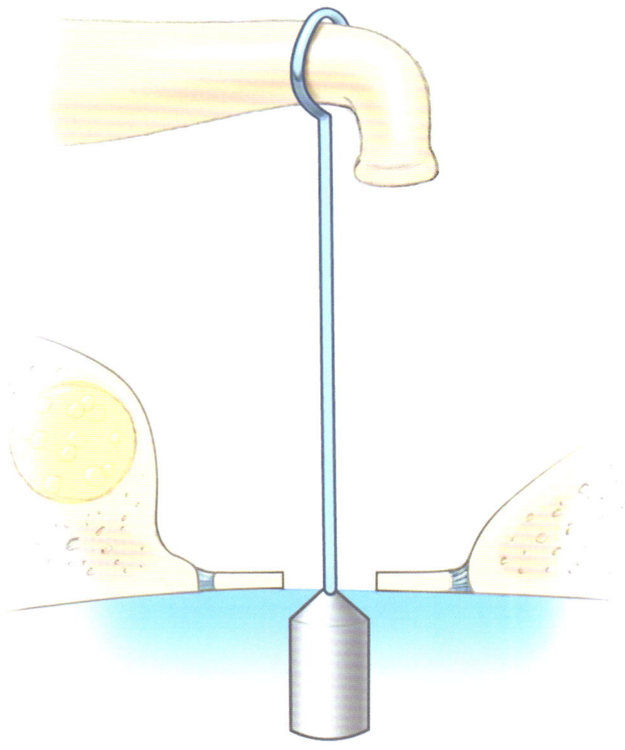

Figure 20-135. An overly long prosthesis may cause vestibular symptoms, especially vertigo triggered by loud sounds (Tullio's phenomenon).

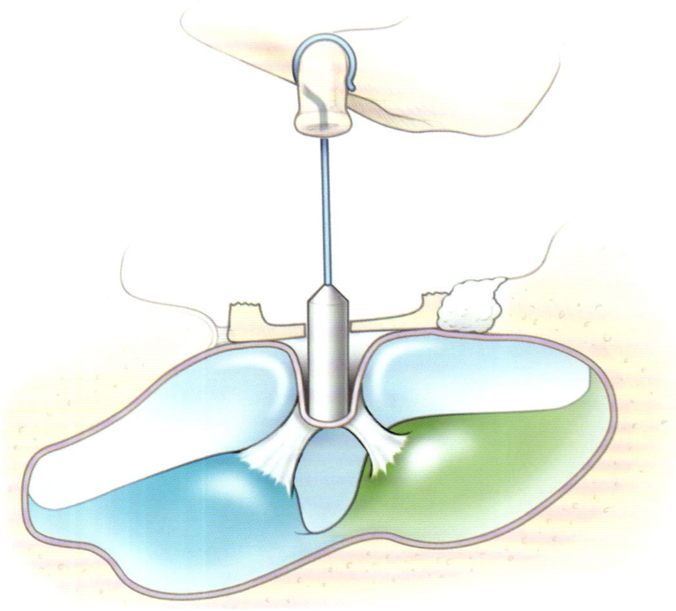

Figure 20-136. Due to adhesion with the endolymphatic membranes, removing an overly inserted prosthesis carries a risk of inner ear damage.

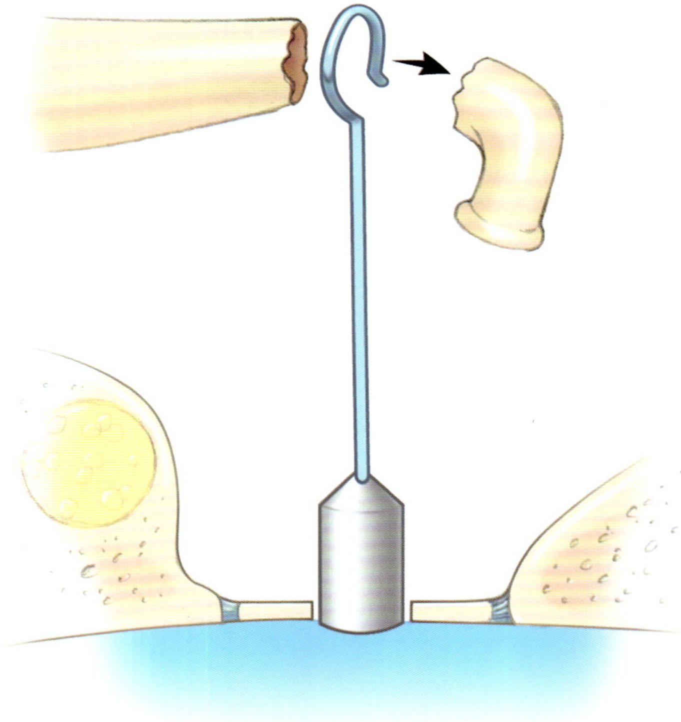

Figure 20-137. Fracture of the long process of the incus. This may occur due to a movement of a loose prosthesis, an overly hermetic crimp resulting in devascularization of the lenticular process, or fragile incus as in osteogensis imperfecta.

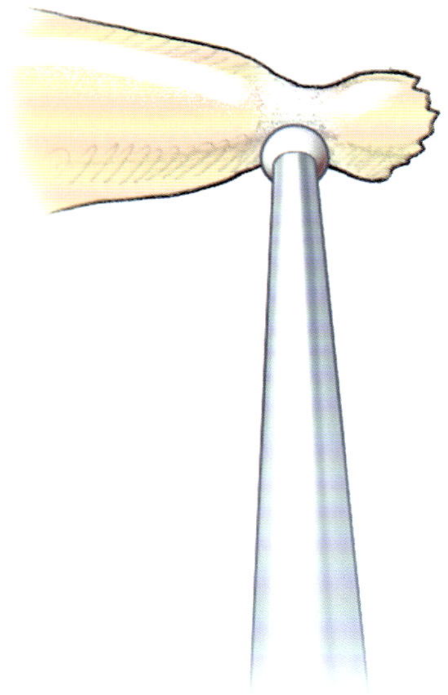

Figure 20-138. Because a fractured incus will not retain a wire without modification, a groove is created to anchor the crimp.

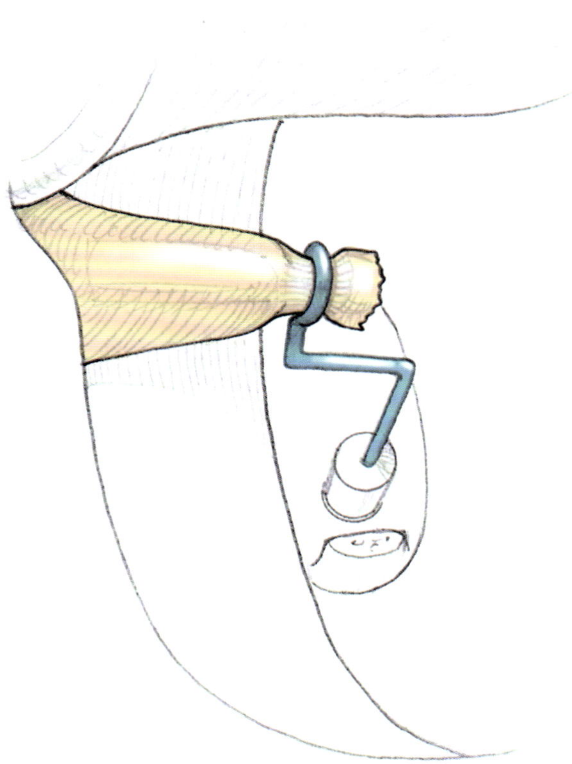

Figure 20-139. A longer prosthesis using a double-bend technique and restoring continuity. A malleus to footplate prosthesis is an alternative solution.

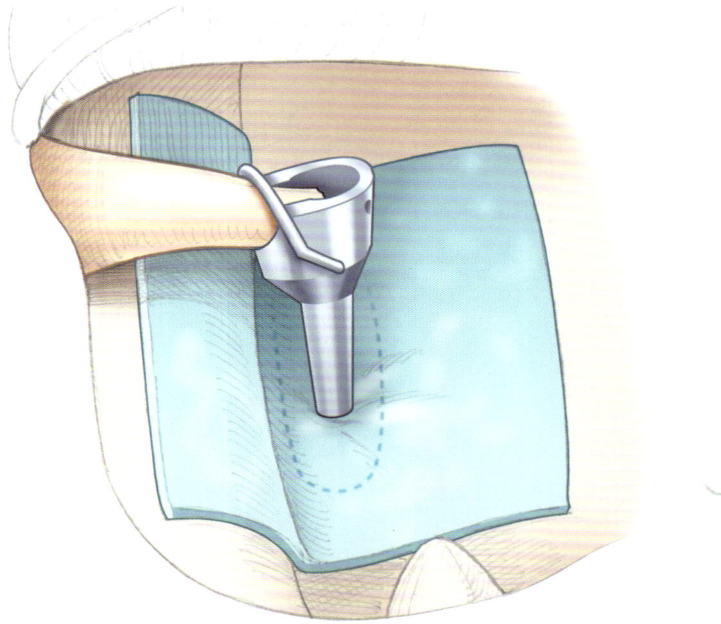

Figure 20-140. A Lippy-modified prosthesis with an elongated bucket is designed to accommodate a deficient incus.

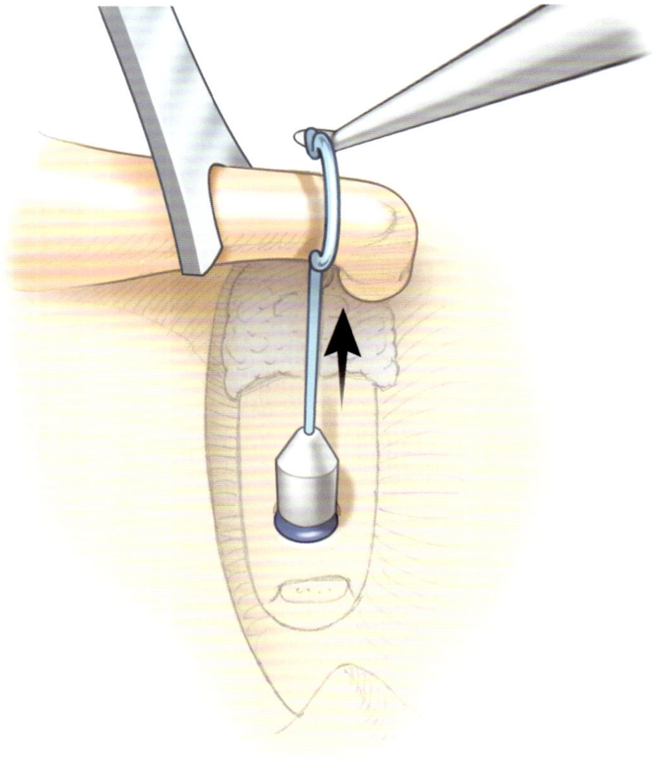

Figure 20-141. Removing a stapes prosthesis during revision surgery requires a two-handed maneuver with stabilization of the incus (shown here with a notched chisel also known as a strut guide). A hook is used to pry the prosthesis from the stabilized incus.

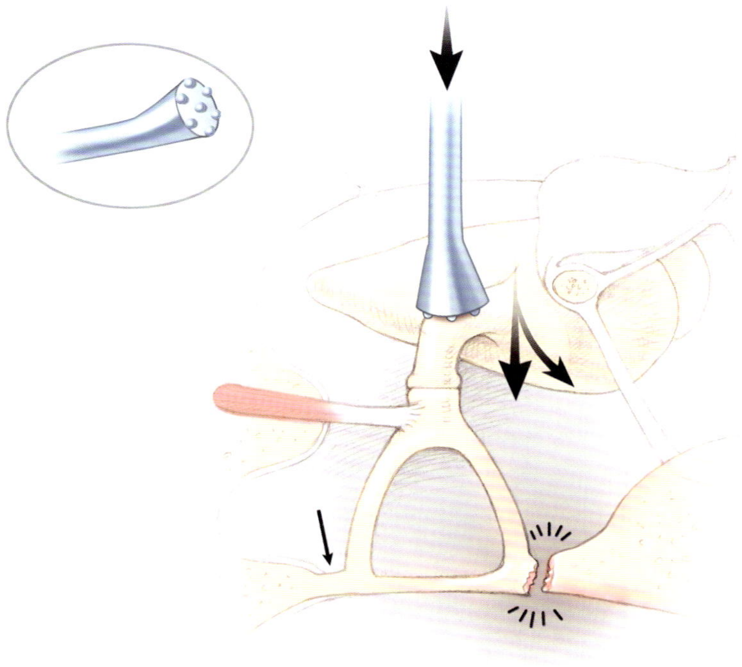

Figure 20-142. In stapes mobilization, an elephant's foot ("Derlaki mobilizer") is used to rock the superstructure. Mobilization should always be attempted during surgery for congenital stapes fixation, but is not often successful due to lack of an annular ligament. Should mobilization be achieved there is no need to proceed with stapedotomy as, in the absence of active bone disease such as otosclerosis, the stapes will not refix.

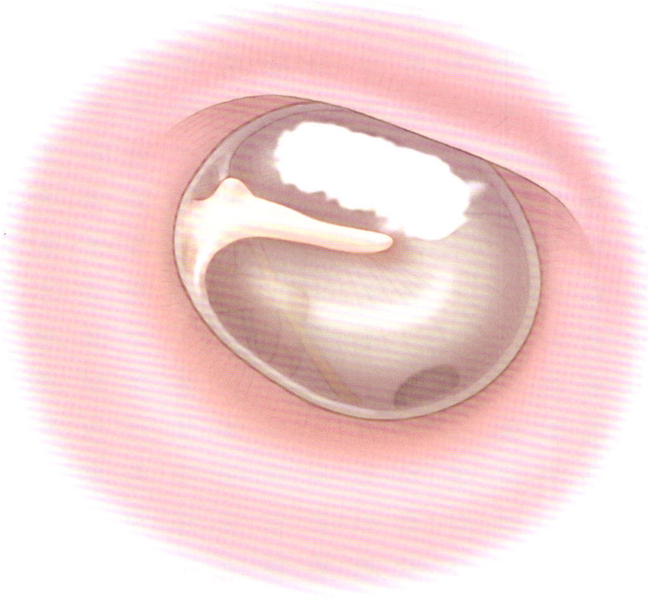

Figure 20-143. The finding of myringosclerosis should raise suspicion of tympanosclerotic ossicular fixation.

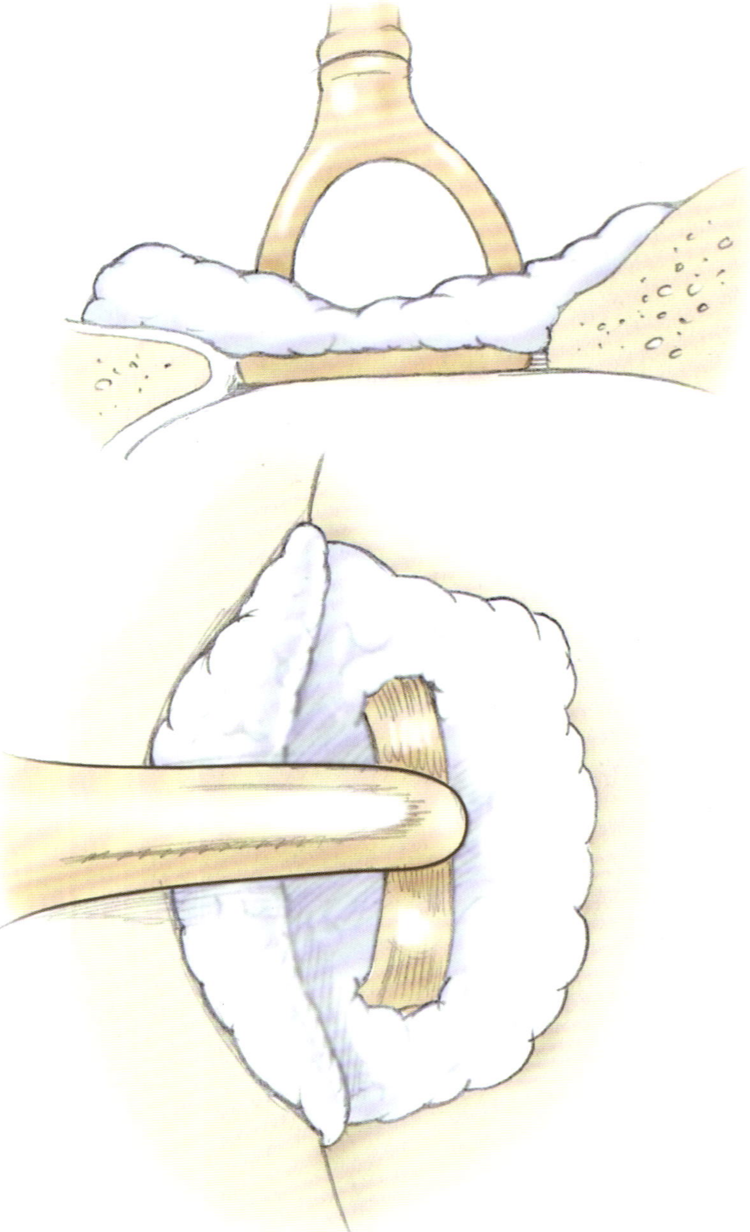

Figure 20-144. Extensive, circumferential tympanosclerotic stapes fixation. Stapes surgery is generally not effective with such extensive disease.

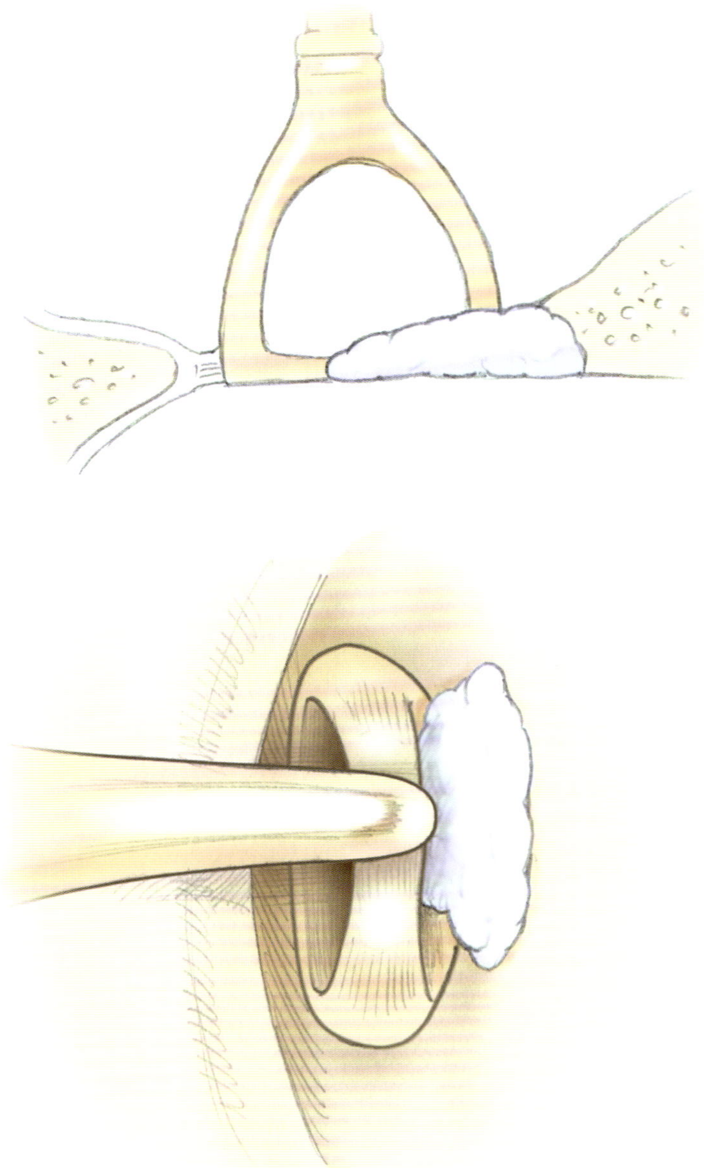

Figure 20-145. Focal tympanosclerotic stapes fixation s more amenable to surgical correction.

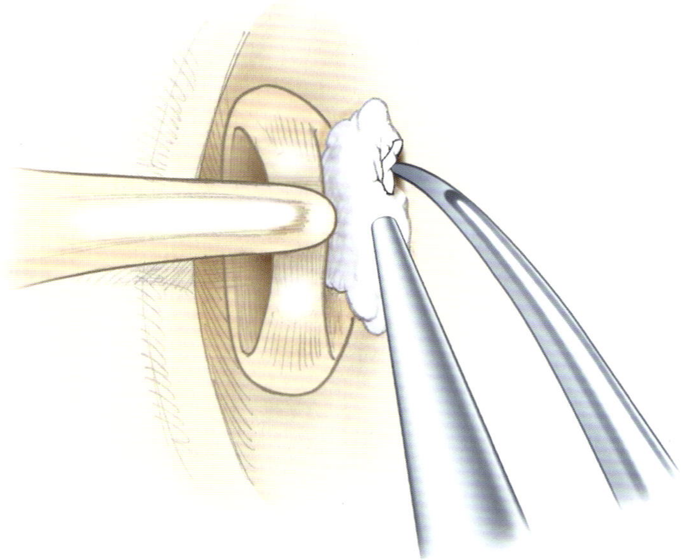

Figure 20-146. Attempt should be made to chip away the fixing bridge of tympanosclerosis. When thoroughly removed, the stapes has a good chance of retaining mobility.

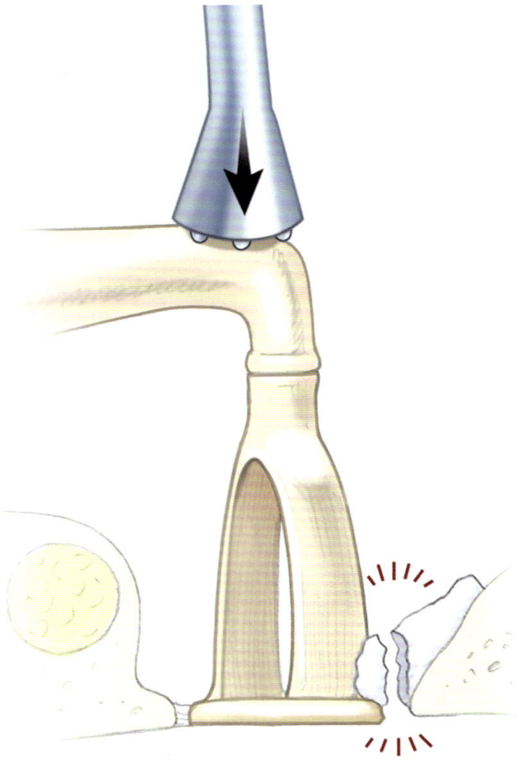

Figure 20-147. Mobilization is also possible in tympanosclerotic fixation, but the fixation tends to recur. Stapedectomy is usually avoided in tympanosclerotic fixation unless the ear has a long infection-free period, the middle ear mucosa is mostly healthy, and the tympanic membrane is not prone to retraction.

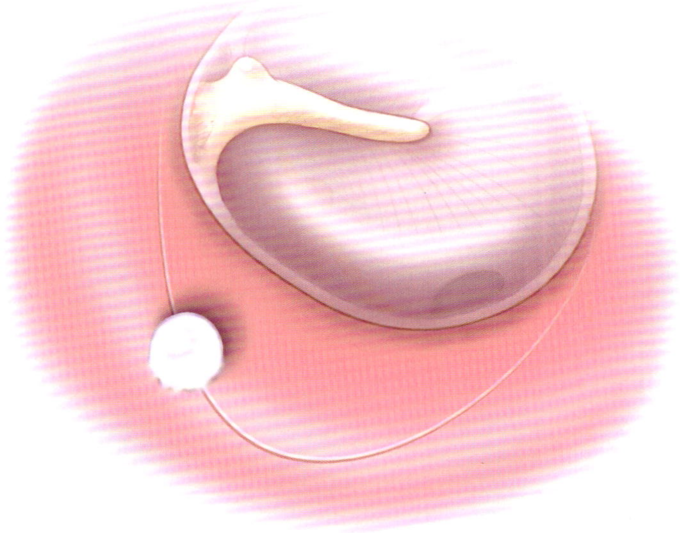

Figure 20-148. Infolding of the tympanomeatal flap edge can lead to formation of a keratin pearl.

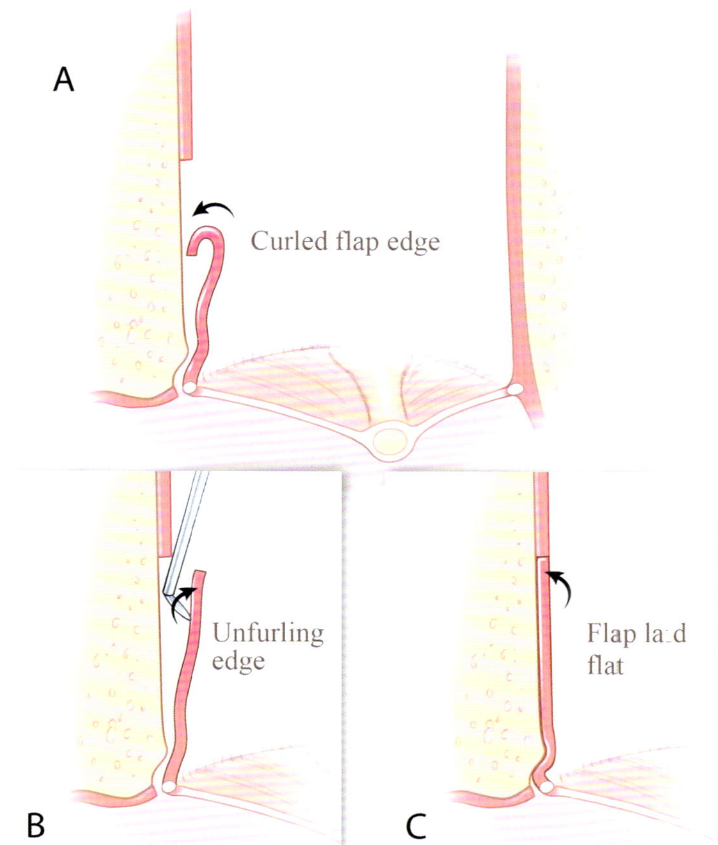

Figure 20-149. A–C. After repositioning the flap, a joint knife may be used to unfurl the curled edge to ensure the flap lies flat against the bony canal.

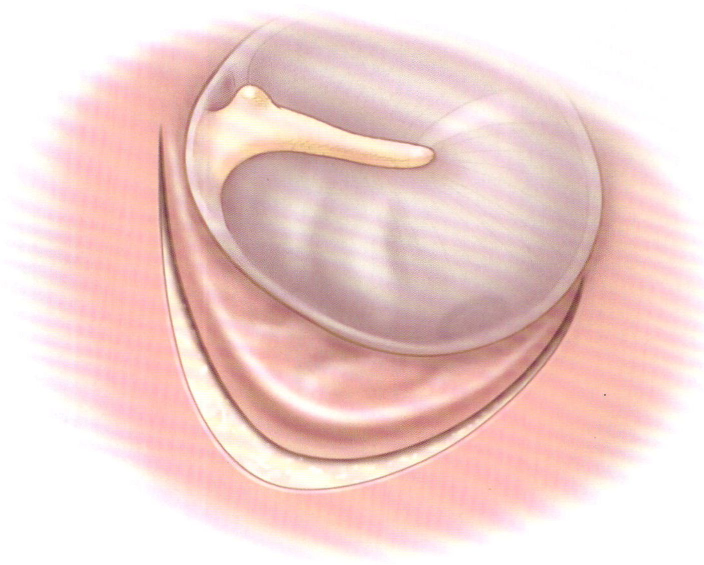

Figure 20-150. The edge of the tympanomeatal flap is curled under.

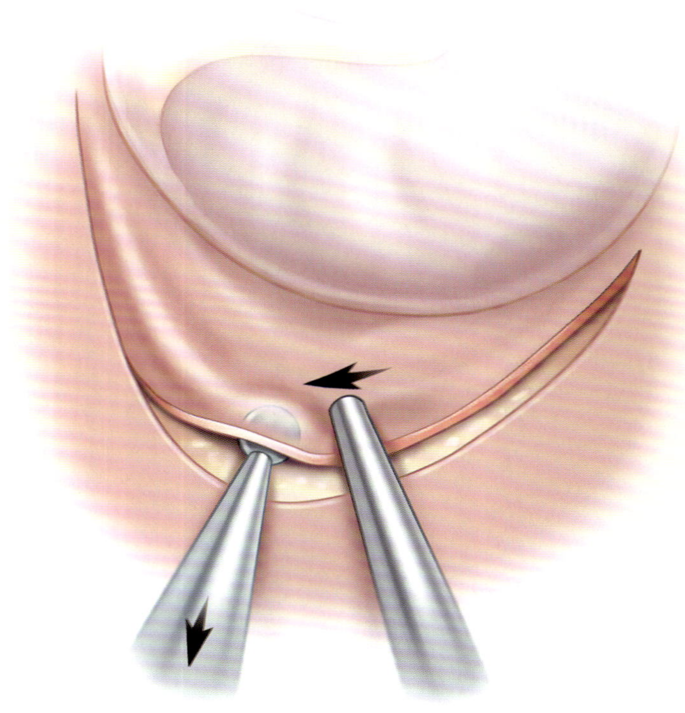

Figure 20-151. A joint knife may be used to unfurl the edge to ensure the flap lies flat against the bony canal.

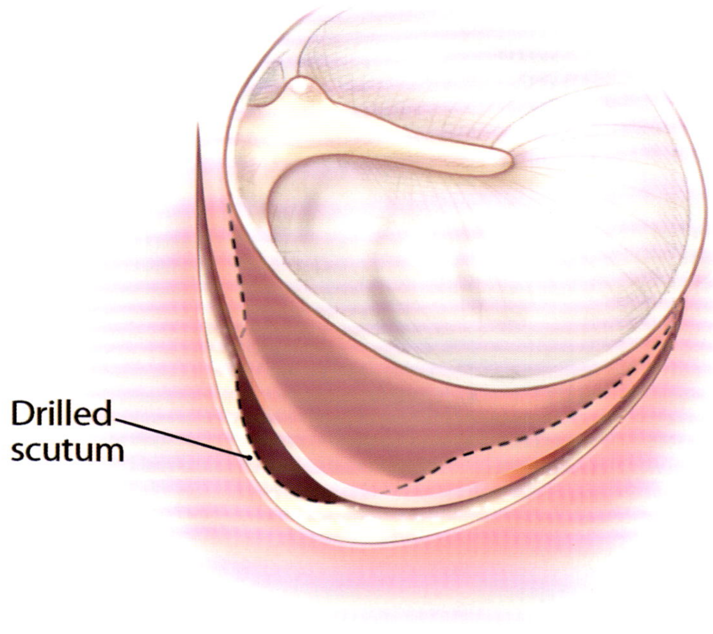

Figure 20-152. Marginal dehiscence of the flap due to either too short of a flap design or a long scutum necessitating more extensive bone removal than the flap can cover.

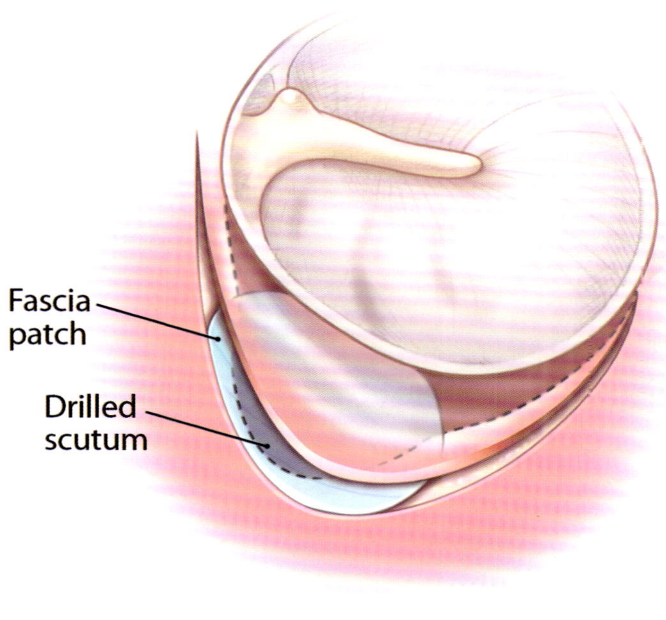

Figure 20-153. Marginal dehiscence should be repaired with a perichondrial or fascial graft.

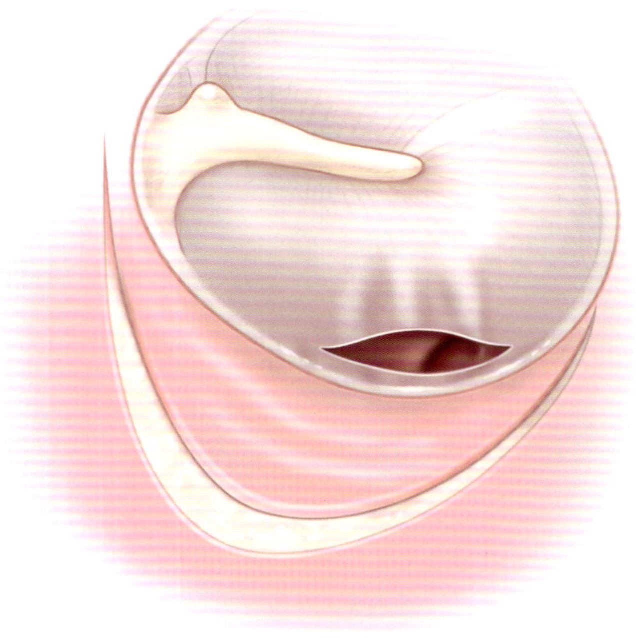

Figure 20-154. Tympanic membrane tear sustained during flap elevation.

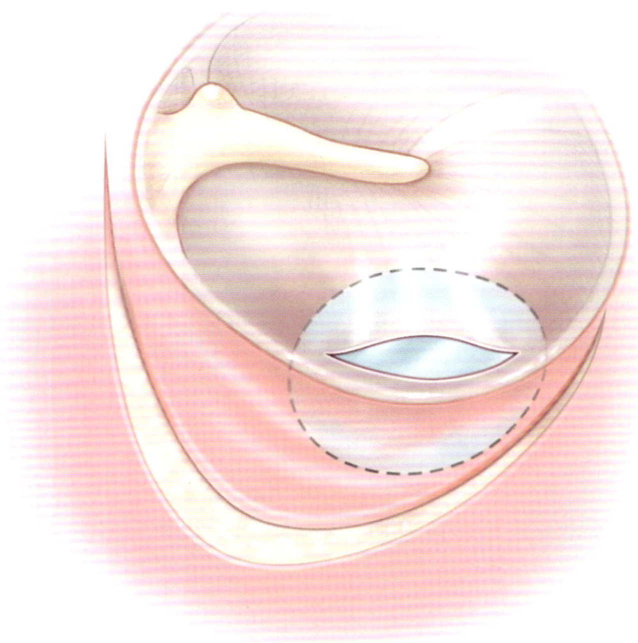

Figure 20-155. As the incision has devascularized the posterior aspect of the tympanic membrane, spontaneous healing is not ensured. The tympanic membrane is best repaired with a perichondrial or fascial graft placed medial to the tear.

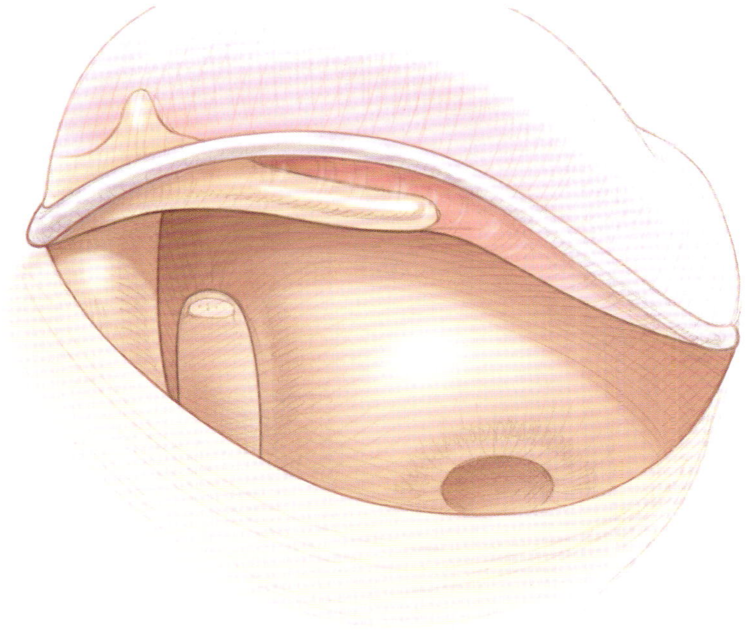

Figure 20-156. An absent or insufficient incus represents a technical challenge in stapes surgery.

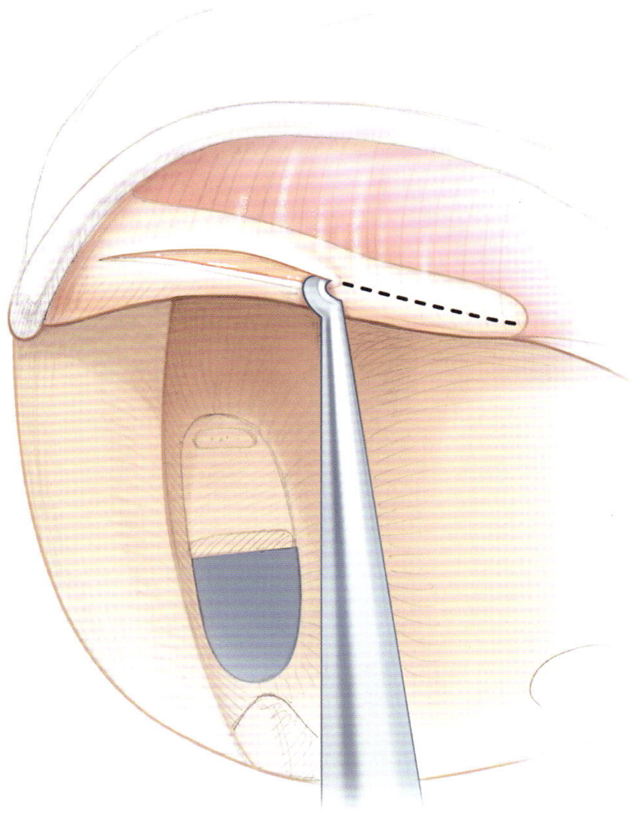

Figure 20-157. Incision is made in the posterior aspect of the umbo with either a myringotomy knife or laser.

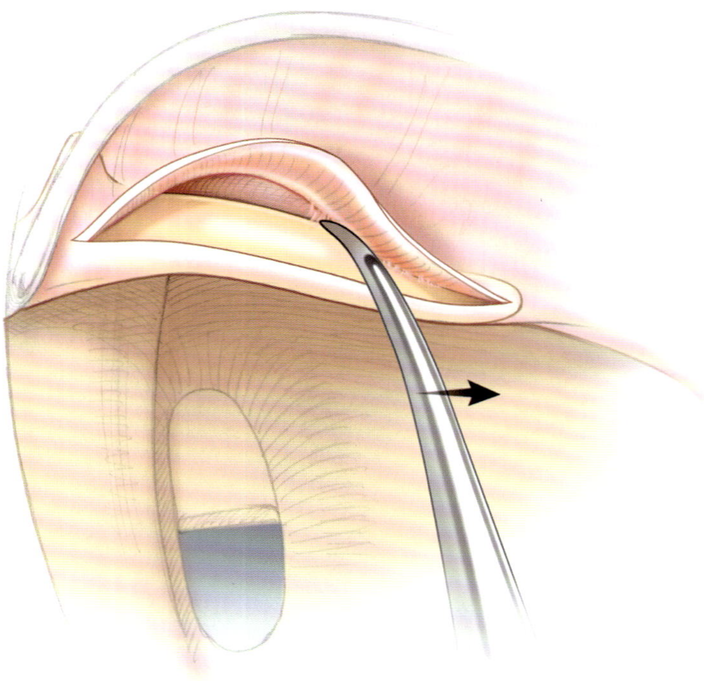

Figure 20-158. A pocket is raised from the malleus short process to the umbo to accommodate the prosthesis. Exercising care to avoid tympanic membrane disruption.

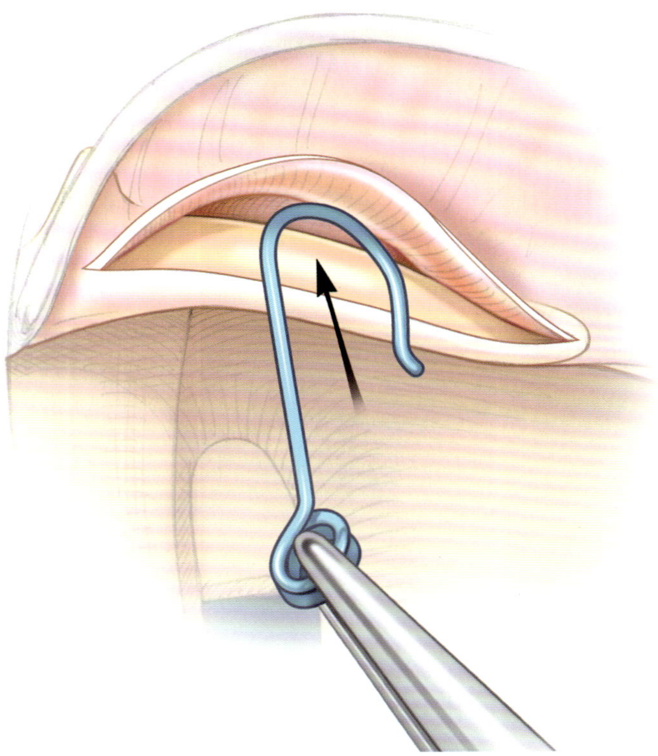

Figure 20-159. Technique of inserting an incus replacement wire (Sheehy IRP).

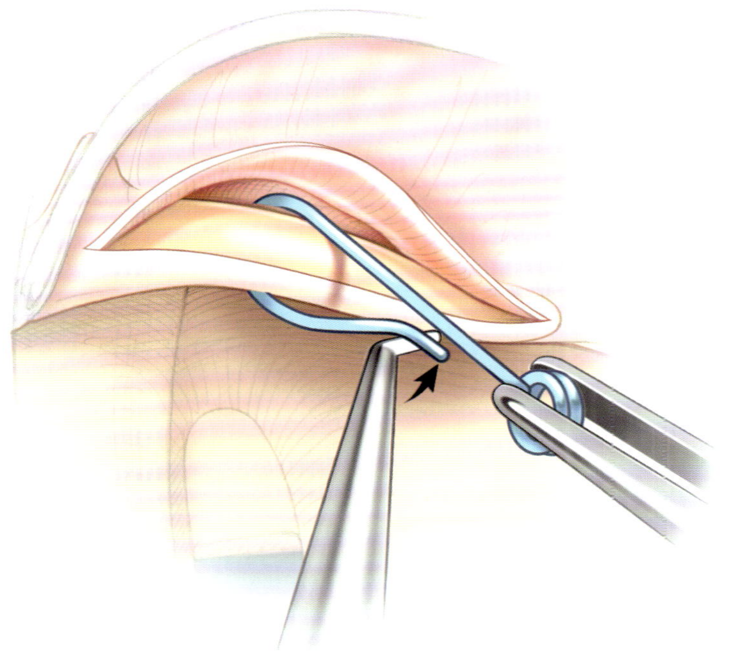

Figure 20-160. The IRP is tied around the malleus with a hook while the prosthesis is stabilized with an alligator.

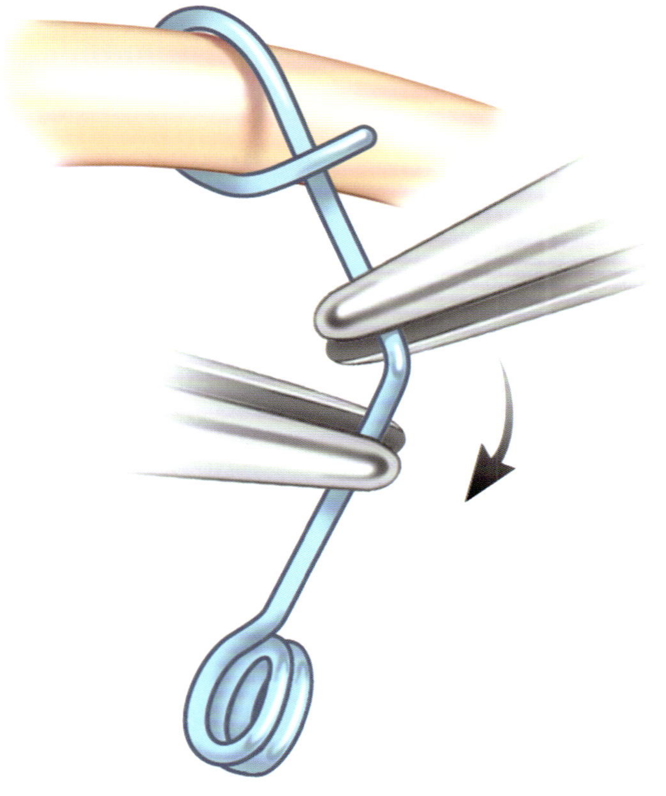

Figure 20-161. To avoid the need for various lengths, a long prosthesis is used, which is bent before positioning above the oval window.

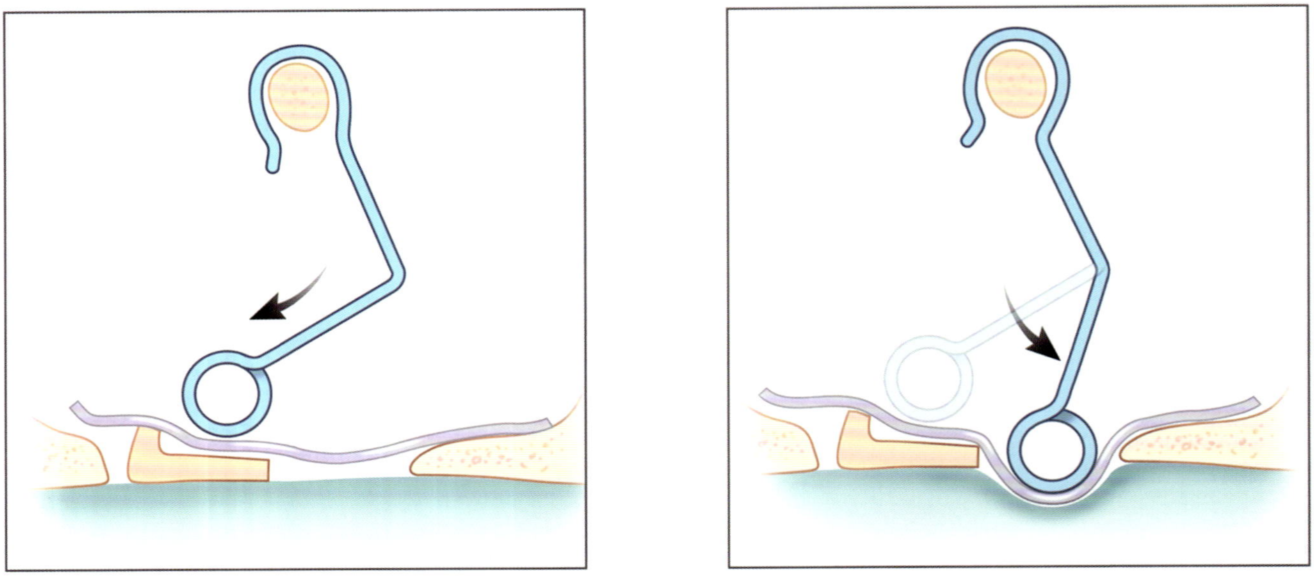

Overbend Unbend

Figure 20-162. The bend is progressively straightened until the desired tension is achieved.

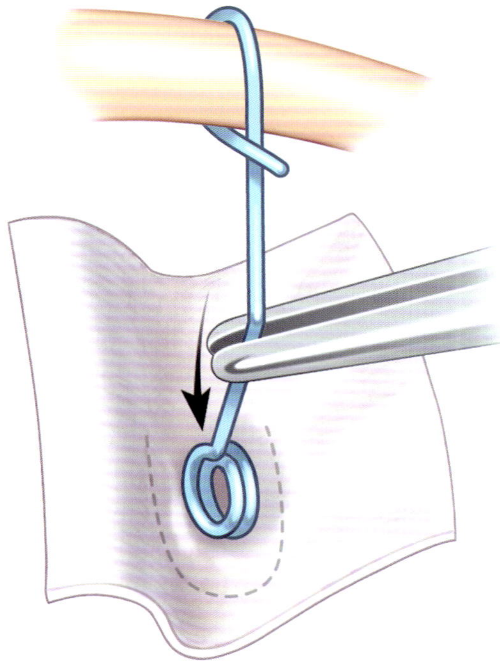

Figure 20-163. The malleus to footplate prosthesis seated into position.

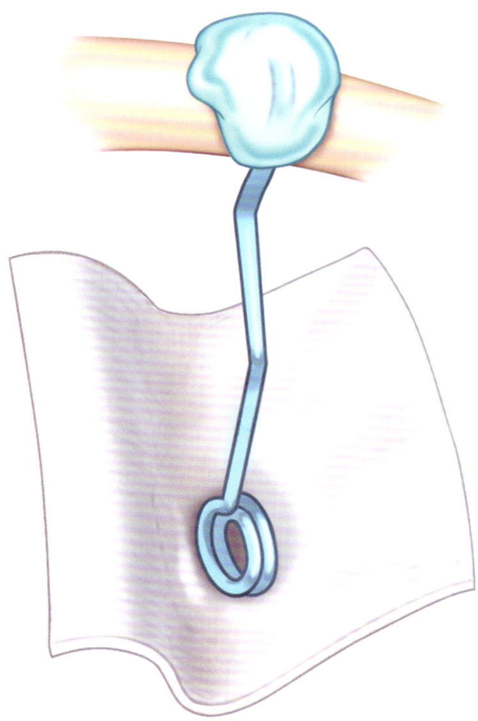

Figure 20-164. A drop of cement may be placed to reinforce the stability of the malleus crimp

CHAPTER 21

Otosclerosis: Clinical Considerations*

Richard James Wiet

INTRODUCTION

The young surgeon expecting to learn stapes surgery will find this one of the more difficult otologic procedures he or she attempts to perform.

Study with a known and recognized expert is recommended, with a period of observation before one attempts the first case. Nevertheless, by temporal bone study and with a slowly increasing surgical volume, mastery of this skill is certainly possible. The author did such a type of observation many years ago with J. Bernard Causse, MD, of Beziers, France, as well as many others. Additional tips on refinement of technique came from time spent with George Shambaugh Jr, author/originator of "Surgery of the Ear."[1]

HISTORY

Our predecessors have documented most of the history of stapes surgery. Shambaugh Jr, after returning from a trip to observe Gunnar Holmgren in Europe, began tinkering with the microscope. It was Holmgren who in 1923 first applied the binocular microscope to otosclerosis surgery. Sufficiently impressed, Shambaugh Jr, made a concerted effort to introduce the microscope to American otologic surgeons by cooperating with the Zeiss optical company. Later, William House introduced the microscope to neurosurgeons, which began to change surgery. Its origin under the influence of otolaryngologists has been recognized by the American College of Surgeons as one of the most significant advances in the history of all surgery.

About 1938, Shambaugh paid a visit to Dr. Julius Lempert of New York. He studied his management of the one-stage fenestration operation for otosclerosis. Initially successful, Lempert had patients flocking to him to correct their hearing from all over the United States. But Lempert never accepted the microscope and eventually lost much of his practice to those who quickly adapted the new technology of the day. (It is a lesson to those who have a blind eye to new technological developments.)

Shambaugh Jr also visited Rosen in New York, who in 1952 first mobilized the stapes footplate and created a rush of new interest in stapes surgery. Rosen's famous question to his patient while performing stapes surgery was: "How do you like your eggs, fried or scrambled?" The patient, hearing more clearly for the first time, responded appropriately, "Fried."

However, it was not until John Shea Jr, in 1956, used a prosthesis after removing the stapes utilizing the microscope. After Shea's success, the era of stapes surgery truly blossomed. Considering that this method was a little more than a half-century ago, stapes surgery is still a young science.

*Funded in part by: The Center for Hearing Restoration and Ear Research of Hinsdale Hospital.

ACADEMY GUIDELINES

The American Academy of Otolaryngology[2] has published reports of recommendations for surgery. These serve as reasonable, but not absolute guides, in assisting the surgeon in his or her recommendations. They consist of the following:

1. Physical exam: absence of chronic infection, and normal tympanic membrane and ear canal.
2. Audiometric testing.
3. Pure tone average: air 25 dB or greater; bone . . . 10 to 15 dB. In addition, there should preferably be good word recognition scores.
4. Tuning forks: 512 cps. Weber and Rinne; lateralization to the ear proposed for surgery. The author wipes the stem of the tuning fork with alcohol and has the patient bite it for more accurate sound lateralization.

The tympanogram should be normal, and *absent* acoustic reflexes, support the diagnosis.

CASE SELECTION

The proper case selection is of paramount importance in stapes surgery. The patient afflicted with otosclerosis typically begins to lose hearing in late 20s and early 30s. Although Mendel Robinson wrote a classic paper[3] that contends otosclerosis may occur even in the juvenile state, this is rare. With children, one must be more cautious, distinguishing between congenital fixations, which comes on from birth, from those individuals who have a latter, rapid onset of conductive loss due to juvenile otosclerosis. These juvenile patients have a tendency to advance rapidly in conductive hearing loss, and early surgery may be preferable.

Satisfactory results can be obtained by first checking the audiologic diagnosis, verifying normality with high-density CT scans. Instruct the radiologist to have a thin section (0.5 mm) CT, and to observe the cochlear duct aperture to prevent operating on a potential CSF gusher patient. Also, it was the opinion of J.B. Causse, MD, that subtle malformations of the stapes cura may signal a potential gusher.[4]

These gushers are more common in X-linked disease and wide vestibular aqueduct yndrome. Conductive hearing loss with wide vestibular aqueduct, while rare, is often confused with otosclerosis and is a congenital problem.

In the adult population, most cases of stapes fixation are bilateral, and there is a female preponderance. When bilateral, and the individual has a mature conductive loss, there may be a phenomena of paracusis of Willis, the ability to hear best, in a loud din. The afflicted person speaks softly because the skull acts as a volume conductor.

Furthermore, we emphasize that the proper audiogram is performed with masking, and verify the conductive hearing loss using tuning forks. An ideal case is the patient who has more than a 20 dB conductive hearing loss, and a negative 512 Rinne's test. Preferably, the tuning fork lateralizes with the Weber to the worst hearing ear. Because of the landmark contribution of Minor (1991),[5] an alert physician always requests stapedial reflexes on all patients going through stapes surgery to avoid the conductive hearing loss caused by a third window. Several years ago this was referred to as "inner ear conductive loss" by Howard House and is the reason for a failure in stapes surgery to correct the conductive loss.

The audiological evaluation is key in helping to diagnose otosclerosis. This evaluation not only includes air conduction and bone conduction thresholds, but also tympanometry, acoustic reflex thresholds, and otoacoustic emissions.

When otosclerosis is present, the audiogram traditionally reveals a conductive hearing loss with an increase in the bone conduction threshold at 2000 Hz, commonly referred to as the "Carhart notch." This threshold may be up to 15 dBHL worse than the bone conduction thresholds at other frequencies in the same ear. The theory behind this notch is that 2000 Hz is the resonant frequency of the ossicular chain; therefore, the effect is stronger at that frequency.

When otosclerosis is progressing in both ears, there will be a bilateral conductive hearing loss. For this reason, it is important to be cautious when masking for bone conduction. The use of insert earphones is recommended. Insert earphones have a higher interaural attenuation than traditional headphones, therefore a less chance of the masking noise crossing to the test ear. Interaural attention values vary based on frequency, but many clinicians use an average value for masking purposes. To be very conservative, a 50-dB HL value may be used for interaural attenuation when using insert earphones to test for bilateral conductive hearing loss.

In addition to the audiogram, immittance testing should be completed. Although tympanometry results for a middle ear with otosclerosis may be within normal limits, it is not considered a reliable predictor of otosclerosis. However, in advanced otosclerosis, the tympanogram may have a low peak, or static admittance, due to the stiffness in the middle ear. Hence, acoustic reflex thresholds are more useful in trying to predict otosclerosis. In early stages of otosclerosis, an upward deflection may be present at the onset of the sound, followed by a downward movement (the typical reflex pattern), then ending with a slight upward deflection as well. Due to the conductive nature of the hearing loss, acoustic reflexes may be elevated as the otosclerosis progresses. If the stapes becomes fixed, reflexes will be absent in that ear. Finally, if the patient has a hearing loss that is mild or severe, otoacoustic emissions are expected to be absent.

OTHER CLINICAL CONSIDERATIONS

Older age onset of conductive hearing loss in an individual may more often be a malleus fixation. This is more typical in an individual who has suffered from chronic infections. Fixation of the malleus may be detected in the office visit by carefully touching the malleus gently with a standard instrument. If it is fixed, it feels like cement and does not move. Similarly, tympanosclerosis is another type of fixation developed in chronic infections that may give the same clinical presentation. The stapes surgeon should be prepared to handle both conditions.

Stapes surgery is possible, but often more challenging in the case of tympanoslcerosis causing conductive loss. I have been successful in mild cases but, when it is massive, it is best not to operate on these individuals.

Another form of conductive hearing loss is Paget's disease,[6] typically more commonly seen in males than females. It has an onset later in years than otosclerosis, usually in the fourth decade. One commonly will see an enlarged skull, and the hearing loss is typically mixed.

Authors have also cautioned that during a hydropic state of Ménière's, there is an enhanced risk of neurosensory hearing loss because the saccule dilates under the footplate. Thus, there may be a more favorable time to operate after the hydropic state abates.

Other types of osteodystrophies of the temporal bone causing conductive hearing loss can include, for example, osteogenosis imperfecta. Its origin is probably in a collagen defect. In these individuals hearing loss is also seen in the second decade of life. It may be similar to the presentation of the otosclerotic patient. There is commonly a history of multiple fractures and, on physical exam, short stature and blue sclera of the eyes. Sillence has given a classification of multiple types of this disorder and one can review that in our monograph.[4,7]

The recognition of this osteogenosis imperfecta is important because the surgery may be more difficult, and the potential for complications are greater than those of the otosclerotic case. Typically, these individuals have a blue sclera of the eye. Furthermore, it has also been reported that the progression in sensorineural hearing loss is faster than the otosclerotic population.

There is a large list of other osteodystrophies, which may cause conductive hearing loss; these include rare disorders such as familial expansile osteolysis, osteopetrosis (Albers-Schonberg disease), and fibrous dysplasia.

As we mentioned previously, the typical patient has a noninfected ear canal. But in some cases, in which the patient has worn a hearing aid for some time (especially when there is a discharge), there can be a threat to bacterial infection, and it is a relative contraindication to surgery. These patients are told to stop using a hearing aid for 2 weeks before surgery and bathe their ear canal in typical otic antibiotics.

Although the majority of patients with otosclerosis have a normal canal and tympanic membrane, there is a rare variation. The Schwartz's sign is a pinkish blush seen through the tympanic membrane in a patient who has active otosclerosis. Once thought to be a troublesome sign, with the onset of laser technology, the active phase of otospongiosis is no longer a reason to postpone surgery. Findings such as secretory otitis, tympanosclerosis, osteogenesis imperfecta, and exostosis may be the reason for other conductive pathologies.

INFORMED CONSENT

All patients who go through the evaluation for conductive hearing loss from otosclerosis may be candidates for hearing aids. This is certainly an option for patients who are risk adverse. I have the custom of discussing this with them, and stating simply if they do not want to accept the risks of surgery, then hearing aids are a satisfactory option.

If the patient is more inclined to accept some reasonable risk, we put into simple terms what those risks are, such as failure to correct the hearing loss, worse hearing, or even total hearing loss in the operated ear. Rarely, tinnitus and dizziness are worsened in stapes surgery, so this should be mentioned. In extreme cases, the facial nerve can be injured, so this should also be discussed.

Additionally, some patients' hobbies or professions may be adversely affected. We advise patients not to scuba dive after stapes surgery for instance. If they are devoted to that hobby, they should consider having no surgery and use a hearing aid. Instead, other patients, notably those who are professional food tasters, should be warned about potential changes in taste due to the chorda tympani nerve. Occasionally, patients will inquire about the possibility of a late complication or late onset hearing loss due to a change in the prosthesis. To reassure them, we state our rate of revision surgery, which is estimated to be only 5% to 8% of our caseload.

IMAGING

Rarely is CT scan imaging requested for confirmation of otosclerosis and is not the standard of care in the United States. However, we use it to evaluate the cochlear capsule as originally suggested by Valvassori.[8] Today, more detailed 0.5-mm scanners are available to detect the spread of otosclerosis throughout the cochlea, evaluate cases such as advanced otosclerosis (Figure 21–1), osteogenosis imperfecta, or with the addition of the Poschel views, the third window abnormality causes of conductive hearing loss.

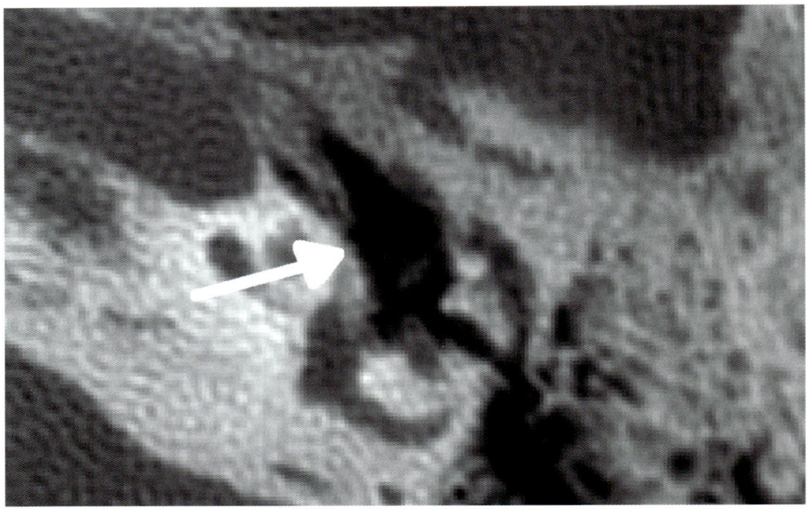

Figure 21–1. Arrow points to otospongiotic focus on cochlea.

Rare Variations of Pathology/Anatomy

It is well known that obliterative otosclerosis can exist, both in the oval and round window. It may be impossible to detect it in the round window, except for checking the round window reflex after stapes surgery is completed. Such cases present a more difficult challenge to the stapes surgeon. Hearing gain is generally unsuccessful. Second, overhang of the facial nerve is a known potential challenge to the novice surgeon. Generally speaking, if the nerve overhangs the view of the oval window by more than 50%, there is nothing wrong with closing and advising the patient to get a hearing aid. Abnormalities of the stapes itself include conditions such as a single cura, osteogenosis involving the ossicles, and congenital fixation, all of which may be more prone to CSF gusher phenomena.

"Far advanced otosclerosis" is a topic unto itself, and exists in the patient who has been wearing a hearing aid for years, speaks softly because of a severe bilateral conductive hearing loss, and presents with an audiogram that appears to be a dead ear. This has to do with the limits of a bone conduction audiometer; consequently, the patient appears to have a false, neurosensory hearing loss. Patients are often the subjects of debate if they have clear indications for a cochlear implant vs. stapes surgery. For a reference to these pathologic states, and others, the reader is referred to "Pathology of the Ear" by the late Hal Schuknecht and his successors.[9]

PRE-OP DISCUSSIONS

For stapes surgery, one must be clear with the patient regarding the surgeon's experience and outcomes. It is a difficult surgery and requires a learning curve to master it. Frequently, a patient will ask if I recommend the surgery, and I do not hesitate, provided they meet standard guidelines of our Academy. However, no matter what the skill level of the surgeon, appropriate risks must be discussed as previously mentioned.

Again, a forthright presentation of risks, including a "dead ear" after surgery, partial hearing loss, failure to correct the condition, dizziness, tinnitus, and taste disturbances are presented to the patient. For the patient with mixed hearing loss, care must be taken to avoid unrealistic expectations and to explain possible outcomes with the sensory component of the hearing loss.

Patients should not exhibit any medical contraindications to surgery requiring general anesthesia. Local anesthetics are chosen for patients undergoing the occasional case of revision. This is to predict a problem of sacular injury, as patients will signal dizziness when attempting the removal of the prosthesis. This presents potential negative consequences of further sensory hearing loss.

SURGICAL TECHNIQUE

Positioning of the patient: I have used a Derlacki head holder for years, which allows the head to be moved back and forth to position the required view of the upper posterior superior quadrant of the tympanic membrane. If that device is not available, further measures must be taken to ensure the correct positioning for surgery. Especially in the case of the patient undergoing general anesthetic, it is vital to tuck the chin down toward the contralateral clavicle, and flex the table down (Figure 21–2). Also, the natural break in the table (at the head) will provide a type of Trendelenberg position. The patient's head should be angled almost 30 degrees downward and then secured.

All patients undergoing stapes surgery are given an antibiotic and Decadron intravenously, prior to the start of the operation. Proper injection is critical for good hemostasis (Figure 21–3). The ear is then injected with a dental syringe and preloaded 1:50,000 xylocaine and epinephrine in separate carpules. I recommend watching for a blanch in skin color, then using the speculum to press inward to the skin of the ear canal with the fluid using a 27-gauge needle.

Although I do not use a speculum holder in every case, I encourage the young surgeon or residents in training to begin to use it. This will allow a two-handed technique. It also gives the surgeon a sense of balance against a solid object as one works through a "test tube"-like environment—the ear canal.

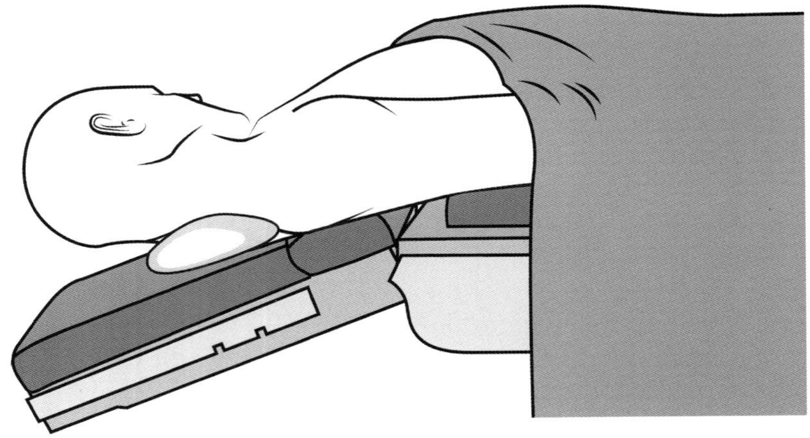

Figure 21-2. Shown is the proper positioning to operate this individual's right ear.

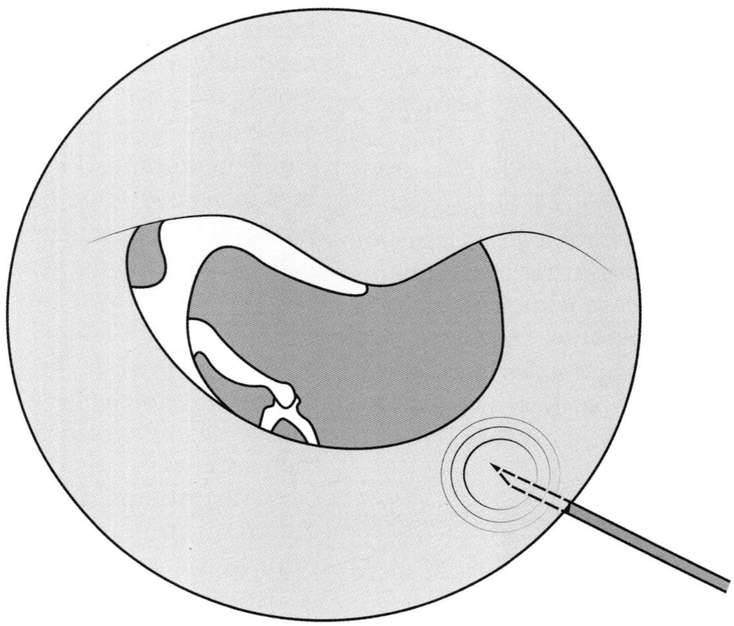

Surgical Position

Figure 21-3. Initial injection with dental syringe; 1 to 50,000 xylocaine and epinephrine in prepared carpules.

The light of the microscope must ride down the axis of the instrument longitudinally. One must be conscious of placement of his or her fingers, so as not to block light while holding the instrument. Finally, the proper diopter setting on the microscope should be adjusted preoperatively if there is any intraocular inequality in visual acuity. All these features improve the technique of the surgery and become a routine habit for an experienced surgeon.

Incisions in the Typanomeatal Flap

I begin every surgery with two instruments handy, the "roller," or pizza cutter knife, and a new 72 Beaver single blade mounted on its handle. I have devised an instrument set for the Medtronic Corporation for that purpose. This is known as the Wiet-Chronic Ear/Stapes set.

Using one or the other the typanomeatal flap is a gentle or broad "V" shape. This is lowered down with a #2 knife (Sheehy weapon or #2 knife) to the level of the annulus. If that is unavailable, the duck-bill or round knife will suffice. The aim is a smooth flap progressing to or toward the annular indentation. When teaching residents, I tell them to imagine a wave of canal skin. Keep this flowing and do not chop or shred the skin. First, take "the wave" of the flap down to the annulus and stop. Next, carefully elevate the annulus with a sharp-tipped angled instrument, for it is easy to disrupt the annulus inferiorly while lifting it. In the same process, try to keep the chorda typmani nerve intact.

Chorda Tympani

The chorda is delivered by fracturing outward the posterior iter. Then, by inserting a curved Rosen needle into the rim, it is carefully delivered toward the folded tympanic membrane. More room for the flap may be gained with the alligator scissors, extended, with one blade in the skin of the ear canal, and one out. The direction is anterior toward the malleus neck. This is especially important in cases where you suspect malleus fixation. Now cut the skin.

Curetting

While in some countries it is more common to use a chisel, the American tradition of curetting the canal bony overhang is typical. Curetting starts just above the annulus of the canal at the scutum (Figure 21–4). Try to make the incision just above the short process of the incus, not extending too far upward. Digging inward is safer, to prevent slippage and consequent subluxation of the incus. The final curetting then exposes the edge of the scutum, and the aim of the technique is to "imagine" the short process of the incus just below the curetted point. In other words, do not curette too closely to the malleus, because in the event the patient has malleus fixation, the incision will need to be extended, and in the event of negative pressure the TM will indent toward the malleus.

IS Joint Management and the Ossicular Chain

Before dividing the joint, the malleus is uplifted gently with a straight or curved Rosen needle to ensure that there is no fixation of the bone. Next, attention is turned to the incus.

The typical patient can have the IS joint disarticulated by first wiggling the joint's synovial capsule (Figure 21–5). Look attentively with high magnification at the joint. Here insert the Harrison knife (joint knife) and divide the joint carefully. Failure to do so could result in subluxation of the incus and the need for an incus replacement prosthesis or malleus to oval window prosthesis.

Management of the Stapes Itself, Footplate

Using the microprobe with the Omniguide laser set at 4.0 watts at 100 microseconds, bursts of laser light are used to divide the stapedial tendon. Next, the same wavelength is used to char the posterior crus. The crus are divided by touching the char to make sure that the crus are dissolved. When a laser is not available or when excessive footplate thickness is present, a Synergy drill may be all that is needed. If accessible, the anterior crus are divided in a similar manner. The cura is removed and submitted to the pathologist for "gross" examination, leaving the footplate to manage. Lastly (Figure 21–6), we make a rosette formation of laser bursts in the posterior one-half of the footplate, with a Farrior rasp, this char is removed to prepare for the prosthesis (see video).

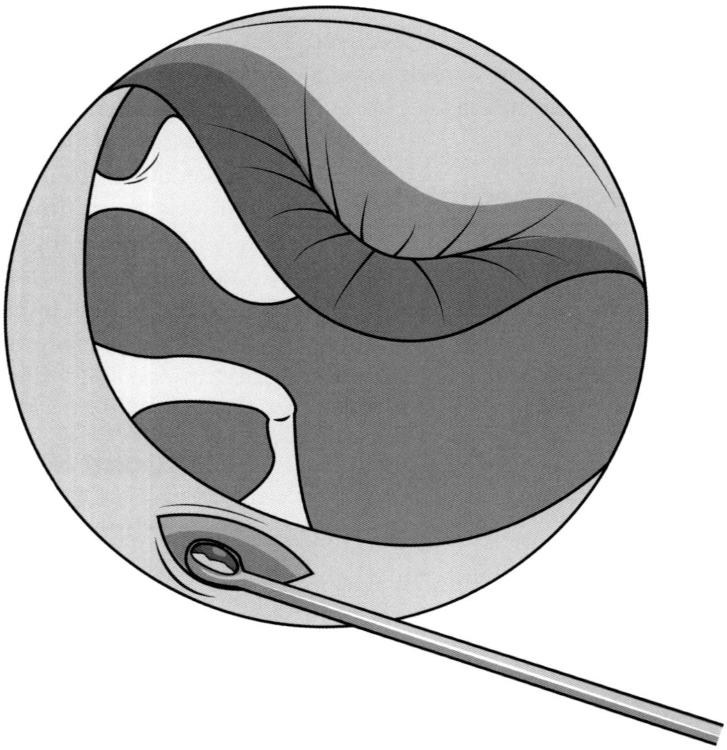

Figure 21–4. Beginning to curet, above annulus, right ear.

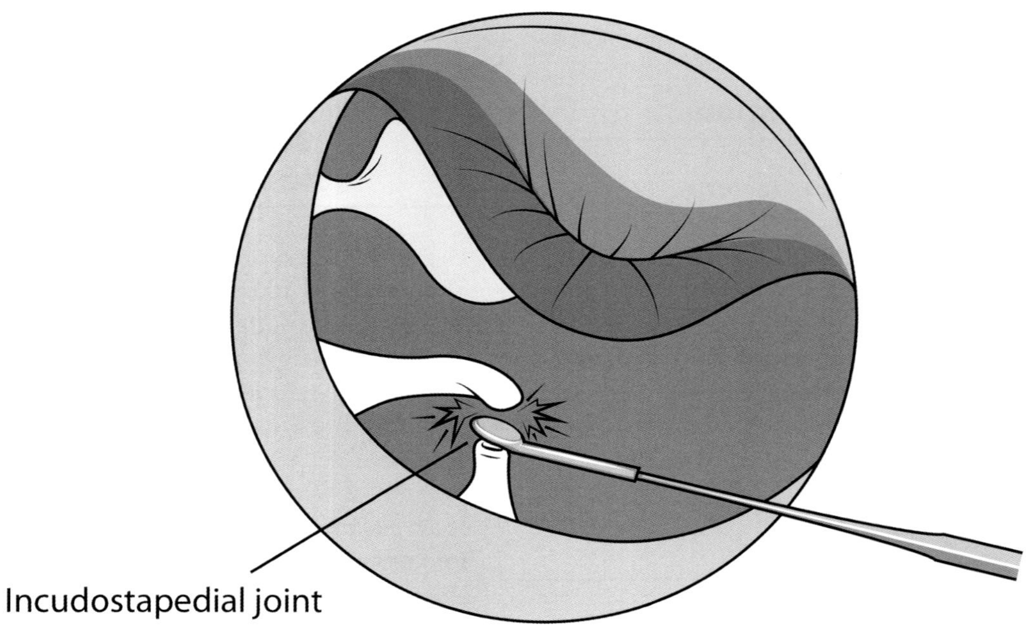

Figure 21–5. Division of IS joint.

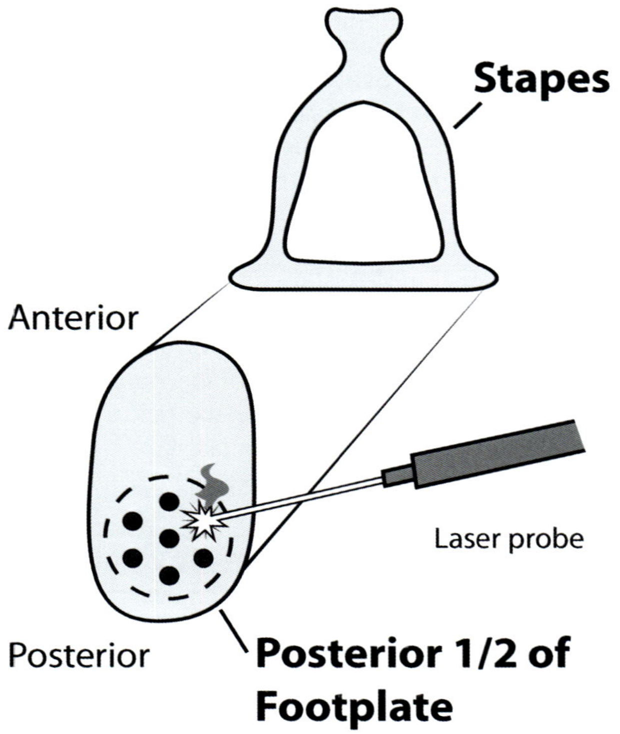

Figure 21–6. Posterior 1/2 stapedectomy, initially with laser at footplate (see text).

Much has been written about footplate management by key authors. Descriptions of biscuit deformities, bifid footplates, mono cura status, and obliterated footplates—all are found in medical literature. The typical footplate is permeable with the laser set at 3.0 watts, for 100 microseconds. Suffice it to say, if the footplate is too thick to be lased, it should be drilled. One must have a most delicate touch with the proper drill to perform a "drill-out, stapedectomy."

The Obliterative Footplate

This type of footplate will not respond to laser permeation. It needs to be delicately drilled out with a soft touch. We typically use a Synergy drill, in cases where there is excessive thickening of the footplate.

The Proper Grafting Technique

We have recently published our findings that nearly equal results obtained with either fat, fascia, or vein. My colleagues and I have done a study on the use of various materials for grafting the oval window.[10] Ultimately, we concluded that differing materials were all effective in the grafting technique. I prefer fat harvested from the back of the auricle. The smallest fragment of fat will do. It is easily harvested by turning over the ear, avoiding any pierced ear hole. Then, one simply makes a linear incision and closes with one mattress suture.

Variations in Footplate Pathology/Cural Malformations

Although the majority of footplates are thin and easily permeable with laser light, some are much thicker. I prefer the simple classification of Gristwood, who emphasized three types: Type I: minor, thin footplate, posterior focus; Type II: intermediate: may be a bipolar focus, slightly thicker footplate, or even a biscuit deformity; and last, the Type III: always requires a drill due to the obliterative type of thick deformity.[11]

Depending on the aggressiveness of this otosclerotic disease there can be sclerotic changes of the cura. Extra thickness from chronic otosclerosis can demand the need to drill to penetrate the fixation.

ROLE OF THE LASER

We said earlier that the microscope and its introduction to surgery by otolaryngologists was a most significant advance. The second advance was the introduction of the laser by Perkins[12] in otosclerosis surgery. Perkins, an American, was one of the first who began to use lasers in otosclerosis surgery. He published his report in 1980,[13] and I visited him to observe his technique.

For decades, lasers have provided the only no-touch tool available to surgeons. Of these, CO_2

lasers have always been considered the most safe and precise. CO_2 laser energy is readily absorbed in water, the main component of living cells, leading to minimal thermal spread and collateral tissue injury (Figure 21–7). Visible laser energy has lower absorption properties and readily passes through the perilymph to be absorbed by pigmented tissue. Carbon dioxide laser energy is absorbed in water and, therefore, has been shown to be 10 times more effective than KTP for ablation of the ossicular chain. Traditional CO_2 laser energy could not be delivered via a flexible fiber, leading many surgeons to utilize less optimal wavelengths such as the KTP or Argon laser. These required an aiming device called a "joy stick." Beginning in 2007, new technologies became commercially available, enabling the flexible delivery of CO_2 laser energy to the delicate structures of the middle ear. This led to the development of a small, delicate, hand-held laser administration system (Figure 21–8).

One of the fundamental elements for stapedotomy success is the production of a precise, symmetrical 0.6-mm footplate fenestration. A precise stapedotomy can be consistently achieved with laser vaporization. The oval window can then be sealed with clotted blood or fat particles, avoiding the need for a collagen tissue seal, reducing the potential for prosthesis migration. Fracturing the stapes crura or mechanically drilling the footplate may mobilize, dislocate, or fracture the footplate, requiring conversion to a partial or complete stapedectomy and a collagen tissue seal (vein or fat). However, the fiber-enabled delivery of CO_2 laser energy allows for atraumatic, fine dissection without the risk of mechanical trauma from traditional instruments or the risk to the perilymph from visible wavelength lasers.

REVISION SURGERY

Leading the pathology that requires a stapes revision is usually something that involves the proximal (incus side) of the prosthesis or the distal side (stapes

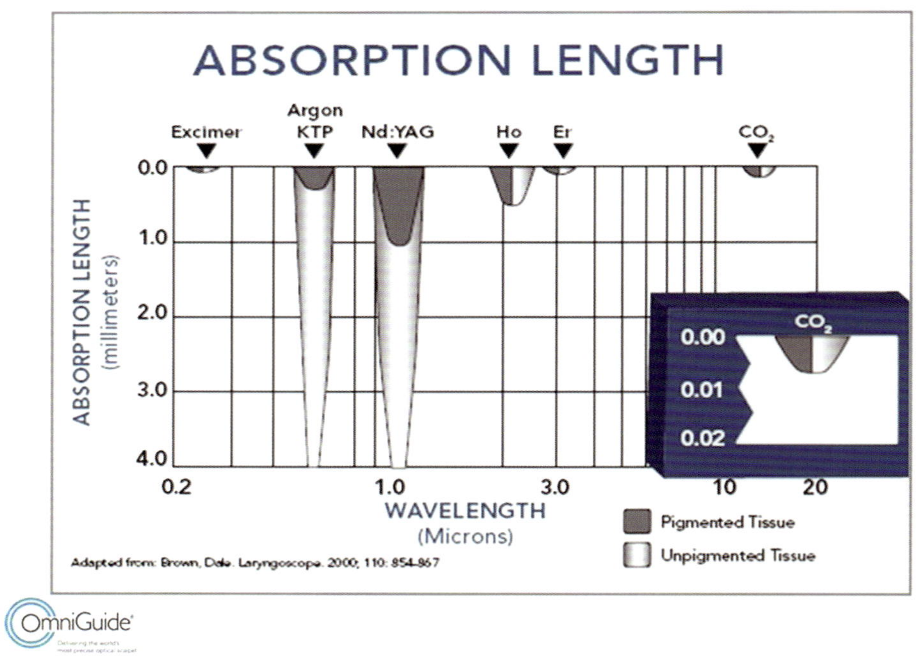

Figure 21–7. The CO_2 laser has a depth of penetration that is 400 times less in unpigmented tissue and 40 times less in pigmented tissue compared to the KTP/Argon laser. Image courtesy of OmniGuide Laser Company.

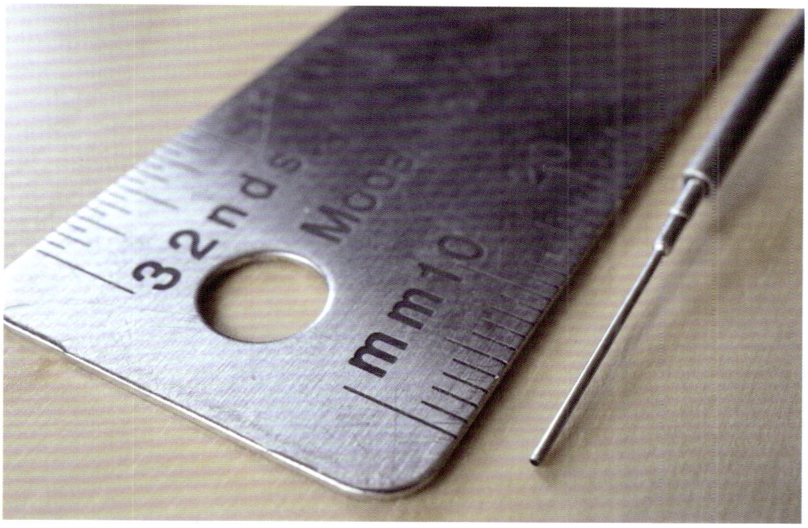

Figure 21–8. Laser probe—hand-held—for footplate ablation, and clearing of adhesions.

footplate). The topic of revision stapes surgery will be a future chapter. Other reasons can include too short, or too long of a prosthesis. I would not operate now without the use of a CO_2 laser in a revision, because the laser has a great advantage in removing collagen tissue or fibrous changes near the distal end of the prosthesis.

CONCLUSION

Our experience now exceeds perhaps 2,000 cases and we are reminded of the incredible number of facts and nuances that come with such practice. The ability to restore excellent hearing to the motivated patient with severe (especially bilateral) conductive hearing loss has been one of the most rewarding joys of my life. Stapes surgery, when one acquires the skill, is dependably predictable. It restores one of the most precious of our special senses: the sense of hearing, and its importance in human communication. So many misunderstandings and hardships can occur without proper hearing. Keeping an open mind to future new developments in otosclerosis surgery, and potential cures through gene therapy, will be forever required if we strive to continue improving our practice "so all can hear."

REFERENCES

1. Shambaugh GE, Glasscock ME. *Surgery of the Ear*. 3rd ed. Philadelphia, PA: Saunders Publishing; 1980.
2. American Academy of Otolaryngology–Head and Neck Surgery. Clinical Indicators: Stapedectomy 2010. http://www.entnet.org/Practice/upload/Stapedectomy-CI.pdf. Retrieved May 1, 2013.
3. Robinson M. Juvenile otosclerosis. A 20-year study. *Ann Otol Rhinol Laryngol*. 1983;92(6 Pt 1):561–565.
4. Wiet RJ, Causse JB, Shambaugh GE, Causse JR, eds. *Otosclerosis (Otospongiosis)*. Alexandria, VA: American Academy of Otolaryngology–Head and Neck Surgery; 1991.
5. Minor LB, Goldberg JM (1991). Vestibular-nerve inputs to the vestibulo-ocular reflex: A functional-ablation study in the squirrel monkey. *J Neurosci*. 1991;(11):1636–1648.
6. Lindsay JR. Otosclerosis. In: M. Paparella, ed. *The Ear*; Vol 2. Philadelphia, PA: WB Saunders Co; 1980:1617–1644.
7. Sillence DO, Morley K, Ault JE. Clinical management of osteogenesis imperfecta. *Connect Tissue Res*. 1995;31:S15–21.
8. Valvassori GE, Dobben GD. CT densitometry of the cochlear capsule in otosclerosis. *Am J Neuroradiol*. 1985;6(5):661–667.

9. Merchant SN, Nadol JB. *Schuknecht's Pathology of the Ear*. 3rd ed. Shelton, CT: People's Medical Publishing House–USA; 2010.
10. Wiet RJ, Battista R, Wiet RM, Sabin A. Hearing outcomes in stapes surgery: a comparison of fat, fascia, and vein tissue seals. *Otolaryngol Head Neck*. 2013;148(1):115–120.
11. Iyer PV, Gristwood RE. Histopathology of the stapes in otosclerosis. *Pathology*. 1984;16(1):30–38.
12. Perkins RC. Preventions in complications in stapes surgery. In: Wiet RJ, ed. *Ear Surgery and Temporal Bone Surgery/Minimizing Risks and Complications*. New York, NY: Thieme; 2006:81–89.
13. Perkins RC. Laser stapedotomy for otosclerosis. *Laryngoscope*. 1980;90(2):228–240.

CHAPTER 22

Obliterative Otosclerosis

Neil M. Sperling and Robert Vincent

INTRODUCTION

Obliterative otosclerosis is a descriptive term for advanced involvement of the stapes footplate and oval window. This has been defined as a greatly thickened footplate and otosclerotic involvement of the annular ligament, such that the margins of the footplate are indistinct.

This condition may render the middle ear anatomy unrecognizable. Histologically, this occurs when the spongiotic growth overwhelms the anatomy of the stapes and oval window region. It has been observed in approximately 5% of surgical cases. And it appears to be bilateral in approximately 30% to 40% of cases identified at surgery. In contrast to the presentation of common otosclerosis, obliterative otosclerosis has been observed more frequently in men than in women.

MANAGEMENT

Obliterative otosclerosis may be considered by some to be a relative contraindication for surgery. Many experienced stapes surgeons, however, have described techniques and outcomes to justify proceeding with stapedectomy. The "drill-out" procedure was first described in the 1960s and has undergone significant refinement with the use of finer microdrills and laser.

There is a small quantity of literature describing the clinical observations of the footplate at stapedectomy. Three footplate patterns have been observed. A "blue footplate" occurs most frequently and refers to a footplate that retains its normal thin bluish appearance at its center and has otosclerotic foci causing fixation at the perimeter of the footplate (most commonly anteriorly). A "white footplate" is less common and refers to foci involving the center of the footplate, with sparing of the annular ligament (biscuit). This morphology may predispose to adverse incidents while doing stapedectomy such as a floating footplate or a footplate fracture. "Obliteration" is an observed morphology described when the footplate is not distinguishable due to extensive otosclerotic involvement of the footplate and annular ligament.

SURGICAL TECHNIQUE

Obliterative changes in the oval window add significant challenge to the surgery. The most important initial step is establishing the position of the oval window and facial nerve. The anatomy needs to be carefully mapped using available landmarks. This includes the round window, chorda tympani, malleus, and incus. The fallopian canal may not be immediately obvious, which adds significant risk to this surgery. It is advantageous to use facial nerve monitoring when obliteration is suspected or, as is the case in some institutions, to use it routinely in all stapes surgeries.

The stapedotomy is created using a combination of sequential laser vaporizations and drilling (Figures 22–1 and 22–2). A wide area is drilled by progressively enlarging the located oval window site. This helps the placement of a vein or tissue graft. It is beneficial to alternate drilling and laser as the vestibule is approached. At the level of the true footplate, laser is used to atraumatically enter the vestibule, and the drill is used to calibrate the size of the fenestration. Because of the depth of drilling required, it is necessary to measure the distance from the incus or malleus to the stapedotomy as progress is made toward the vestibule and again after drilling has been completed.

Ossicular chain reconstruction can be done in most cases from incus to vestibule as in routine primary stapedotomy. If incus erosion is present, bucket handle prosthesis or bone cement or malleus to vestibule prosthesis may be needed.

OUTCOMES

In general, outcomes for stapes surgery in obliterative cases have been reportedly poorer than in routine cases, with air–bone gap closure occurring in 50% to 70% of most series. Some series, however, report excellent outcomes, which may approximate or equal primary stapes surgery. The risk of sensorineural hearing loss appears to be higher possibly as a result of extensive drilling. In addition, some authors have observed regrowth of otosclerosis with decline of good results over time.

SUGGESTED READING

Amedee RG, Lewis ML Jr. Obliterative otosclerosis. *Laryngoscope.* 1987;97(8 pt 1):922–924.

Ayache D, Sleiman J, Plouin-Gaudon I, Klap P, Elbaz P. Obliterative otosclerosis. *J Laryngol Otol.* 1999;113(6):512–514.

Malafronte G, Filosa B, Cantone E. New macroscopic classification of stapedio-ovalar otosclerosis: a simplified rating for training in stapedotomy. *Otol Neurotol.* 2008;29 (7):889–892.

Vincent R, Sperling N, Oates J, Jindal M. Surgical findings and long-term hearing results in 3,050 stapedotomies for primary otosclerosis: a prospective study with the otology-neurotology database. *Otol Neurotol.* 2006;27:S25–S47.

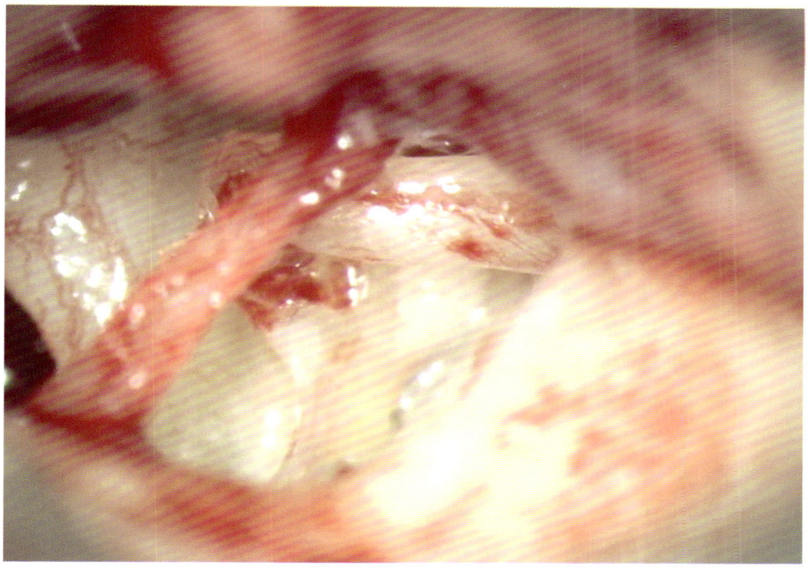

A

Figure 22–1A. Exposure of the ossicular chain revealing obliterative otosclerosis.

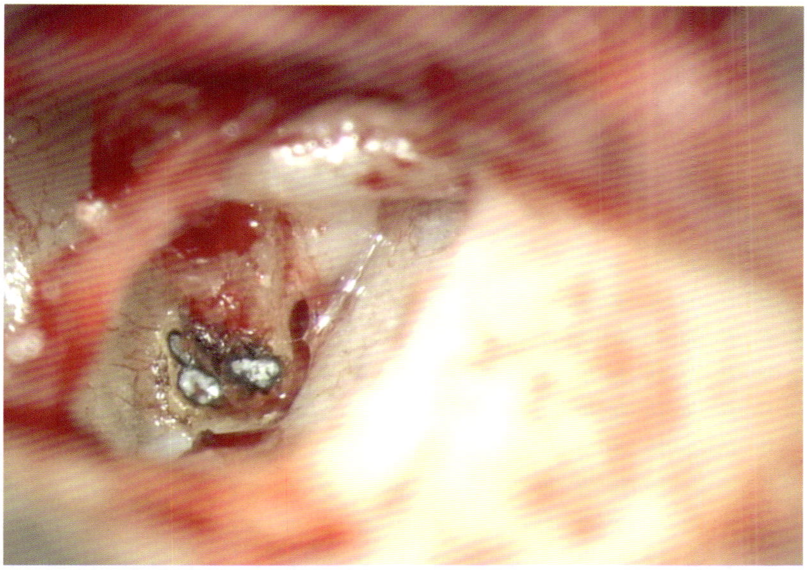

B

Figure 22–1B. Laser removal of the superstructure.

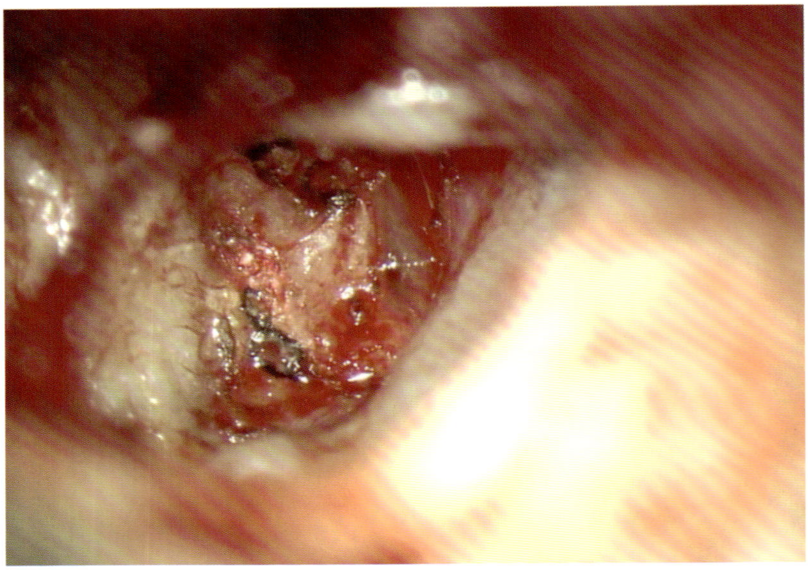

C

Figure 22–1C. Obliterative footplate exposed.

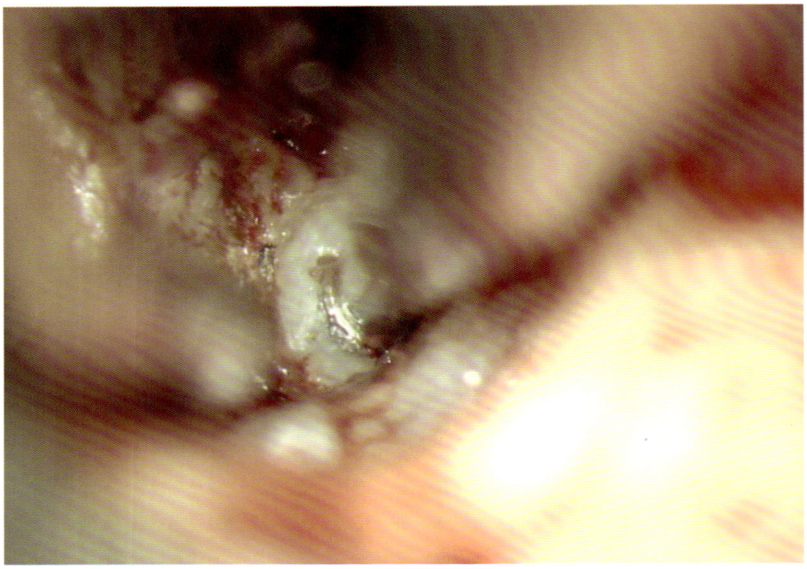

D

Figure 22–1D. Drilling of footplate: part 1.

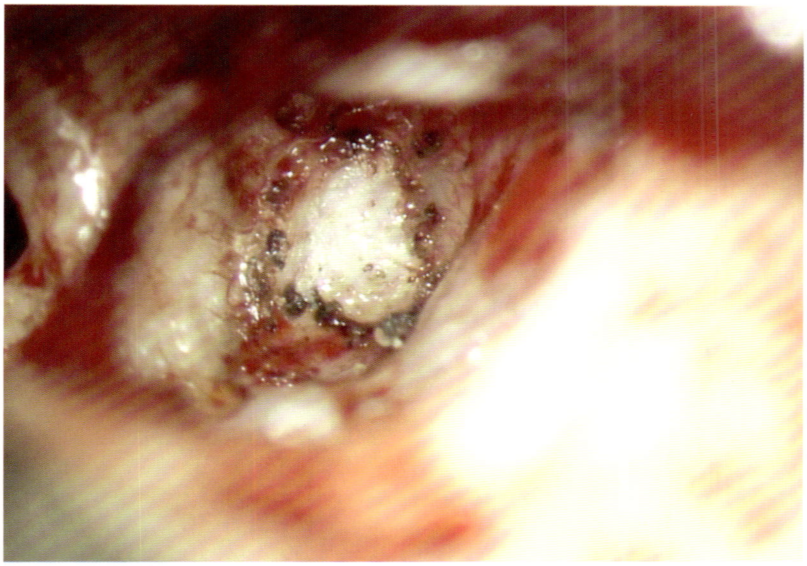

E

Figure 22–1E. Drilling of footplate: part 2.

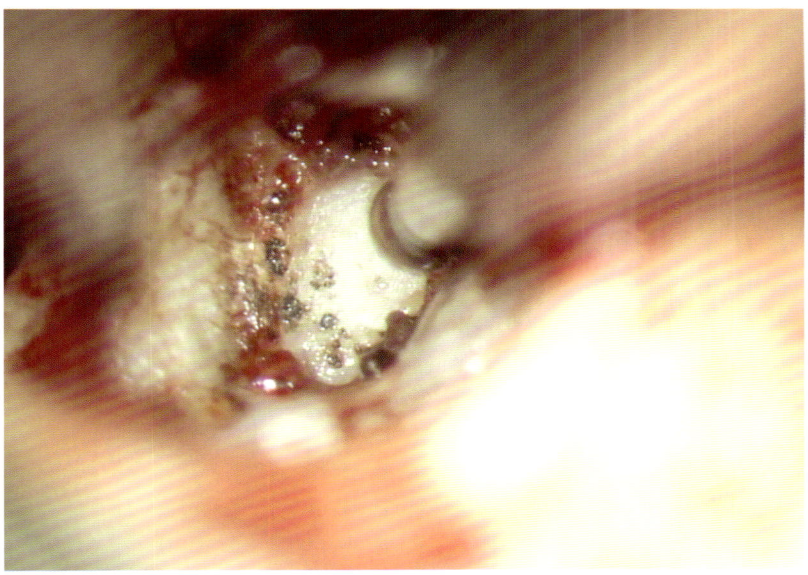

F

Figure 22–1F. Drilling of footplate: part 3.

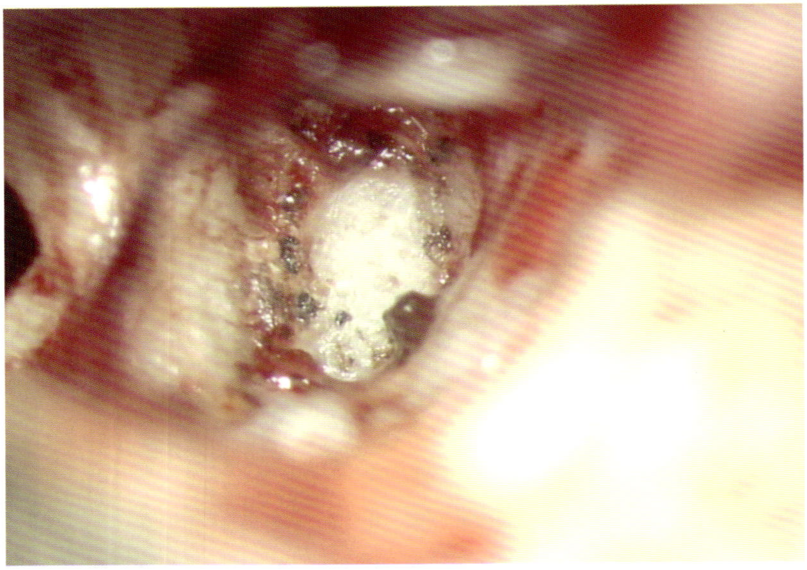

G

Figure 22-1G. Drilling of footplate: part 4.

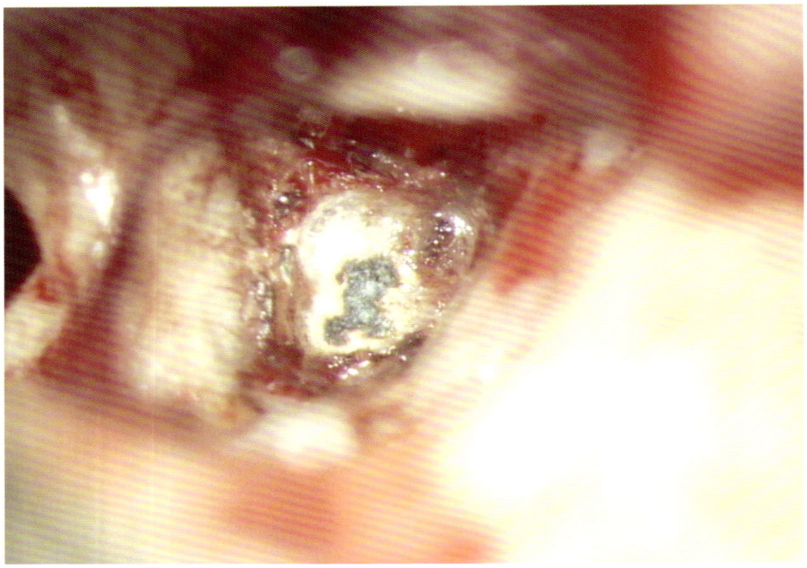

H

Figure 22-1H. Laser of obliterative footplate.

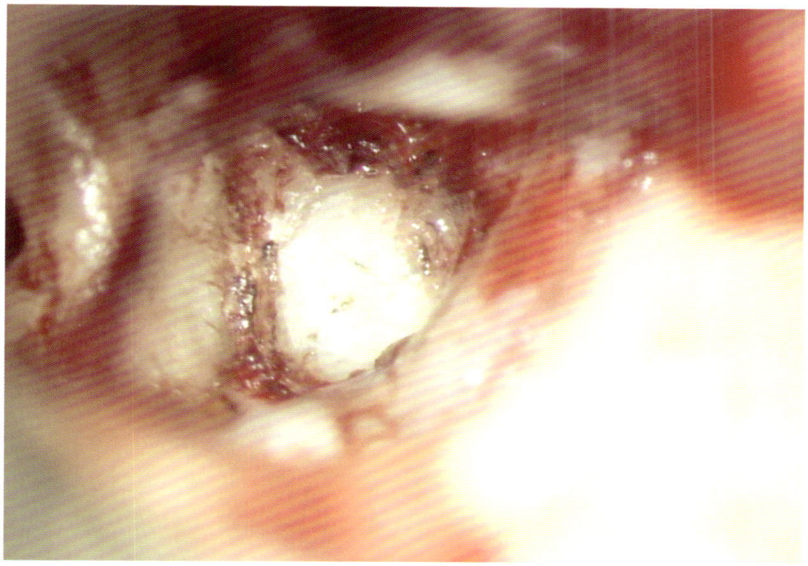

I

Figure 22–1I. Additional drilling of footplate.

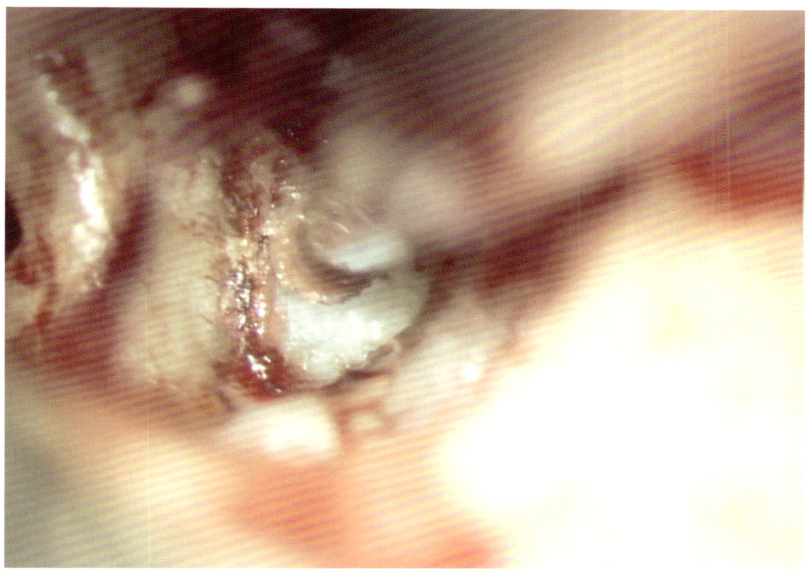

J

Figure 22–1J. Additional drilling of footplate.

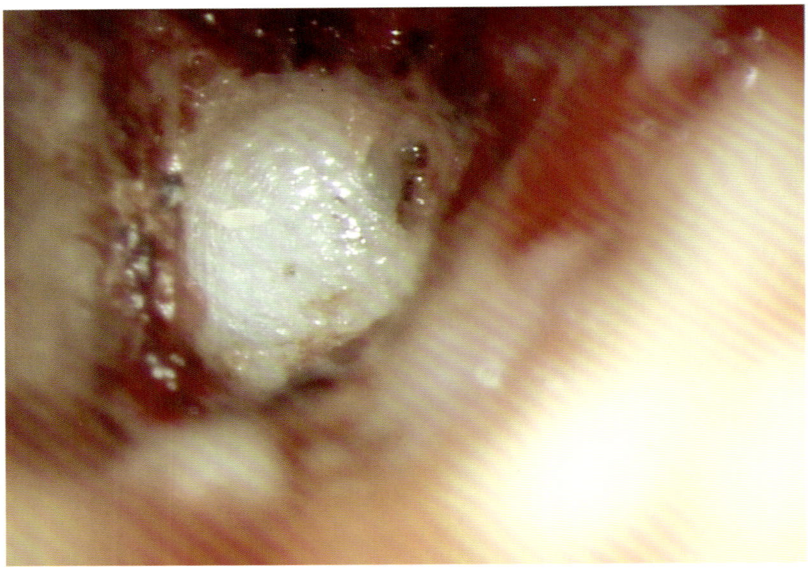

K

Figure 22–1K. Additional drilling of footplate.

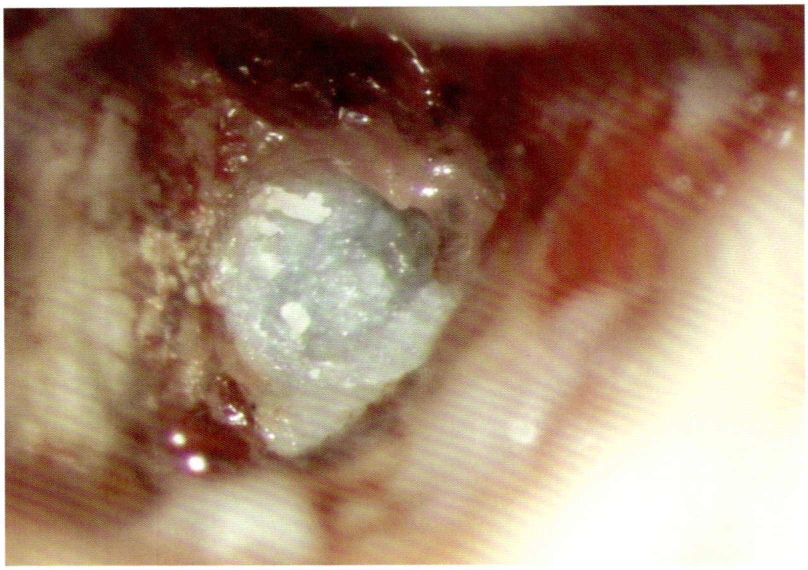

L

Figure 22–1L. Additional drilling of footplate.

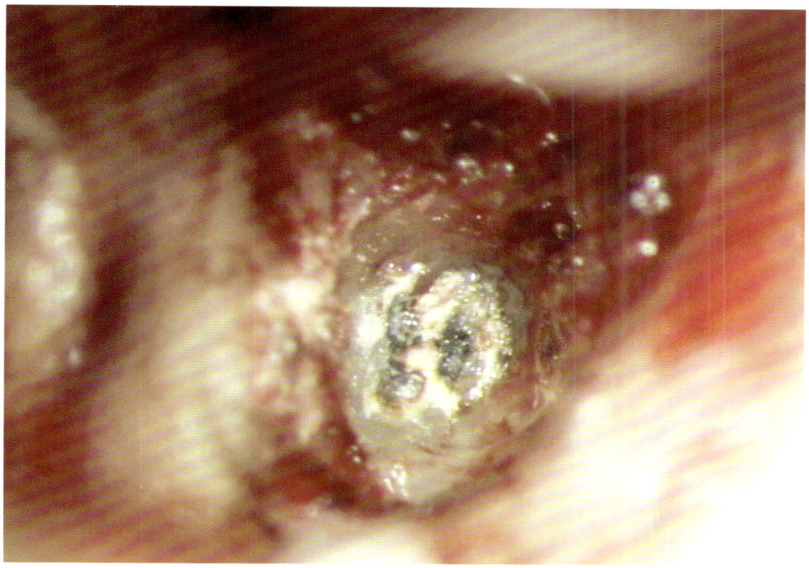

M

Figure 22–1M. Additional laser of footplate.

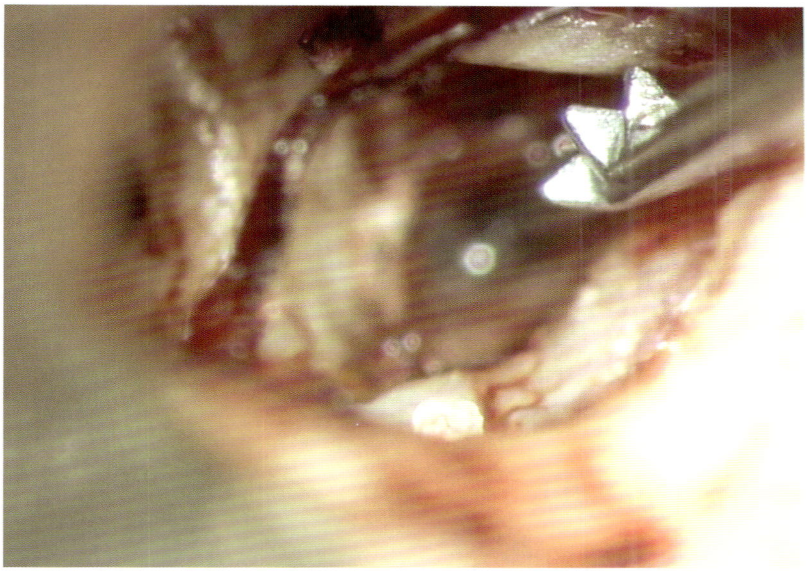

N

Figure 22–1N. Measuring after completing drill-out.

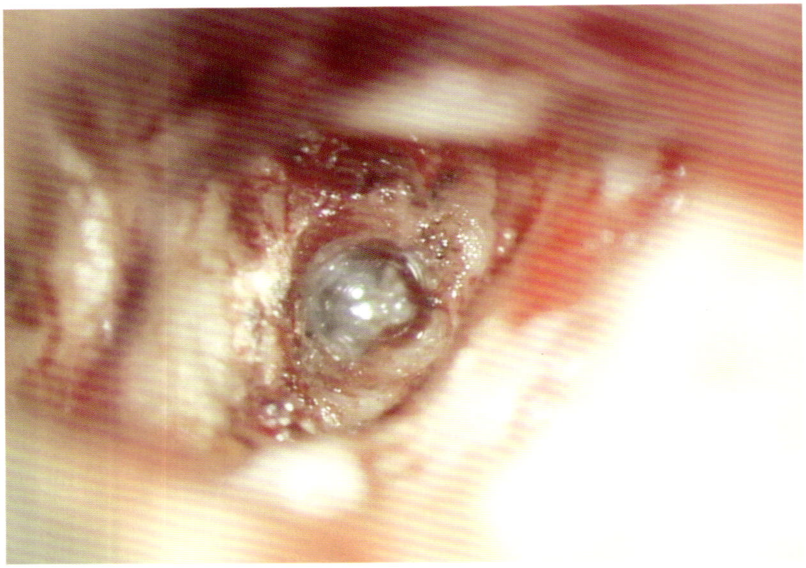

O

Figure 22-1O. Fenestration completed.

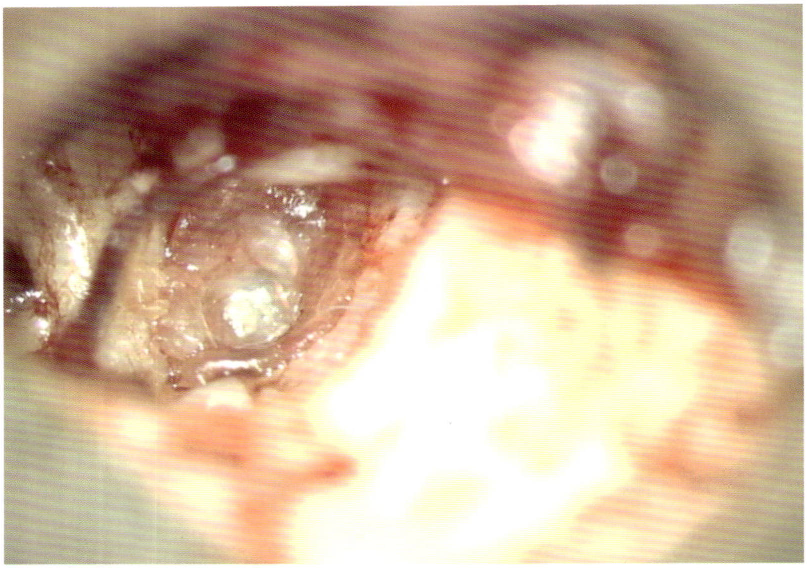

P

Figure 22-1P. Vein graft is positioned.

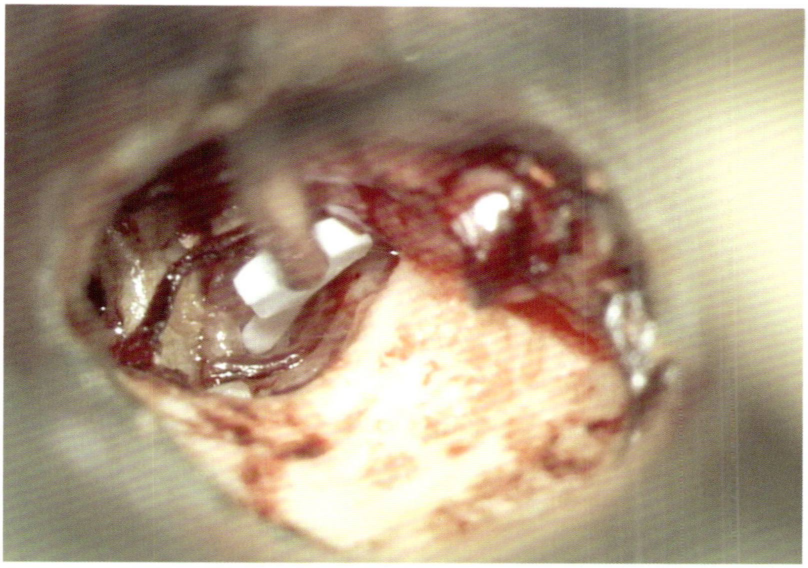

Q

Figure 22–1Q. Piston placement.

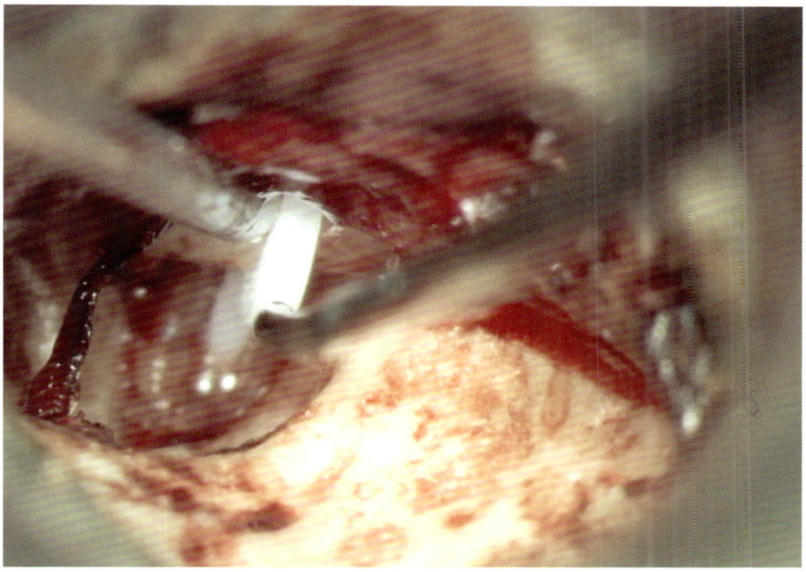

R

Figure 22–1R. Piston positioning.

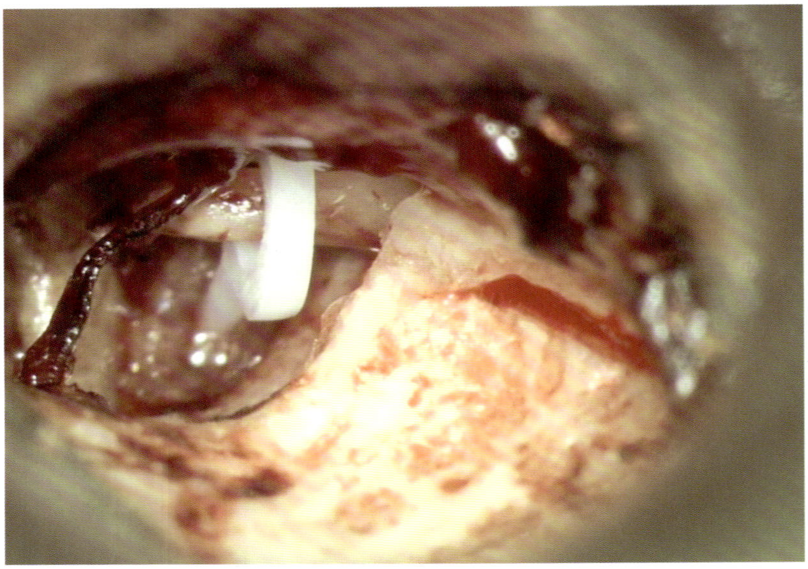

S

Figure 22–1S. Piston in place.

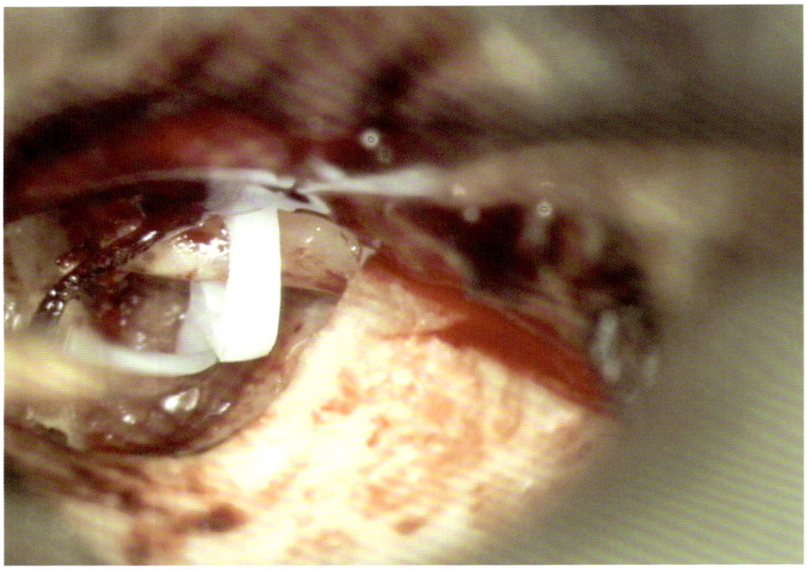

T

Figure 22–1T. Crimping piston with two picks.

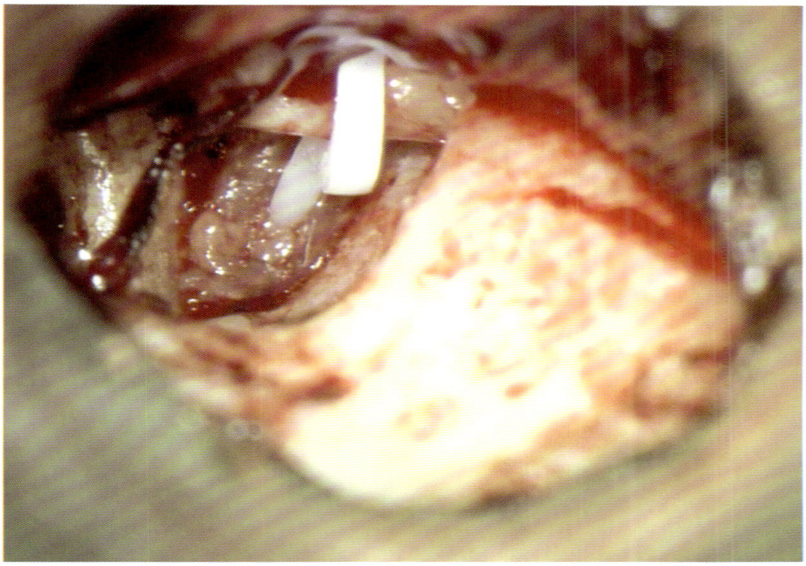

U

Figure 22–1U. Final position of piston.

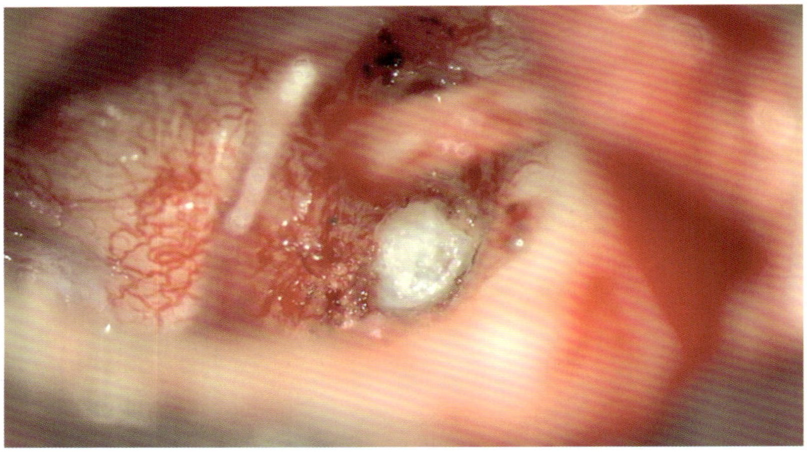

A

Figure 22–2A. Exposure of the footplate.

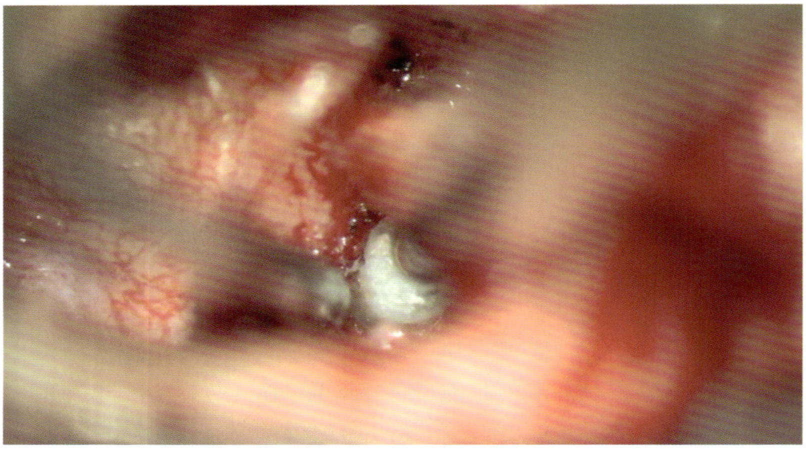

B

Figure 22–2B. Drilling of the footplate.

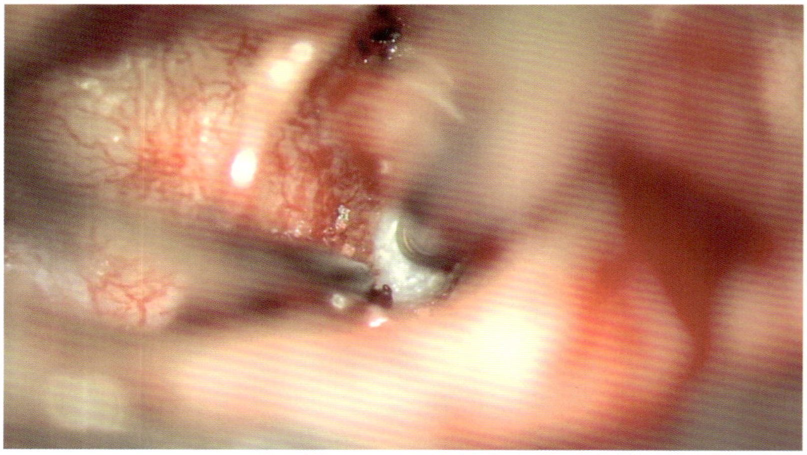

C

Figure 22–2C. Drilling of the footplate.

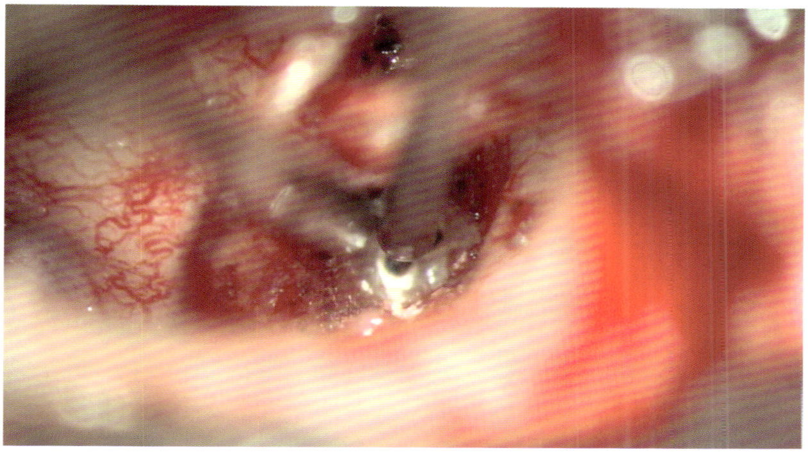

D

Figure 22–2D. Laser use on the footplate.

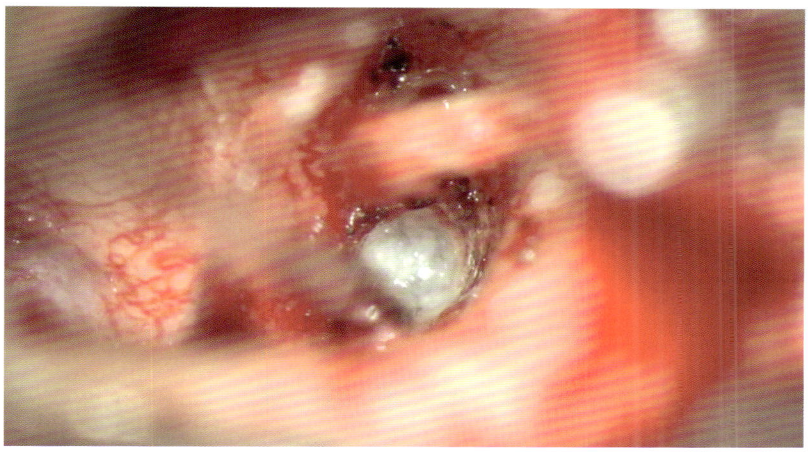

E

Figure 22–2E. Blue lining the vestibule.

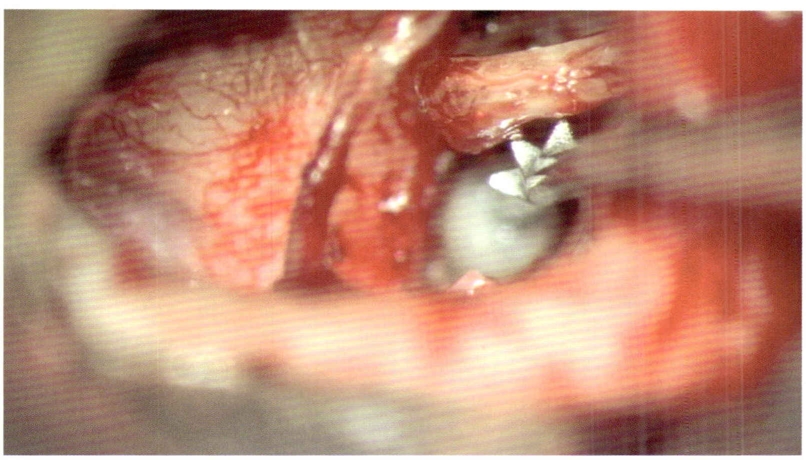

F

Figure 22–2F. Measuring after completing drill-out.

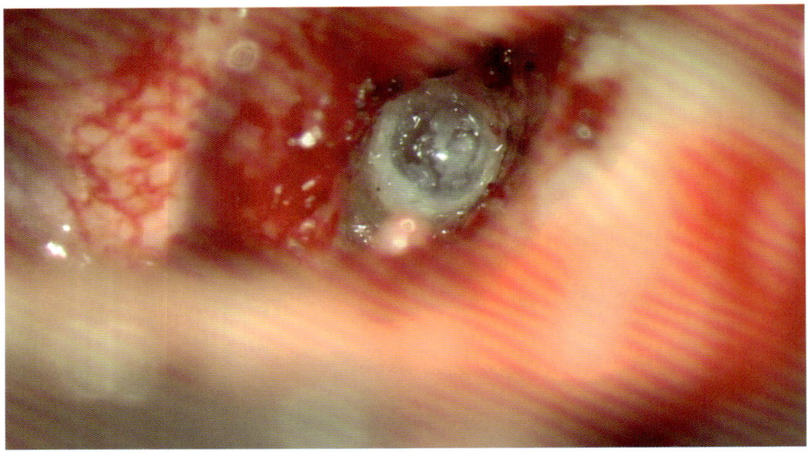

G

Figure 22–2G. Fenestration completed.

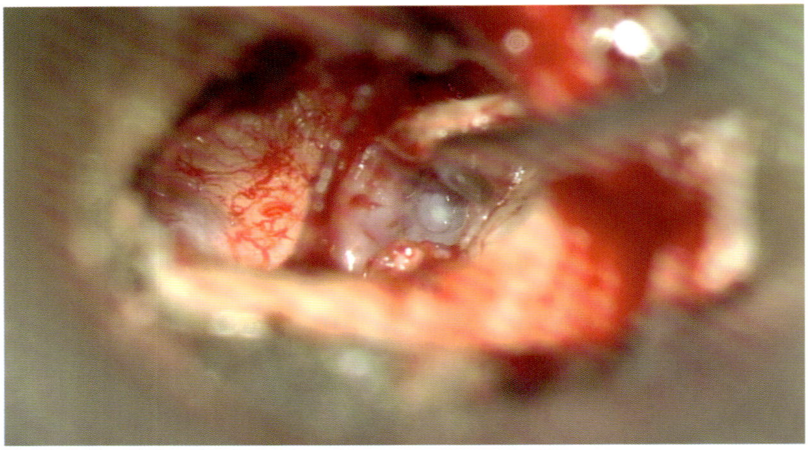

H

Figure 22–2H. Vein graft positioned.

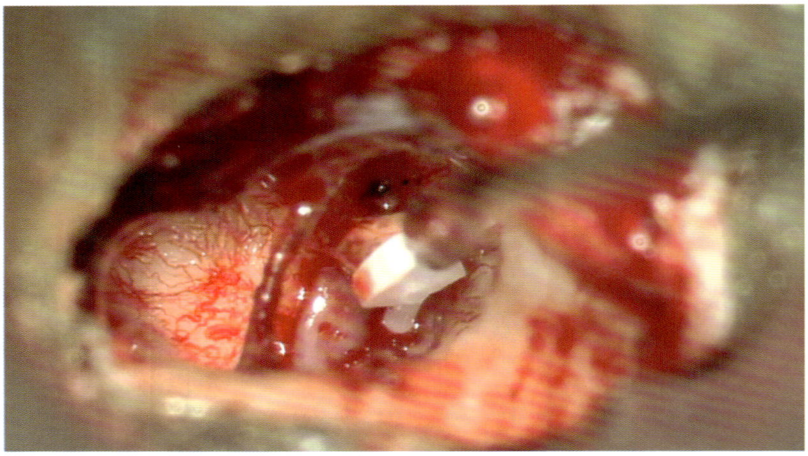

I

Figure 22–2I. Piston placement part 1.

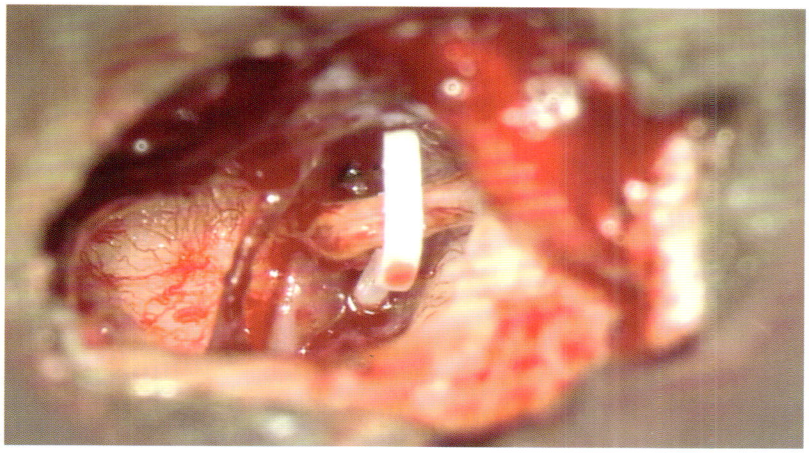

J

Figure 22–2J. Piston placement part 2.

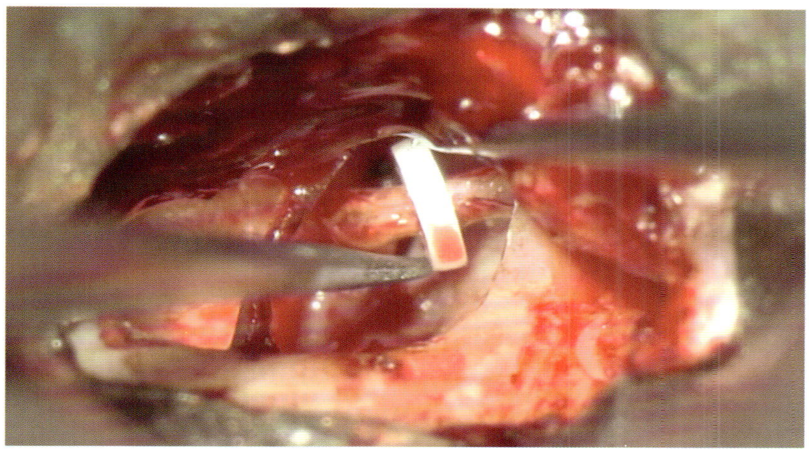

K

Figure 22–2K. Crimping piston with 2 picks.

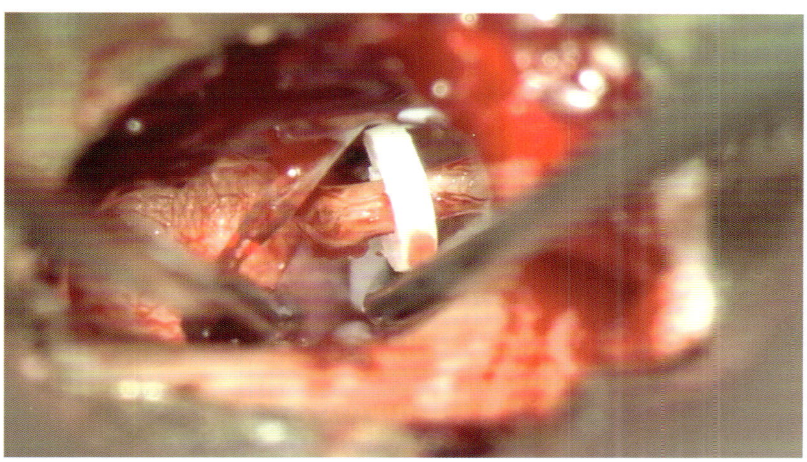

L

Figure 22–2L. Final check of piston placement.

CHAPTER 23

How to Do a Stapedotomy When the Facial Nerve Is Dehiscent

Thomas Linder and Christoph Schlegel-Wagner

INCIDENCE AND IMPACT OF A DEHISCENT FACIAL NERVE IN STAPES SURGERY

A dehiscent facial nerve along the tympanic segment is a frequent finding in middle ear surgery. Its prevalence has been estimated with a wide range of 5% to 57%[1,2] and the most common location is just over the oval window region. Whereas in cholesteatoma surgery its occurrence may not be appreciated initially, because the site is covered by keratin and cholesteatoma matrix, a dehiscent facial nerve is easily appreciated at middle ear surgery for otosclerosis or in other types of ossiculoplasties. If a CT scan has been performed preoperatively, a thorough glance at the coronal section and a second look at the axial cut of the same location should enhance the awareness of this situation in ossiculoplasty. At surgery, the facial nerve appears white and shiny with its vessel running parallel on the surface and a careful palpation with a blunt (!) instrument verifies the condition of a dehiscent facial nerve, not covered and therefore not protected by a thin layer of bone. The most dangerous situation is in tympanosclerosis surgery: The dehiscence cannot be easily appreciated on a preoperative CT scan, and at the time of surgery, the forceful removal of a tympanosclerotic plaque may damage the facial nerve and lead to an iatrogenic lesion of the facial nerve.

In otosclerosis surgery, two types of "dehiscences of the facial nerve" can be encountered and addressed separately:

- A dehiscent facial nerve in its regular course along the tympanic segment.
- A dehiscent facial nerve protruding over the oval window niche: malposition (Figure 23–1).

Whereas a normal course of the facial nerve should not greatly impact the surgical technique, an overhanging and therefore malpositioned facial nerve may pose a surgical challenge. We use in all instances an **endaural approach** and an **enlarged tympanomeatal flap**.[3] The chorda should be left attached to the drum. This will allow pushing of the drum and the chorda inferiorly at the same time, allowing a wider access to the oval window region (Figures 23–2, 23–3, 23–4, and 23–5). Otherwise, the chorda is constantly in the surgeon's view and may be difficult to manage. At a later stage, the chorda can still be detached from the drum, if necessary. All these issues will be highlighted below.

A. Dehiscence of a Facial Nerve in Its Regular Course

If a preoperative CT scan was performed, this frequent situation can be expected before entering the middle ear (see Figure 23–1) and should be verified after careful exposure.

Proper exposure requires sufficient removal of bone posterosuperiorly at the medial end of the external ear canal (see Figures 23–2, 23–3, 23–4, and 23–5). Using the curette with both hands, three landmarks

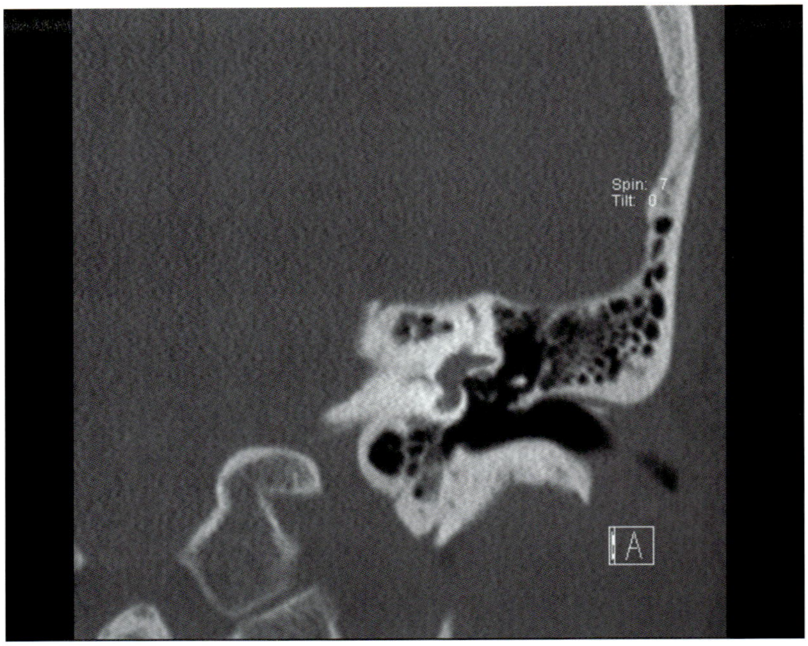

Figure 23–1. Slightly protruding and dehiscent facial nerve over oval window niche.

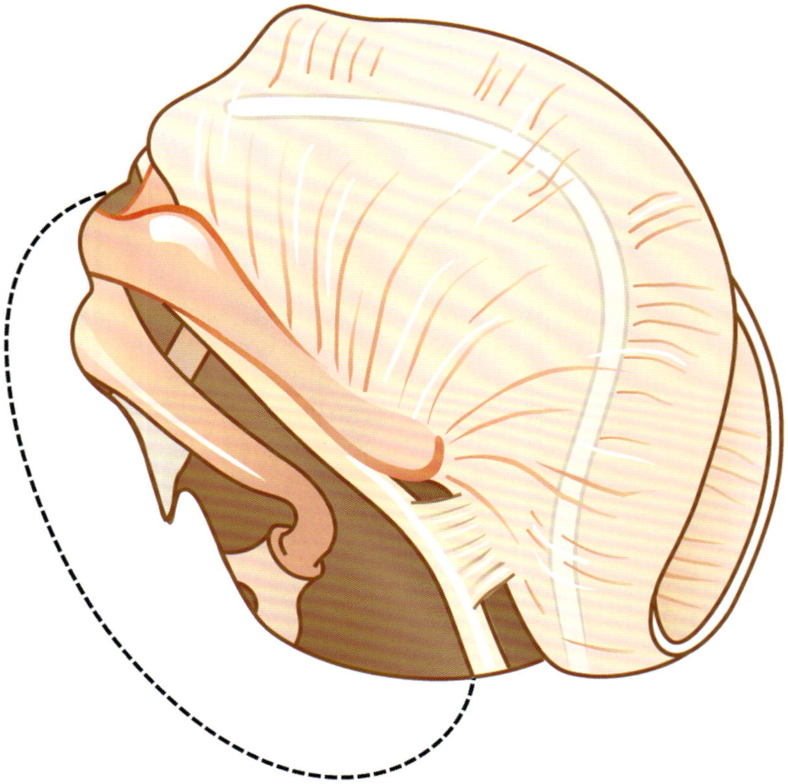

Figure 23–2. Outlined bony enlargement, allowing the direct view over the beginning of the incudomalleal joint, facial nerve, and pyramidal process with the stapes in the center of the field.

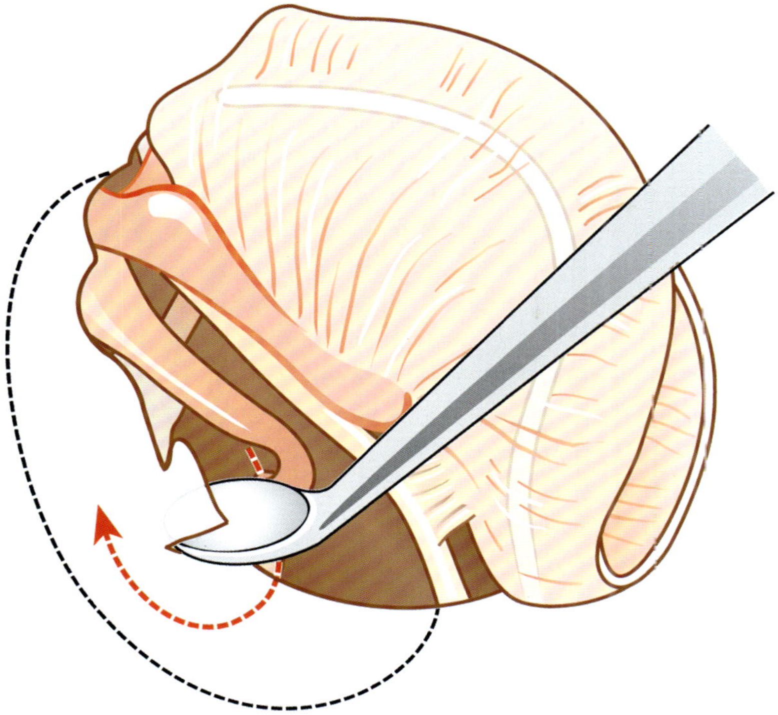

Figure 23–3. Rotation of the curette away from the incus body and chorda.

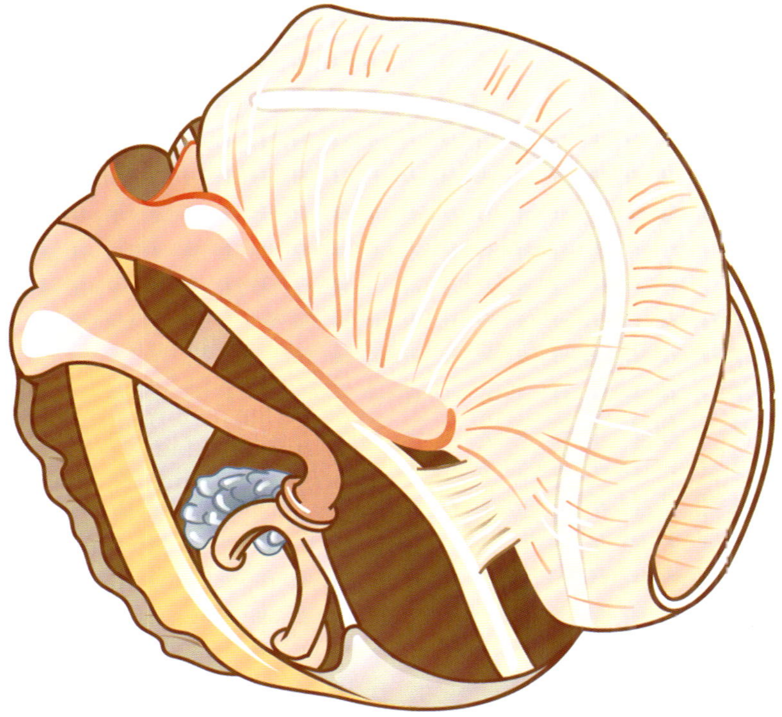

Figure 23–4. Sufficient space has been gained to see the field of action. Note that the chorda is kept attached to the inferiorly displaced eardrum, therefore not obstructing the surgeon's view.

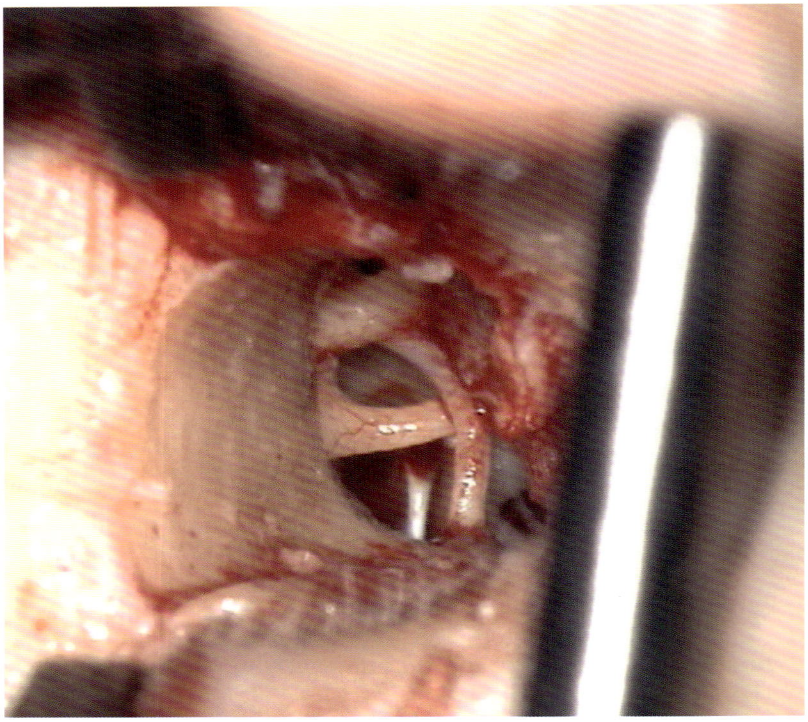

Figure 23–5. Proper exposure before continuation of the surgery. Chorda is gently displaced inferiorly.

should be visible before continuation of the surgery: the beginning of the incudomallear joint anteriorly, the facial nerve superiorly, and the pyramidal process and entire stapes tendon posteriorly (see Figures 23–4 and 23–5). Once the otosclerotic fixation of the stapes has been confirmed, any movements of instruments toward the dehiscent facial nerve segment have to be avoided.

These potentially "dangerous" instruments include:

- The use of lasers directed toward the dehiscent nerve.
- The use of a "too" large drill inadvertently touching the facial nerve.
- The use of a sharp hook accidentally hitting the facial nerve.

The most dangerous "instrument" is the laser. A CO_2 or Erbium:YAG laser mounted on the microscope and guided by a micromanipulator may unintentionally strike the nerve or a handheld probe of a KTP/Argon/Diode/CO_2 laser could collide with a dehiscent facial nerve segment while dissecting the posterior or anterior crus. Therefore, the laser beam should always be directed away from the facial nerve canal and toward the promontory.

The facial nerve may be dehiscent over the oval window and at the same time prolapse inferiorly to occlude the oval window niche. The surgeon's view may further be impaired by a thick and long incus process, a widened chorda tympani, and an obliterative otosclerotic focus. The overlapping facial nerve is only one of several problems to address in these cases. The most conservative way to manage this worst situation is to close the ear and have the patient sent for a hearing aid or bone conduction implant. An inexperienced surgeon should be advised to act prudently, abandon the surgery, explain his decision honestly to the patient, and discuss the intraoperative findings with an experienced colleague. It is best to make a surgical drawing immediately after the middle ear inspection, because most photographs may be darkened in color and do not readily appreciate the narrow situation. We have not encountered a single patient who did not appreciate this treatment strategy upon referral to our tertiary referral center. On the contrary, patients gain respect for the referring physician and appreciate the network of doctors taking care of his unusual problem.

Nevertheless, for an experienced stapes surgeon, it is usually possible to complete the operation on most, but not all cases.

B. Partial Malposition for a Dehiscent Facial Nerve

The primary goal is to improve the exposure (Figure 23–6). This is accomplished by:

- Removing the stapes suprastructure first: This step requires careful transection of the crura, and—as mentioned previously—avoiding a laser beam toward the dehiscent facial nerve. The posterior crus may be cut using "cold" instruments such as curotomy scissors, microdrills, or manual perforators. The anterior crus is crushed toward the promontory using a 2.5-mm angulated hook. Once the suprastructure is removed, a larger surface of the footplate becomes visible (Figures 23–7 and 23–8).
- Drilling a wider access along the promontory: To appreciate the lower edge of the footplate, an overhanging promontorial bony rim can be removed using 0.8-mm to 1.0-mm diamond microdrills. A skeeter drill, a Bienair Osseostap® microdrill, any other drills with a slim handpiece are adequate surgical tools to reach this goal. Irrigation is not possible at the same time as drilling, but the surgeon intermittently irrigates the field manually (see Figure 23–7).

Once a space of at least 0.5 mm is reached between facial nerve and inferior rim of the stapes footplate, a stapedotomy opening for the introduction of a 0.4-mm stapes piston is performed using

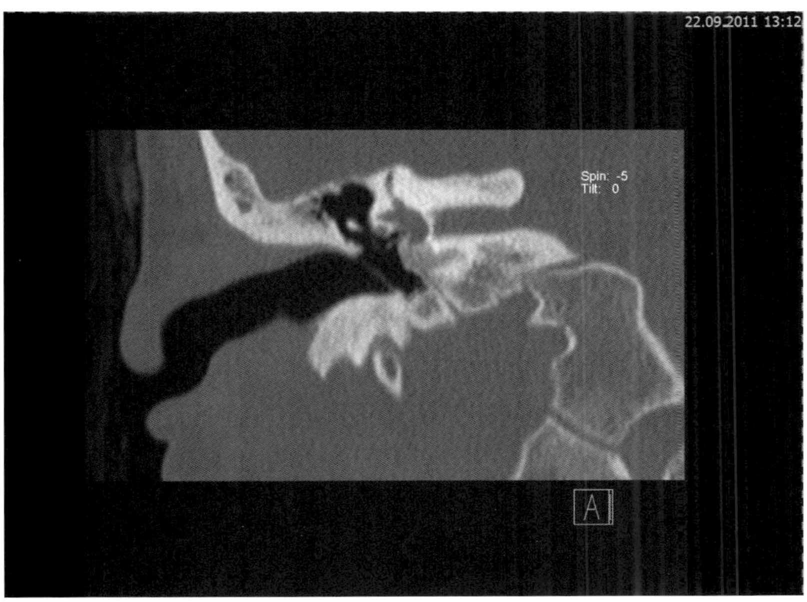

Figure 23–6. Coronal CT scan revealing slightly protruding facial nerve and narrow oval window niche due to a large otospongiotic focus at promontory and basal turn.

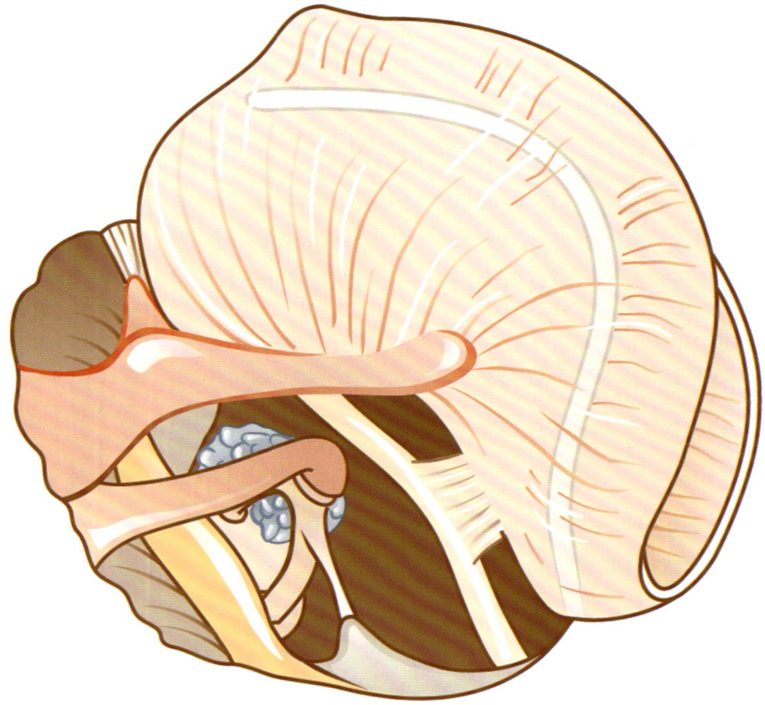

Figure 23–7. Limited view due to protruding facial nerve, otosclerotic focus, and deep oval window niche. Placing a 0.4-mm measuring rod confirms sufficient space on the footplate.

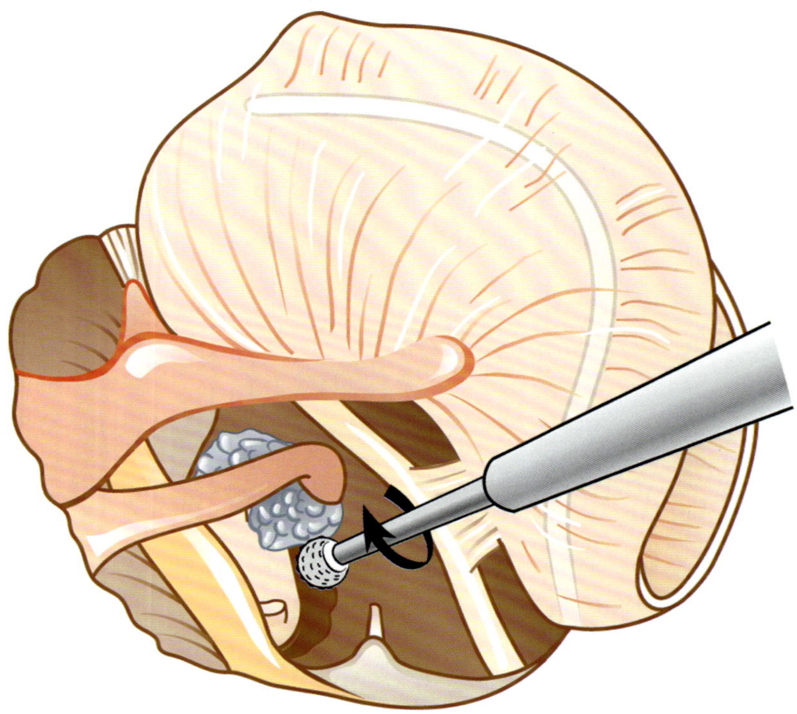

Figure 23–8. Enhanced exposure following removal of stapes suprastructure and drilling of otosclerotic focus toward the promontory.

manual perforators (Figure 23–9). Larger size prostheses are not possible, because the space is truly limited. Slight contact of the prosthesis with the facial nerve will not cause facial nerve dysfunction and does not necessarily impair the functional result.

C. Subtotal Prolapse of a Dehiscent Facial Nerve: Indication for a Malleostapedotomy

In this situation, it is not just the facial nerve, but also incus and stapes suprastructure preventing a sufficient view to continue the surgery. In case a preoperative CT scan was performed, not only the otosclerotic/otospongiotic focus should be appreciated, but also the overhanging facial nerve on the coronal section through the oval window area (Figure 23–10).

If you feel uncomfortable with this anticipated situation, you may refer the patient preoperatively to an experienced colleague.

Once again, gaining exposure is the main goal. As outlined above, all surgeries at our center are performed using the endaural approach and dissecting an enlarged tympanomeatal flap before entering the middle ear (Figure 23–11). All overhanging bone within the external ear canal is removed using drills or curettes to ensure maximum illumination by the microscope and using straight instruments within the middle ear space (Figure 23–12).

The drum is reflected inferiorly below the short process of the malleus. The anterior malleal ligament is inspected and its mobility is verified. The posterosuperior canal wall is enlarged sufficiently to identify the beginning of the incudomalleal joint, facial nerve, and pyramidal process (Figure 23–13).

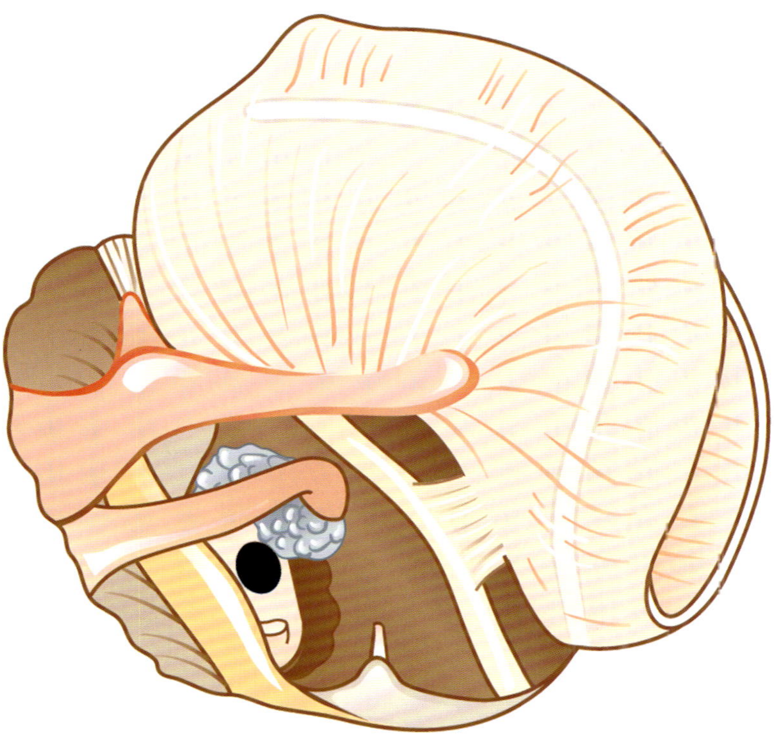

Figure 23–9. An 0.5-mm opening for a 0.4-mm stapes piston has been accomplished.

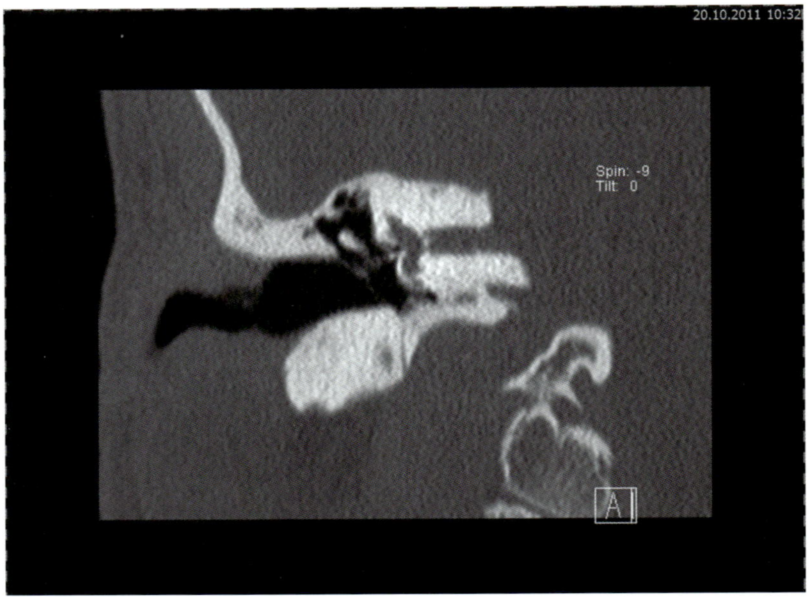

Figure 23–10. Coronal scan reveals overhanging facial nerve and very narrow oval window niche.

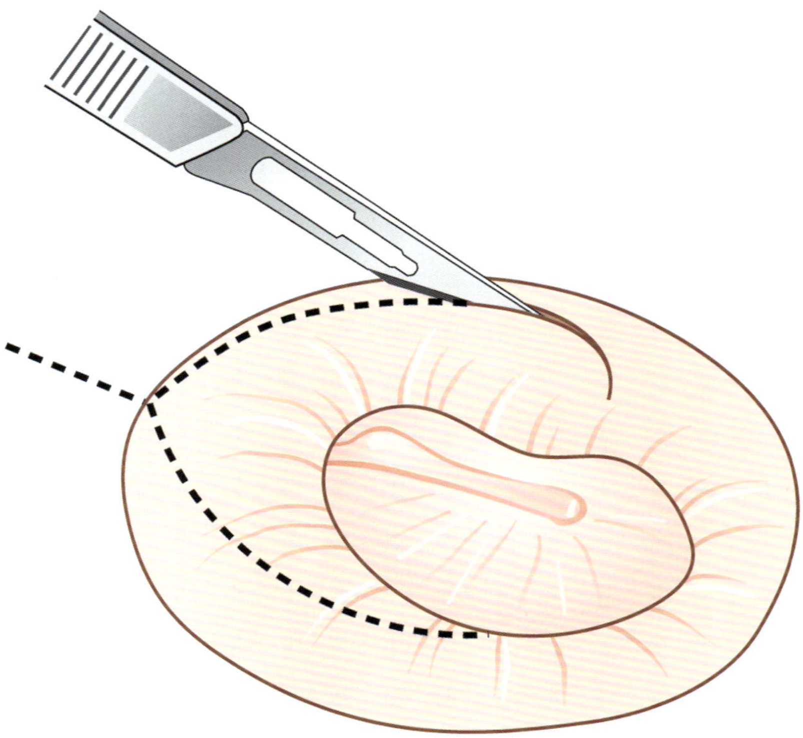

Figure 23–11. Endaural incision with enlarged tympanomeatal flap outlined.

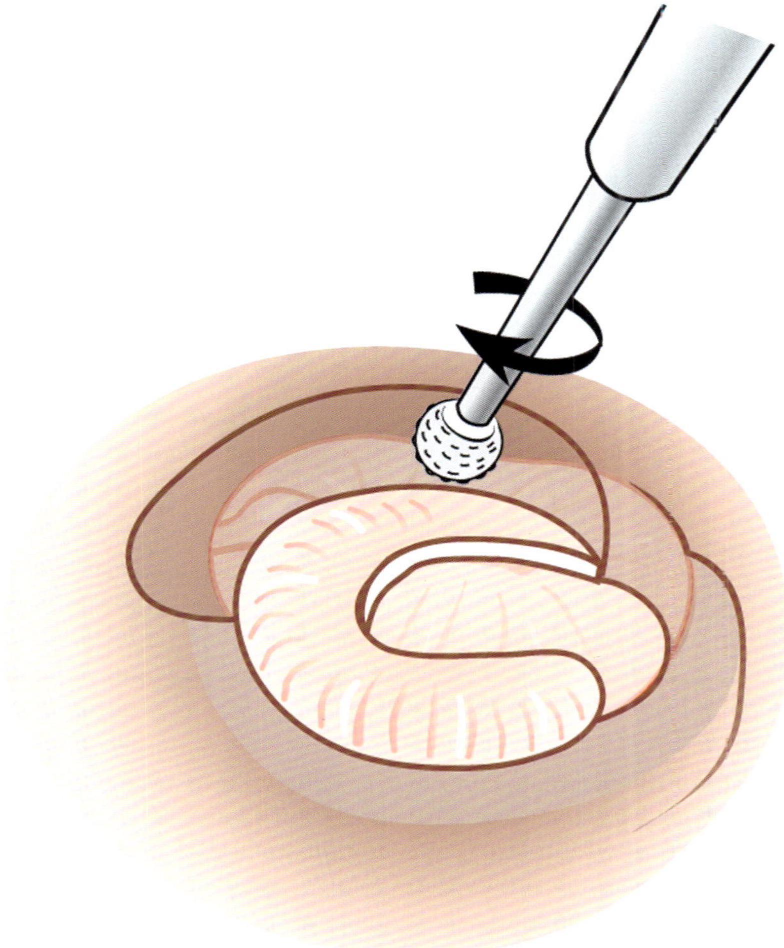

Figure 23–12. Enhanced exposure anterosuperiorly by removing bone within the external ear canal (partial canalplasty).

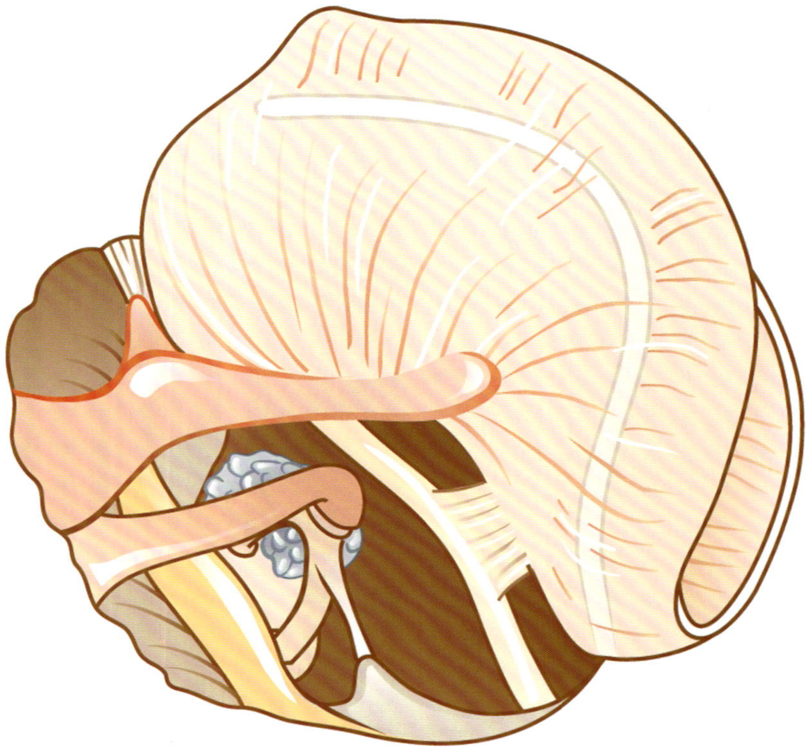

Figure 23–13. Complete exposure reveals direct view over anterior malleal ligament, short process of malleus, as well as "standard stapedotomy exposure" to continue with malleostapedotomy. The chorda will be detached later from the drum.

If only a small segment of the footplate can be visualized and a 0.4 mm measuring rod seems to pass beside the facial nerve onto the footplate (Figures 23–14 and 21–15), but the view is blocked by the facial nerve, incus, stapes suprastructure (and often also due to the chorda), extra space can be gained by removing the incus first. This is an important decision to make, because it is not reversible and the other choice would be to abandon the surgery and provide a hearing aid (or bone conduction implant) preserving the incomplete air–bone gap (usually less than 40–60 dB). If the surgery would be abandoned after incus removal, a total air–bone gap (60 dB) would result!

In situations where a malleostapedotomy can be performed safely, the functional gain is as good as or even superior as in incus-stapedotomy.[4]

The incudostapedial joint is separated using a small joint knife and the incus is removed by opening the incudomalleal joint with a 2.5-mm hook and rotating the incus body out, lifting the long process with the same 2.5-mm hook. If the incus is too long and may therefore rupture the chorda, a malleus nipper is helpful to cut the long process of the incus, allowing it to rotate the body of the incus without disrupting the chorda.

By removing the incus, the entire stapes suprastructure becomes visible and this view allows safe removal of the suprastructure (Figure 23–16). An overhanging promontory or an obliterating otosclerotic focus can also be drilled away with direct vision, as the incus was removed. The surgeon will truly appreciate this better visualization of the narrow space, and it allows the surgeon to continue the surgery.

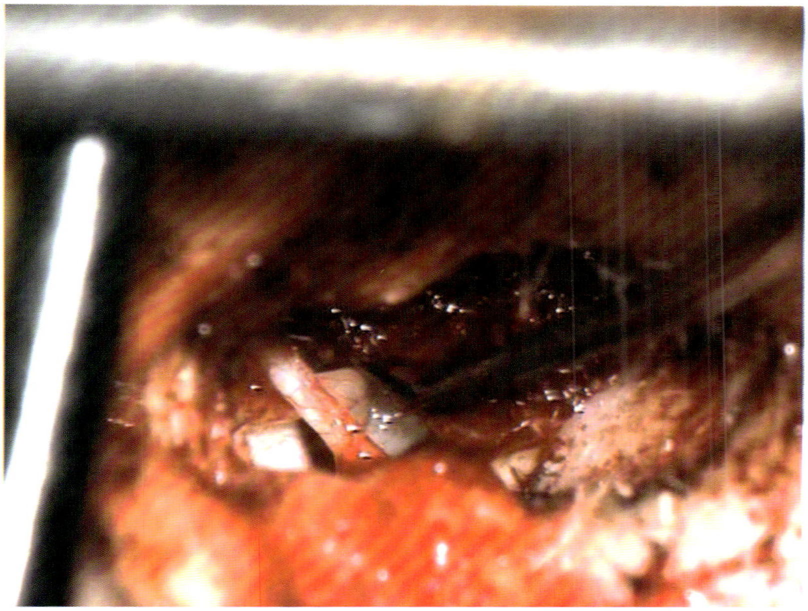

Figure 23–14. Limited view over footplate due to overhanging facial nerve, chorda, thick incus, and narrow oval window niche.

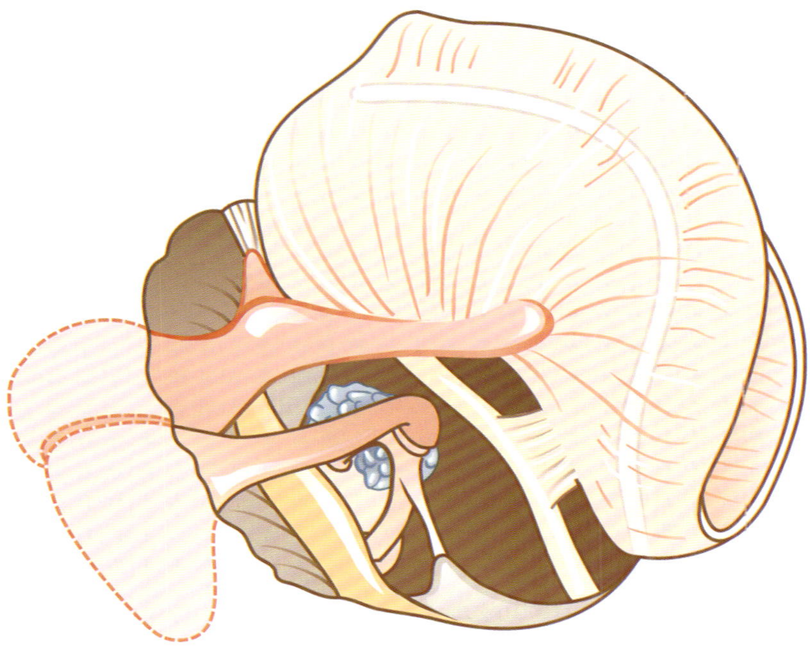

Figure 23–15. Mobile malleus and incus, but limited view onto footplate. Decision is made to remove the incus in order to enhance the surgical space.

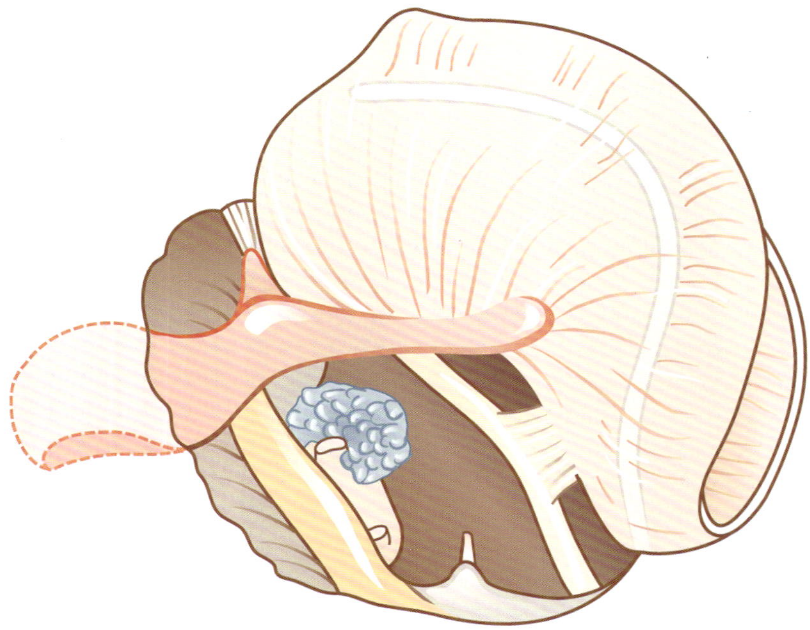

Figure 23–16. Improved visualization over the footplate once the mobile incus is removed. The mobile malleus is kept in place to perform the malleostapedotomy.

Contrary to incus-stapedotomy, in malleo-stapedotomy the steps are slightly different: The prosthesis (0.4 mm in diameter) is measured, angulated, and introduced first, before the stapedotomy opening is performed. Ideal is the Fisch Titanium Stapes Piston (Storz), which allows trimming the length, angulating the shaft, and enlarging the loop of the piston to accommodate the prosthesis next to the overhanging facial nerve perpendicular onto the footplate (Figure 23–17).

In short the individual steps are:

- Measure the length using the measuring rod: Calculate the distance from the lateral surface of the malleus handle (just distal to the short process of the malleus) to the stapes footplate
- Cut the prosthesis to the proper length (adding 0.5 mm to the measured distance).
- Introduce the prosthesis next to the shaft of the malleus (the chorda runs cranially, and therefore needs to be separated at this stage from its attachment to the drum).
- Estimate the correct length and identify a possible angulation between shaft and loop of the piston.
- Remove the piston from the middle ear and adjust its length and angulation to the individual situation. Enlarge the loop—if necessary—by sliding the prosthesis along the shaft of a 1.5- or 2.5-mm angulated hook using watchmaker forceps.
- Reintroduce the piston and verify the perfect placement.
- Place the piston next to the footplate and perform the stapedotomy opening with manual perforators, lasers, or microdrills.
- Introduce the piston into the stapedotomy opening and over the malleus handle.

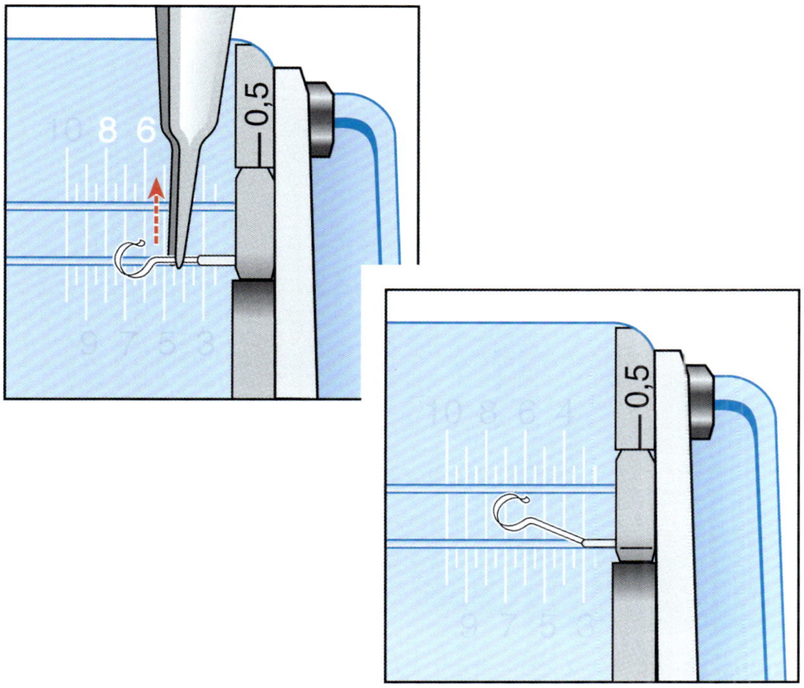

Figure 23–17. Adjustments made on the prosthesis: Cutting the length and angulating the shaft.

- Crimp the loop onto the malleus (Figures 23–18, 23–19, and 23–20).
- Seal the opening using small pieces of soft tissue (form the endaural incision) and some drops of patient's own blood.

There are two important tips to facilitate these steps:

- Make sure that the tympanomeatal flap is pushed inferiorly to the short process of the malleus and stays in that position, allowing access to the proximal malleus handle. If the flap tends to fall back, you will not be able to place and crimp the prosthesis sufficiently.
- Expose the surgical field sufficiently enough to ensure the view with one position of the microscope onto the proximal malleus handle and the footplate.

D. Total Prolapse of a Dehiscent Facial Nerve: Abandon the Surgery

In the rare instance of a total prolapse of a dehiscent facial nerve, completely obscuring the view over any remnant of the footplate, it is best to abandon the surgery. A total conductive block is rarely encountered in these situations, the patient is habituated to this hearing loss and can be fitted with a hearing aid quite successfully. "Nil nocere" is the principle, because any manipulation of the ossicular chain and abandoning the surgery at a later stage will most likely lead to an increased air–bone gap.

If not performed prior to surgery, a CT scan 4 to 8 weeks postoperatively (once the blood is completely out of the middle ear) will help to clarify the entire course of the facial nerve and also reveal the situation of the contralateral ear, in case of bilateral otosclerosis. It is also essential to identify any otosclerotic focus to determine the correct diagnosis of

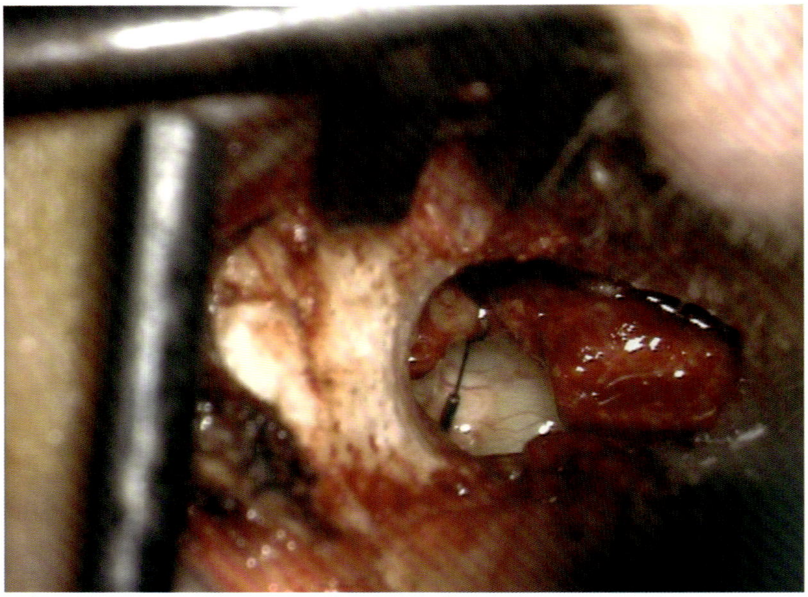

Figure 23–18. View onto the malleus with the prosthesis just distal to the short process of the malleus.

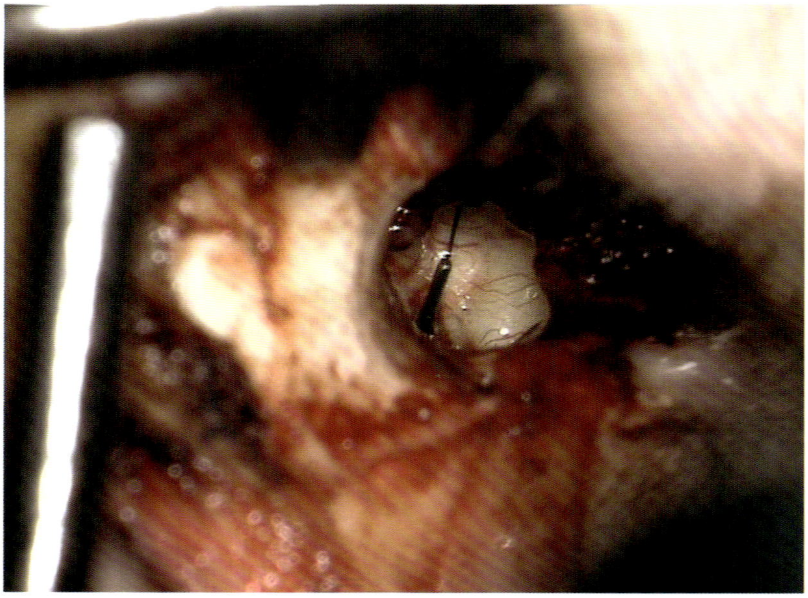

Figure 23–19. View onto the footplate with the prosthesis in place.

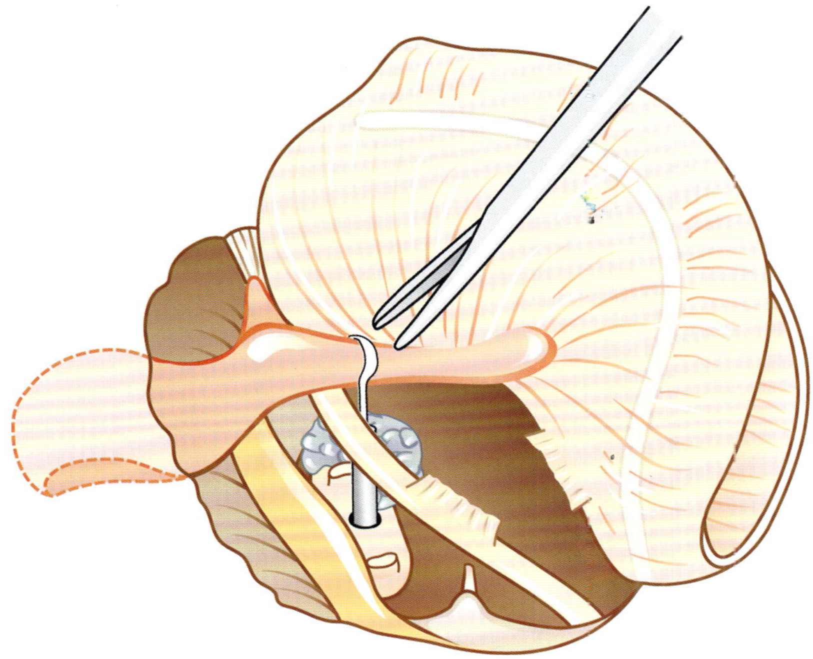

Figure 23–20. Crimping of the piston on the malleus handle, the chorda has been detached from the drum to gain space.

the hearing loss. We do not advise to retract the facial nerve superiorly[5] or to drill an opening into the promontory and to guide a piston from the incus to the cochlea, as it has been suggested elsewhere. One of our patients (Figures 23–21 and 23–22) was indeed very grateful once the situation had been clarified and the possible risks (facial palsy, total deafness, vertigo) explained postoperatively.

SUMMARY

In case a preoperative CT scan has been performed, we strongly advise not only to concentrate on viewing the otosclerotic focus, but to analyze the CT scans using a "virtual" checklist. One item is the appreciation of the position of the facial nerve over the oval window niche. The coronal section is most appropriate to realize a dehiscent and protruding facial nerve. Using an endaural approach, an enlarged tympanomeatal flap and perfoming a partial canalplasty before entering the middle ear in all cases of ossiculoplasties allows maximum exposure and illumination of a potentially narrow surgical field. Sufficient removal of bone posterosuperiorly further widens the surgical access before dealing with the ossicular chain. If continuation of the surgery seems feasible, removal of the incus largely opens the view over the oval window niche, and malleostapedotomy instead of incus-stapedotomy can be the procedure of choice.

Acknowledgments. We greatly appreciate the help of Mrs. Katja Dalkowski, medical illustrator, Hauptstrasse 64, 91054 Erlangen (http://www.meddesign.online.de)

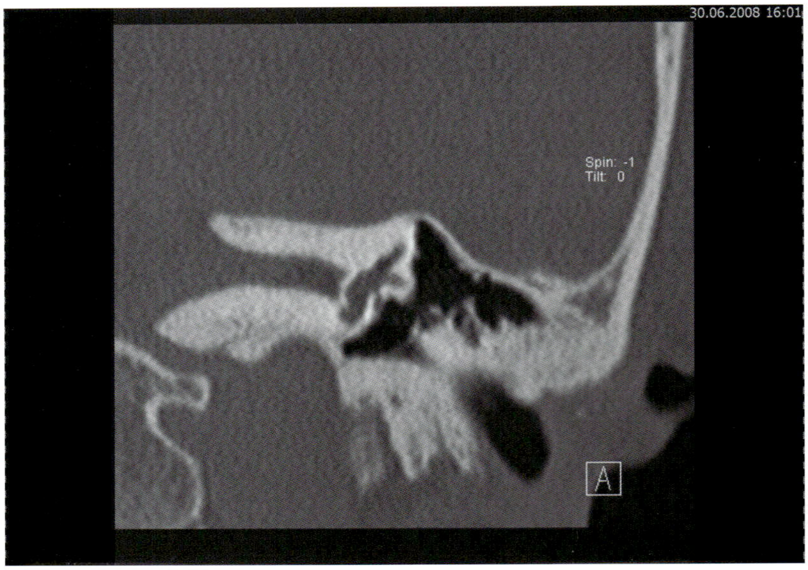

Figure 23-21. Coronal CT revealing the misplaced facial nerve running through the oval window niche.

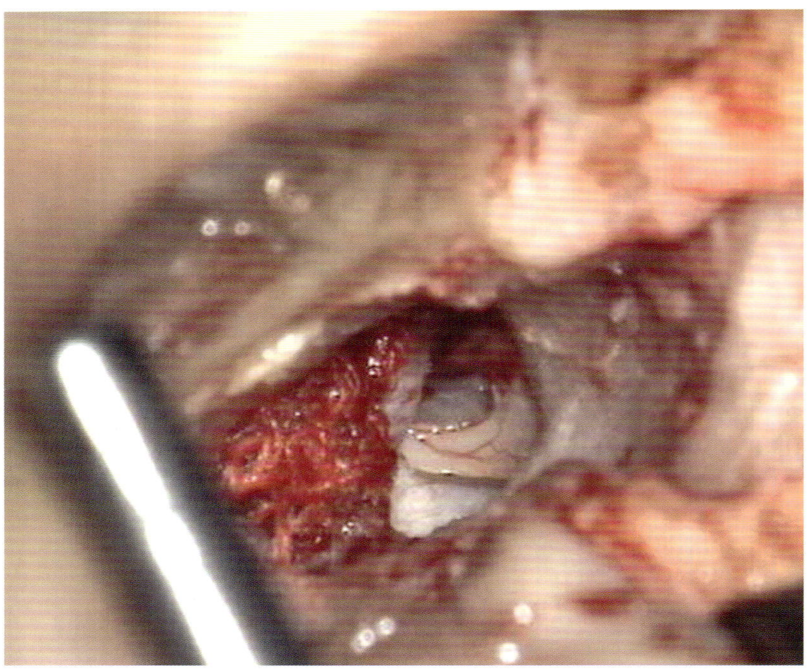

Figure 23-22. Intraoperative view with broad incus and facial nerve running through the oval window area as a flattened white structure.

REFERENCES

1. Althaus SR, House HP. The facial nerve in middle ear surgery. *Otolaryng Clin North Am.* 1974;7:461–465.
2. Baxter A. Dehiscence of the fallopian canal: An anatomical study. *J Laryngol Otol.* 1971;85:587–594.
3. Fisch U, May J, Linder T. *Tympanoplasty, Mastoidectomy and Stapes Surgery.* 2nd ed. New York, NY: Thieme; 2007: 244–245.
4. Rambousek A, Schlegel CH, Linder TE. From incus bypass to malleostapedotomy: Technical improvements and results. *J Laryngol Otol.* 2012;126:995–1002.
5. Brackmann DE, Shelton C, Arriaga MA. *Otologic Surgery.* 3rd ed. Philadelphia, PA: Saunders Elsevier; 2010: chaps 25, 26.

CHAPTER 24

Revision Stapes Surgery: Technique of Neil M. Sperling

Neil M. Sperling

INTRODUCTION

Revision stapes surgery is a significant challenge to the otologic surgeon. Whereas primary stapedectomy requires precision, revision surgery requires the judicious decision making that comes only from significant surgical experience coupled with skillful execution. The stakes are high given the significant benefit a patient may receive and the potential for devastating loss of residual hearing.

ASSESSMENT

Etiologies of recurrent conductive hearing loss are varied. Clinical assessment is inadequate to determine the exact etiology in most cases. Recurrent conductive hearing loss early after primary surgery suggests technique failure, such as improper fit or crimping of a prosthesis. The onset years later suggests prosthesis migration or ossicular erosion/fixation.

A careful physical exam may indicate a malpositioned prosthesis. Tympanic membrane pathology may also indicate other etiologies of recurrent hearing loss such as perforation or retraction. Micro-otoscopic exam, however, may be normal. CT imaging is recommended, but may be of limited benefit. Whereas the grossly displaced prosthesis is easily identified on imaging, incus demineralization or local migration of the prosthesis may be difficult to detect.

ETIOLOGY OF RECURRENT CONDUCTIVE HEARING LOSS

Our knowledge of etiologies is attributed to several published clinical series. We are indebted to these highly experienced surgeons who have reviewed their decade's worth of experience with revision surgery.

Etiologies related to the prosthesis are most common. This may include displacement, lateralization, or improper length (Figure 24–1). Incus erosion is recognized as the second most common etiology. Other etiologies include: otosclerotic refixation/closure of the fenestration, granuloma, and malleus/incus fixation.

Certain materials and designs have been implicated in failures. Schuknecht wire/fat or wire/Gelfoam® prostheses have been reported to have higher failure rates. Gold pistons have been associated with significant granulation formation. Incus necrosis has been reported with all prostheses, but has been more commonly observed with crimped wire prostheses, with fewer cases observed with Robinson and Lippy-modified bucket-type prostheses. Some of the newer heat-activated prostheses have been associated with an increase in displacement. As techniques and prosthetics evolve, these findings are likely to change.

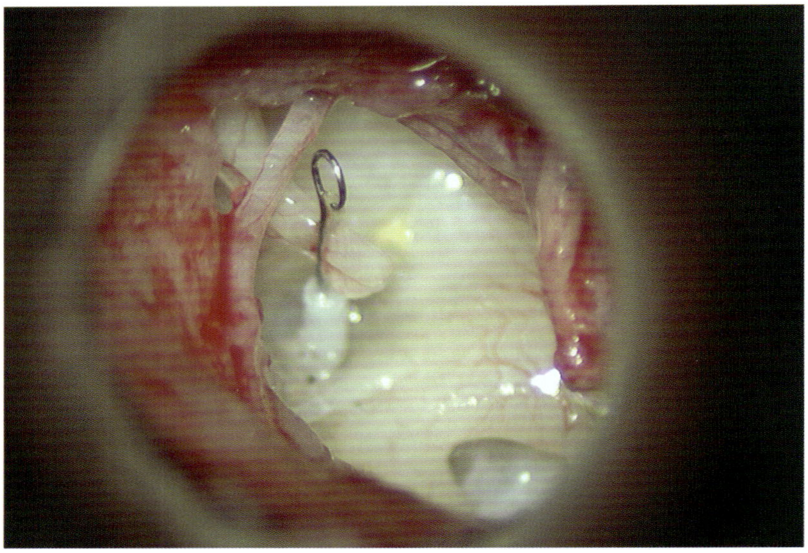

Figure 24–1. Initial findings at revision stapedectomy (prior to prosthesis manipulation). Note lateralized stapes prosthesis with partial incus erosion.

MANAGEMENT

Indications for Surgery

Recurrent Conductive Hearing Loss

The decision to proceed with revision surgery should be a shared decision with an informed patient. Because outcomes are generally not as good as primary surgery, and risk of hearing loss real, the decision to surgically intervene must be made carefully.

Perilymph Fistula

Sensorineural hearing loss after stapes surgery is unlikely to be recovered with revision surgery. If a perilymph fistula is suspected, surgery for repair is indicated to improve vestibular symptoms and may stem the progression of a partial sensory loss. Tissue grafting of the oval window for fistula repair may be combined with replacement of the prosthesis. A prosthesis penetrating deeply into the vestibule may be best left in place in case there are adhesions attached to the membranous labyrinth.

Surgical Approach

The choice of anesthesia has been debated. Local anesthesia is favored by some surgeons to provide patient feedback. Significant vertigo intraoperatively may alert the surgeon of labyrinthine irritation. General anesthesia offers a consistent surgical environment, with minimal risk of patient motion, which is preferred by other surgeons.

Middle ear exploration should be done in a methodical fashion to determine the reason for failure and to determine what technique will most likely resolve the defect. Successful revision stapes surgery depends on precise determination of the underlying etiology.

Lasers have been advised for revision stapes surgery to reduce trauma to the inner ear. The laser offers a method to dissect adhesions and fibrosis in the oval window using minimal mechanical energy. This has received considerable support by experienced surgeons who believe that outcomes are significantly improved using the laser routinely.

Analysis of Etiology

The cause for recurrent conductive hearing loss can be obscure and only careful investigation will reveal it. Each component of the ossicular chain is palpated for mobility. The interface of incus and prosthesis must be inspected and palpated to assess for appropriate crimping, demineralization, or bony erosion. Gentle dissection (preferably with laser) removes the adhesions surrounding the prosthesis until the actual oval window is reached. The patency of prior fenestration is assessed by removing the adhesions to the level of the footplate. The prosthesis is not removed until the position of the distal end of the prosthesis is identified.

Decision-Making and Surgical Options

Several surgical repair options exist for revision surgery and are dictated by the pathology found. If the incus remains intact, any preferred stapes prosthesis may be chosen. Often, however, the incus is compromised. The following solutions can be considered in revision surgery:

1. It may be possible to use an eroded incus to place a crimped prosthesis above the level of the erosion. However, this may not be feasible and may be associated with recurrent failure.
2. The Lippy-modified Robinson (bucket) prosthesis can be used successfully (Figure 24–2, video).
3. When incus erosion is severe, or the incus is subluxed, or when malleus or incus fixation is encountered, a malleostapedotomy can be done. This is done by exposing a portion of the malleus handle, notching it, and placing an extended-length prosthesis. This can be technically difficult.[1]
4. An elegant adaptation of malleostapedotomy utilizes the malleus relocation technique described by Vincent in 2004. Positioning the malleus directly over the oval window greatly improves the geometry for placement of a prosthesis between the malleus and vestibule (Figure 24–3).[2]

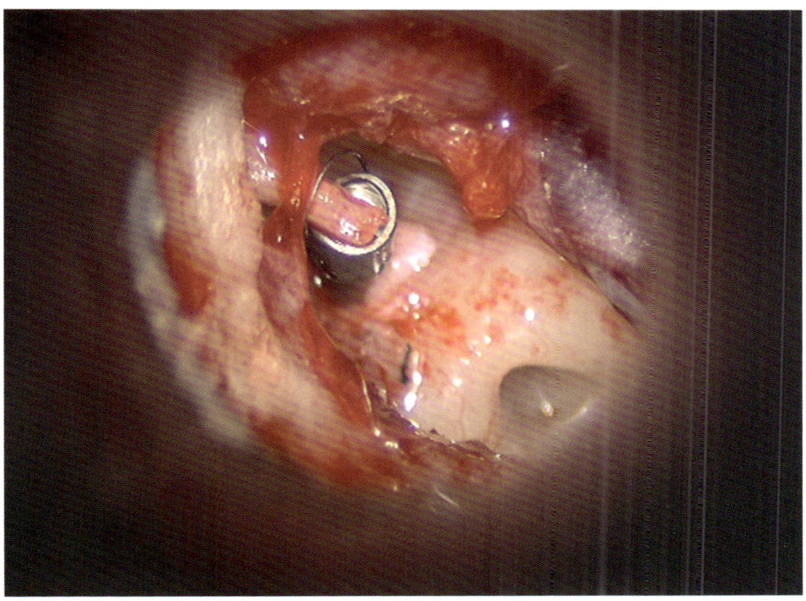

Figure 24–2. Bucket-handle prosthesis placed on eroded end of the long process of incus.

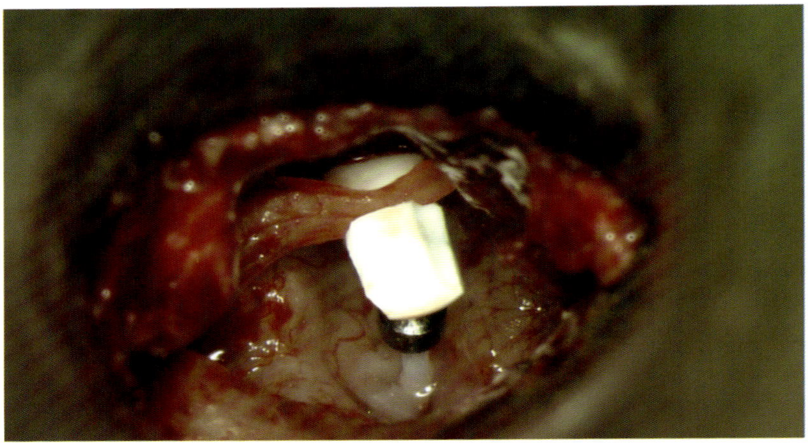

Figure 24–3. TORP prosthesis used with relocated malleus and vein graft. Image courtesy of Dr. Robert Vincent, Beziers, France.

5. Bone cement repair of the incus long process with placement of a standard stapes prosthesis.

Outcomes

Case series from experienced surgeons report approximately 50% to 70% rate of excellent results (air-bone gap ≤10 dB) and 60% to 80% of good results (ABG ≤20 dB). Early reports of revision surgery reported a 20% risk for hearing degradation. This was later repudiated in the 1990s with dead ears reported at a much lower rate (similar to primary surgery 0.5%–2%) and partial sensory hearing loss occurring 1% to 8% after revision surgery.

REFERENCES

1. Posada R, Fisch U. Stapedotomy and malleo-stapedotomy: the Fisch technique. In: Goycoolea MV, ed. *Atlas of Otologic Surgery*. New Dehli, India: JP Brothers; 2012:897–922.
2. Vincent R, Oates J, Sperling NM, Annamalai S. Malleus relocation in ossicular reconstruction: managing the anteriorly positioned malleus: results in a series of 268 cases. *Otol Neurotol*. 2004;25(3):223–230.

SUGGESTED READING

De La Cruz A, Fayad JN. Revision stapedectomy. *Otolaryngol Head Neck Surg*. 2000;123:728–732.

Fisch U, Acar GO, Huber AM. Malleostapedotomy in revision surgery for otosclerosis. *Otol Neurotol*. 2001;22:776–785.

Lesinski SG. Causes of conductive hearing loss after stapedectomy or stapedotomy: a prospective study of 279 surgical revisions. *Otol Neurotol*. 2002;23:281–288.

Lippy WH, Battista RA, Berenholz L, Schuring AG, Burkey JM. Twenty-year review of revisionstapedectomy. *Otol Neurotol*. 2003;24:560–566.

Schimanski G, Schimanski E, Berthold M. Diagnostic findings in stapes revision surgery: a retrospective of 26 years. *Otol Neurotol*. 2011;32:373–383.

Vincent R, Rovers, M, Zingade N, et al. Revision stapedotomy: operative findings and hearingresults: a prospective study of 652 cases from the otology–neurotology database. *Otol Neurotol*. 2010;31(6):875–882.

CHAPTER 25

Revision Stapedectomy: Technique of John C. Goddard

John C. Goddard and Audrey P. Calzada

INTRODUCTION

Revision stapes surgery represents one of the most challenging procedures that otologists perform. Proper patient selection is critical and begins with a thorough history and physical examination with particular attention to details surrounding the initial operation. Accurate audiometry confirmed by tuning fork examination is required in all cases. General anesthesia is avoided to allow for adequate feedback from the patient during the operation. The following series of images will examine the basic steps in revision stapes surgery as well as several potential problems that one might encounter. Finally, a variety of surgical solutions to these various problems will be depicted.

SURGICAL STEPS (Figures 25-1 through 25-7)

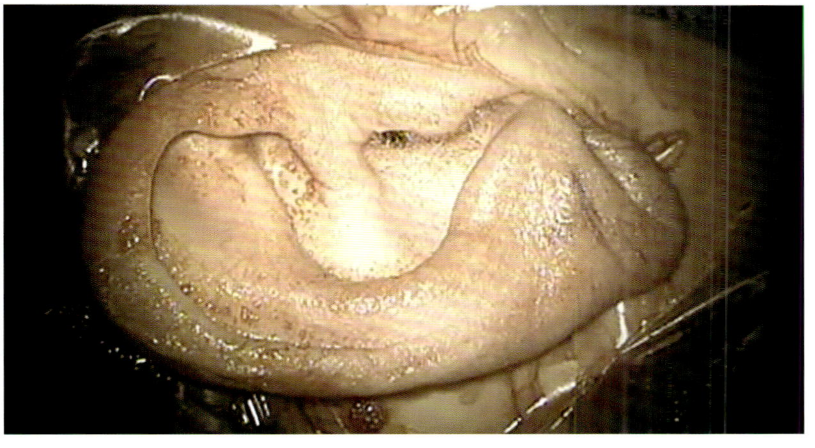

Figure 25-1. The ear is prepped and draped in a standard fashion, keeping the entire auricle, tragus, and a small area of postauricular skin exposed. (*Right ear*)

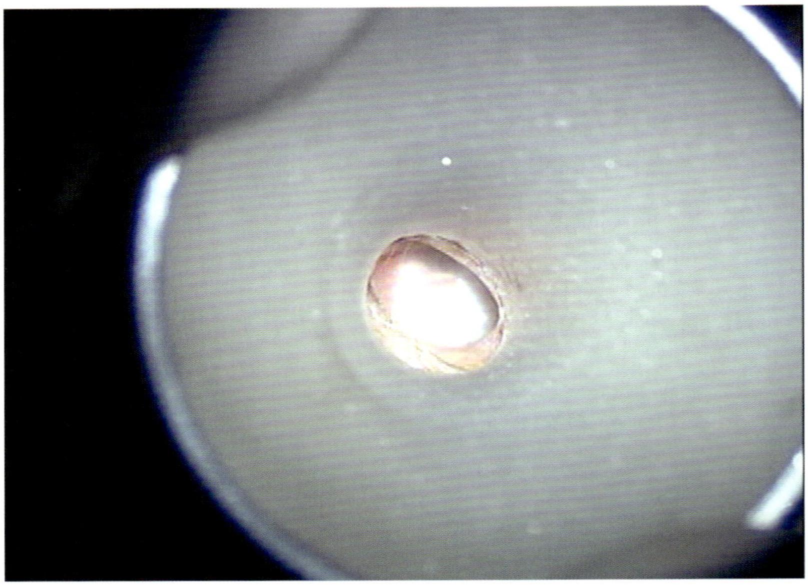

Figure 25-2. The largest, securely fitting speculum is used to expose the ear canal and tympanic membrane. The meatus is injected in a four-quadrant fashion, using local anesthesia buffered with bicarbonate (not shown). (*Right ear*)

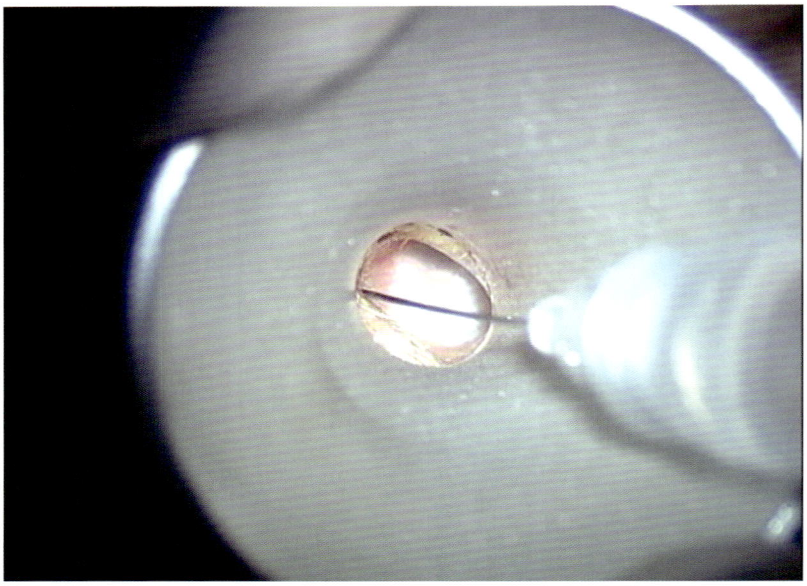

Figure 25-3. The vascular strip region is slowly injected with local anesthesia until blanching of the vascular strip and vessels along the tympanic membrane occurs. (*Right ear*)

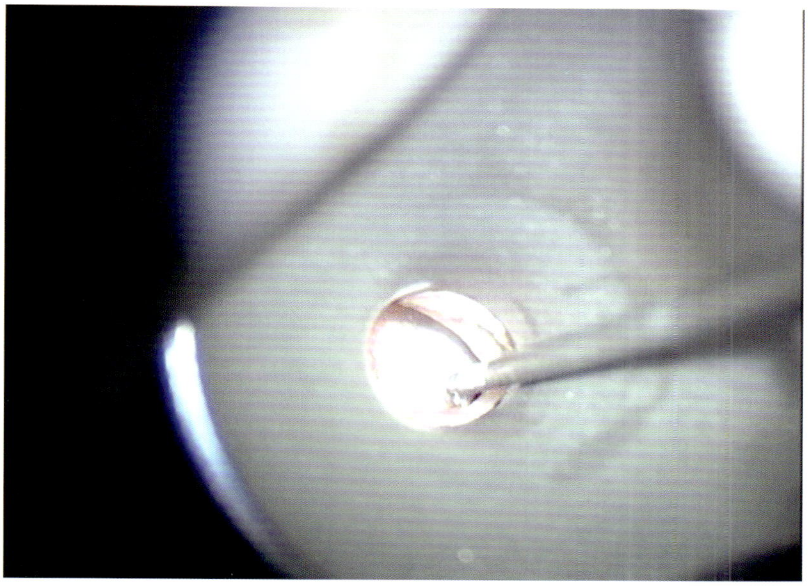

A

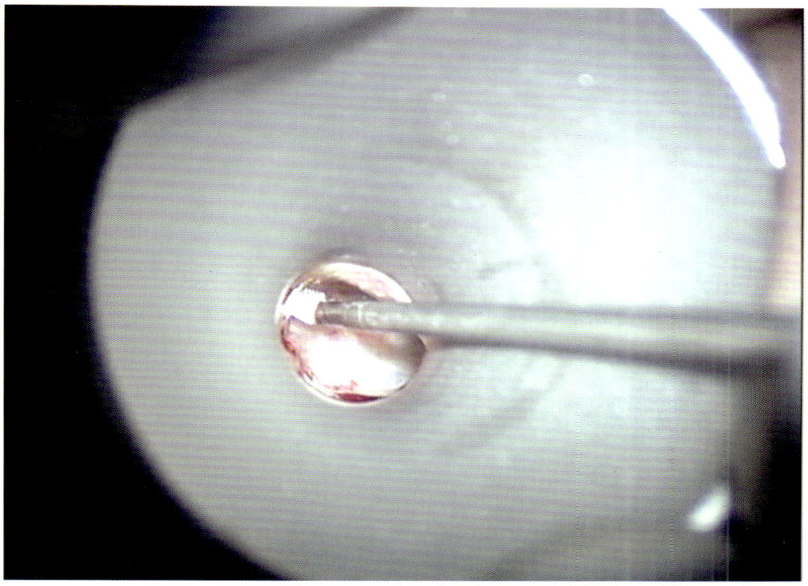

B

Figure 25-4. A–B. Elevation of the tympanomeatal flap begins inferiorly near the annulus and is carried laterally and superiorly into the vascular strip region. (*Right ear*)

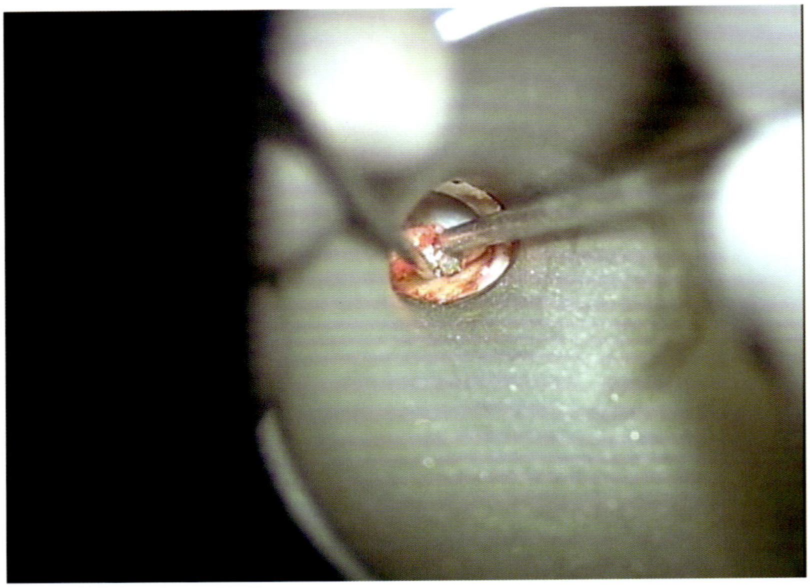

A

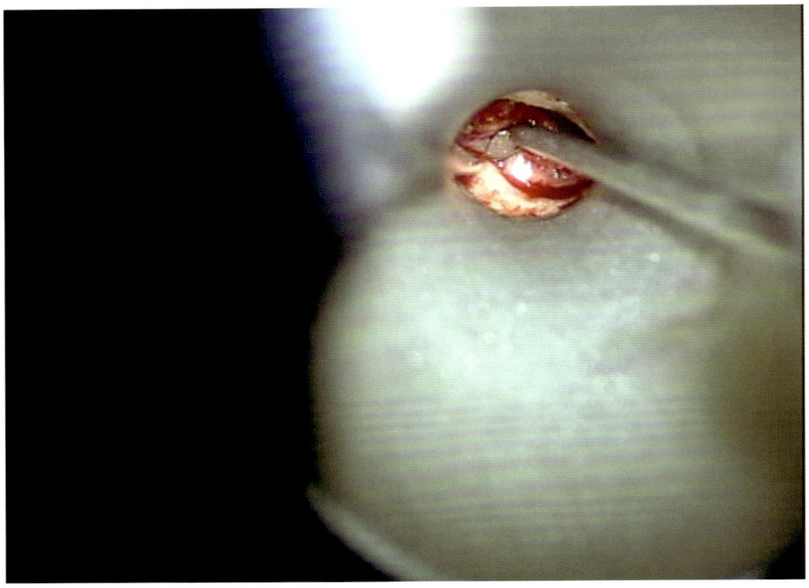

B

Figure 25–5. A–B. Because of prior surgery, the skin of the vascular strip is often thinner and more susceptible to injury. Consequently, flap elevation should be performed with a #22 Baron needle suction to minimize trauma. (*Right ear*)

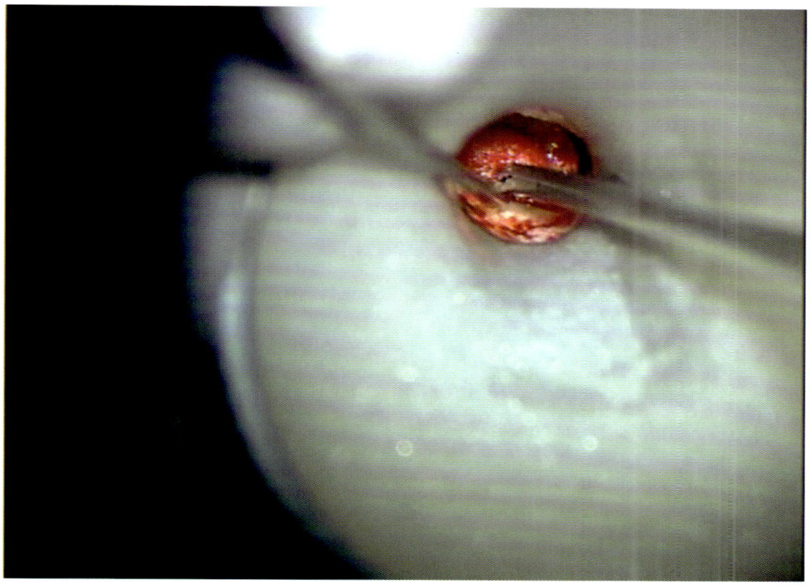

Figure 25-6. Prior to entering the middle ear space, a cotton ball, soaked in 1:1000 epinephrine, should be used to aid with hemostasis and to bluntly dissect the flap near the bony annulus.

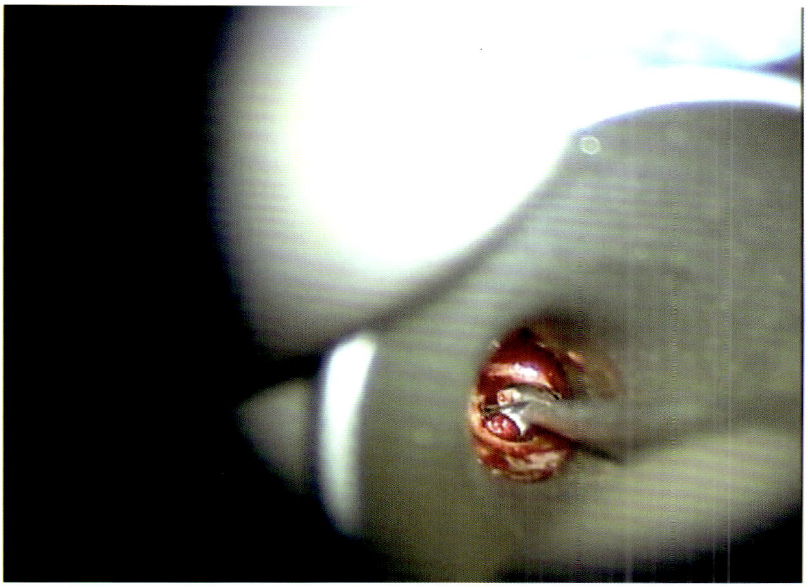

Figure 25-7. Depending on the adequacy of bone removal from the original operation, curetting of additional bone from the scutum may be required. The pyramidal eminence and tympanic portion of the facial nerve should be visible. (*Right ear*)

Once the middle ear space is entered, a variety of conditions may be encountered. The following images depict commonly encountered problems and various solutions (Figures 25–8 through 25–21).

Problem: Displaced Prosthesis (Figures 25-8 to 25-10)

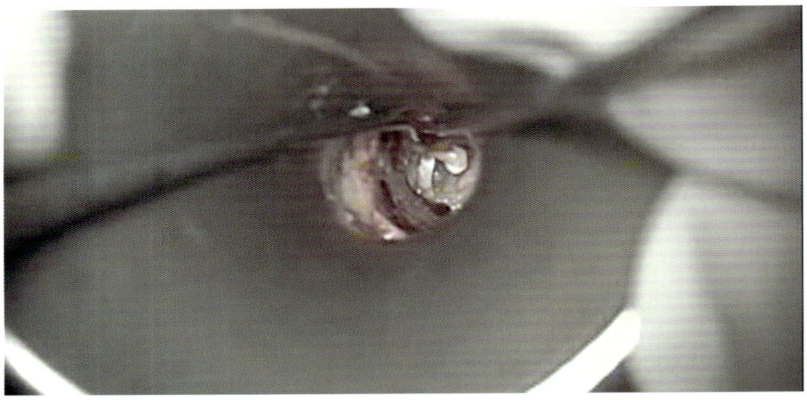

Figure 25-8. The previously placed stapes prosthesis may become displaced. Displacement can occur at the level of the incus, the footplate, or both. (*Right ear*)

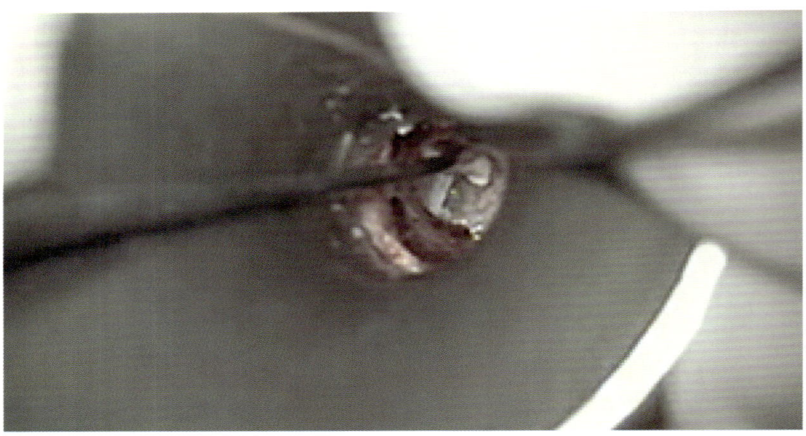

Figure 25-9. For displaced prostheses, the old prosthesis is carefully removed, using a combination of hand-held laser, for vaporization of scar tissue/adhesions, and sharp right-angled hooks. (*Right ear*)

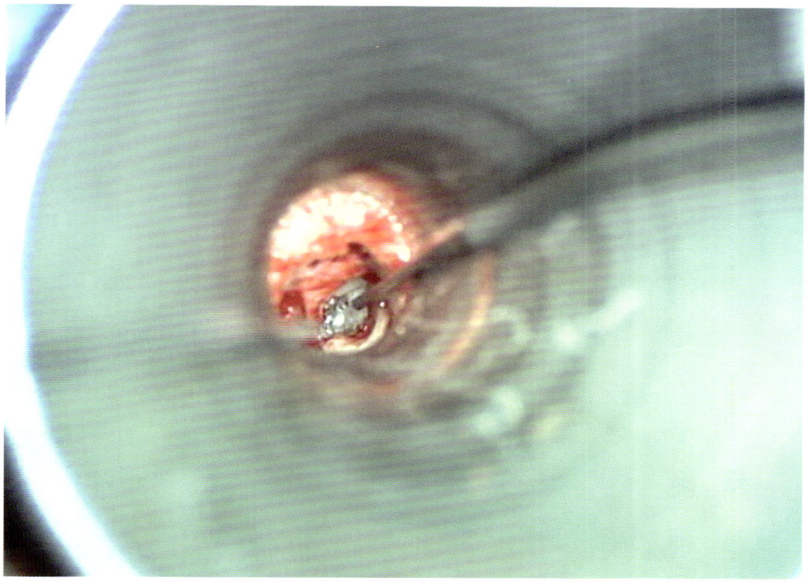

A

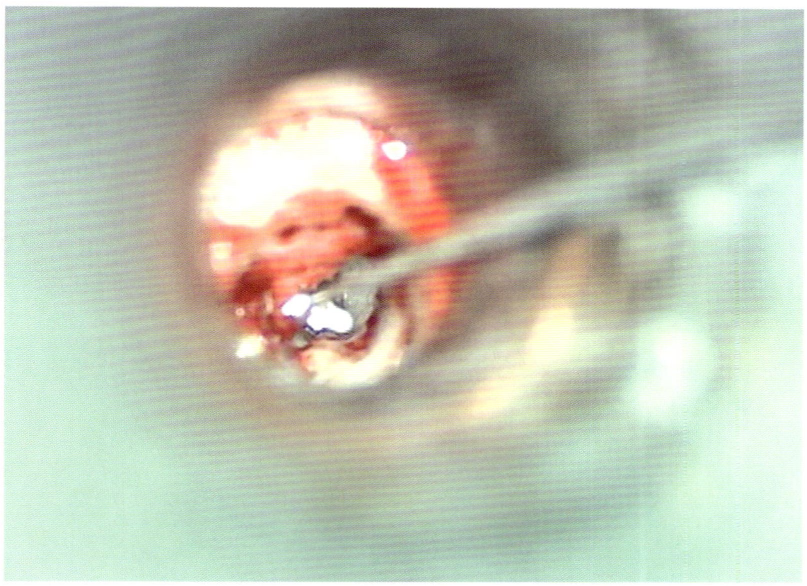

B

Figure 25-10. The CO_2 laser is used to facilitate adhesion removal (**A**) and a footplate (right-angled) hook is used to gently remove the prosthesis (**B**). (*Left ear*)

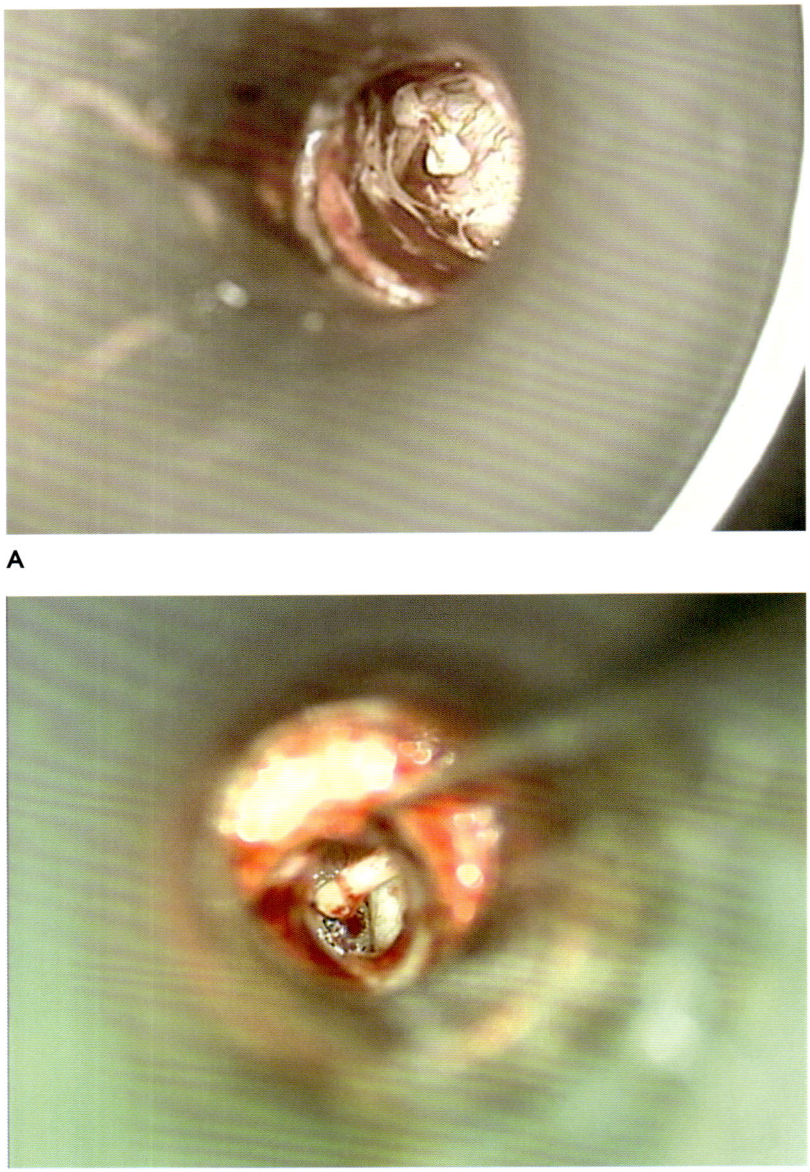

A

B

Figure 25-11. Incus necrosis, to varying degrees, is commonly encountered in revision stapes surgery. (**A.** *Right ear*; **B.** *Left ear*)

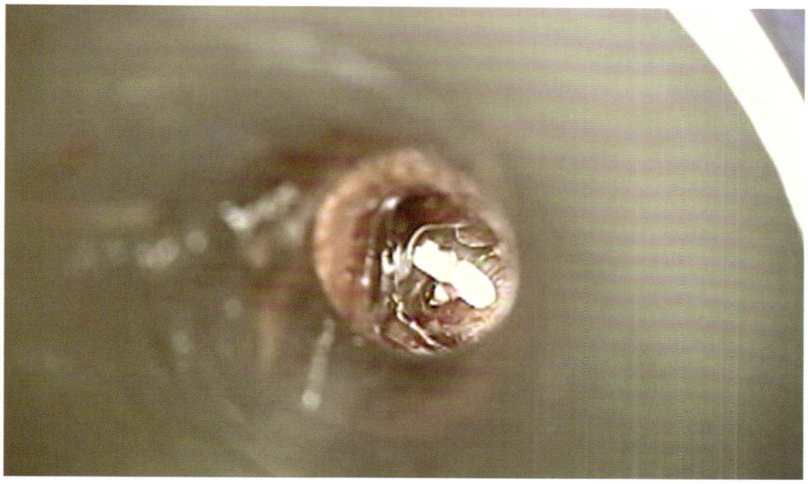

Figure 25–12. In cases of incus necrosis, bone cement may be used to recreate the long process of the incus and secure the prosthesis in position. (*Right ear*)

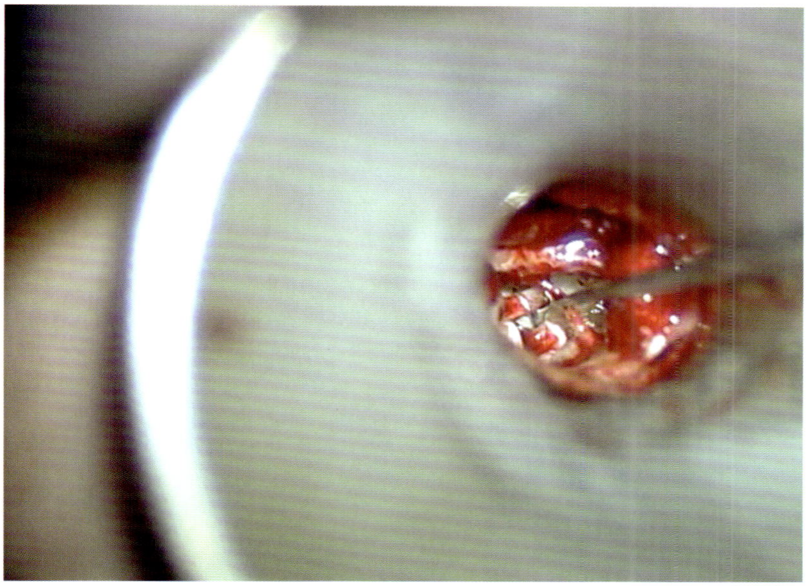

Figure 25–13. A notched, bucket-handle prosthesis may be used in cases of incus necrosis. The use of this type of prosthesis requires a tissue seal over a footplate that has undergone a partial or total stapedectomy. (*Right ear*)

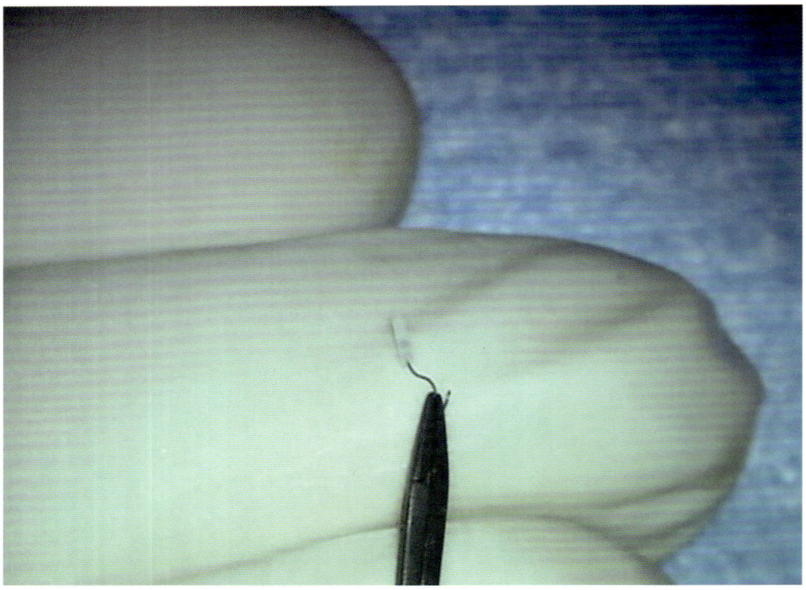

Figure 25-14. A slightly longer than normal piston prosthesis may be used and "bent" in two places to allow for attachment more proximally to an eroded long process.

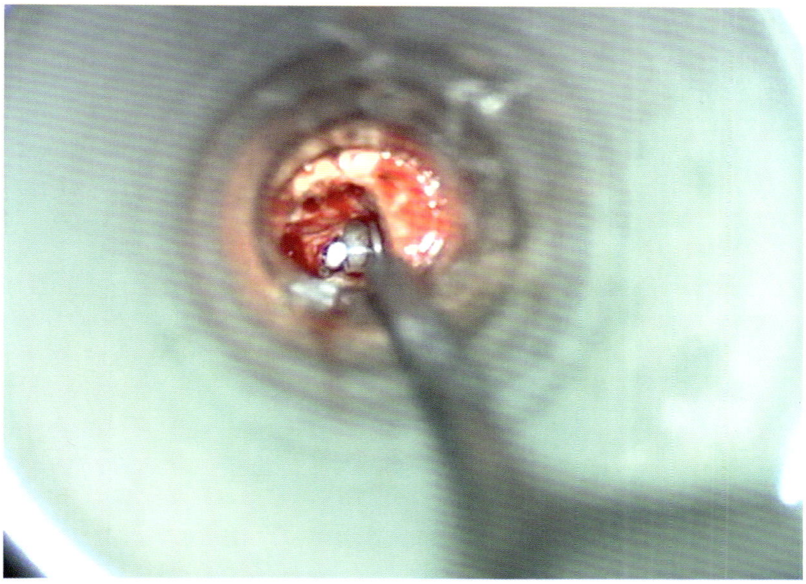

A

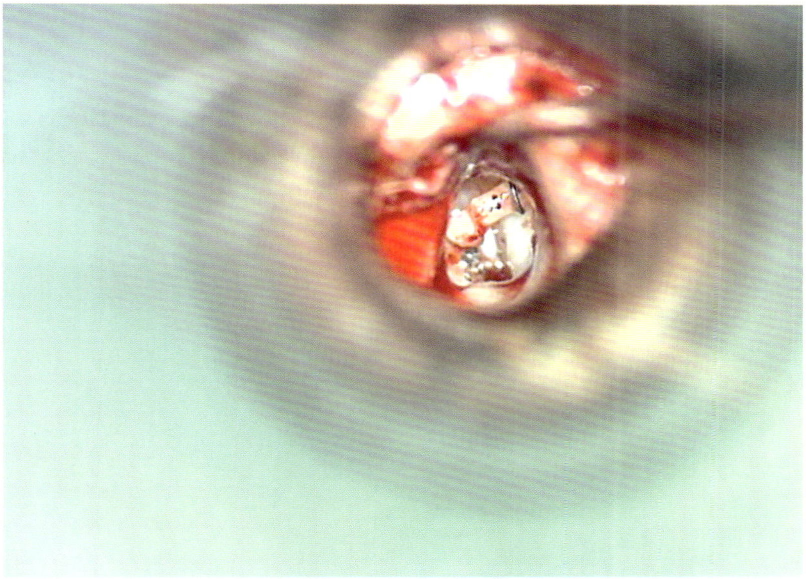

B

Figure 25-15. A–B. Placement of the "double-bent" prosthesis is similar to standard prosthesis placement, though the crock of the prosthesis is able to sit well away from the necrotic portion of the incus. (*Left ear*)

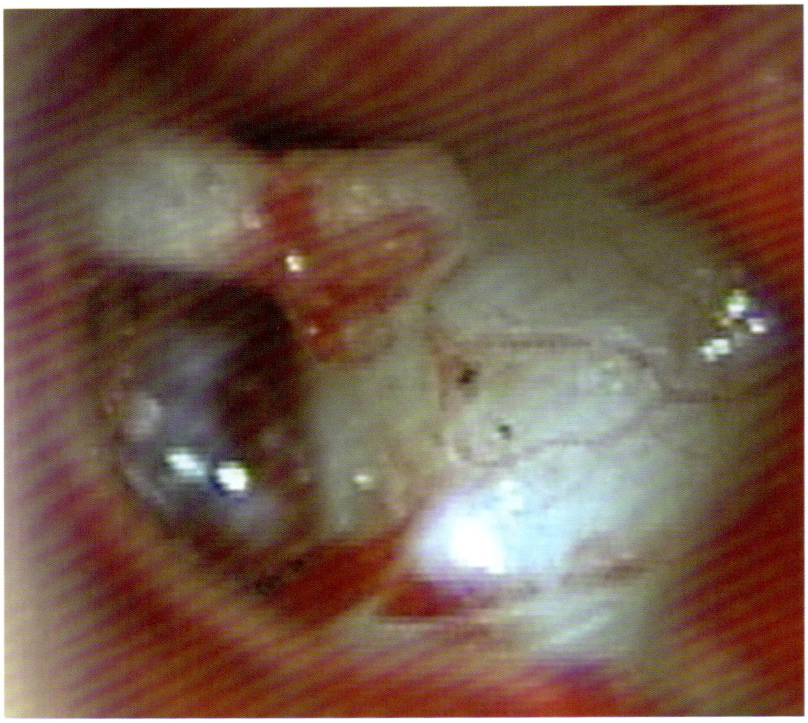

Figure 25-16. Regrowth of bone at the level of the oval window may occur, causing refixation of the footplate. (*Right ear*)

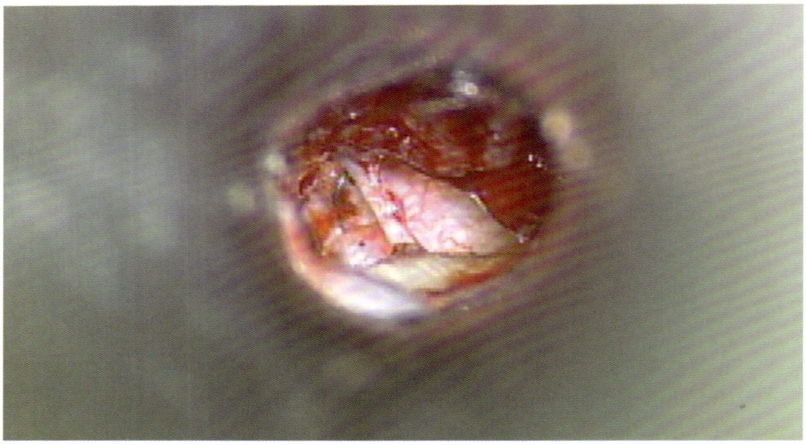

Figure 25-17. Extensive bony regrowth may obliterate the area of the oval window, surrounding the prosthesis, and leading to recurrence of a conductive hearing loss. (*Right ear*)

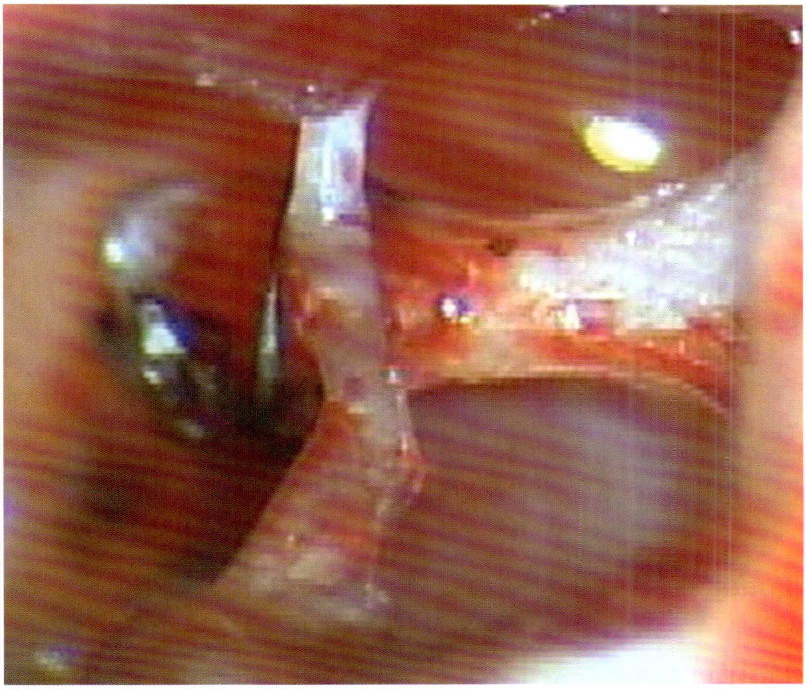

Figure 25-18. Granulomatous tissue around the prosthesis may also limit mobility. The CO_2 laser is useful for vaporizing bone regrowth and associated granulation tissue (not shown).

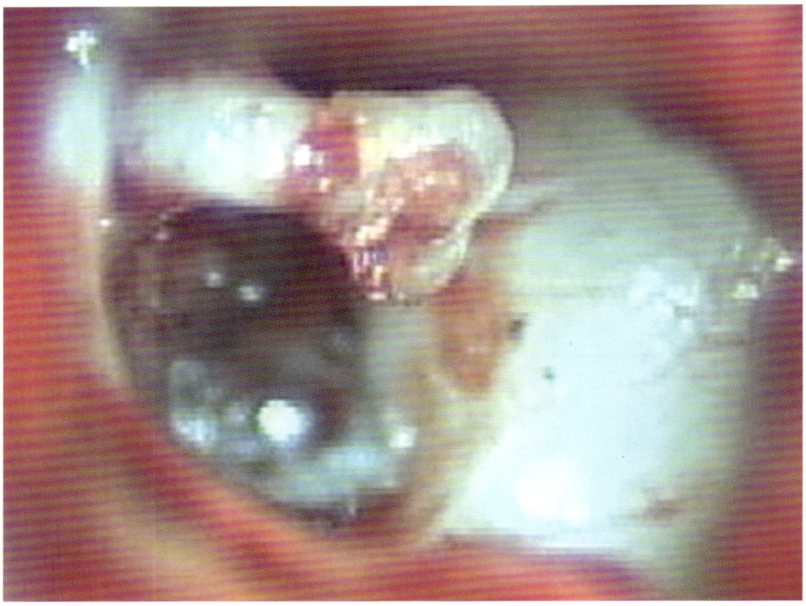

A

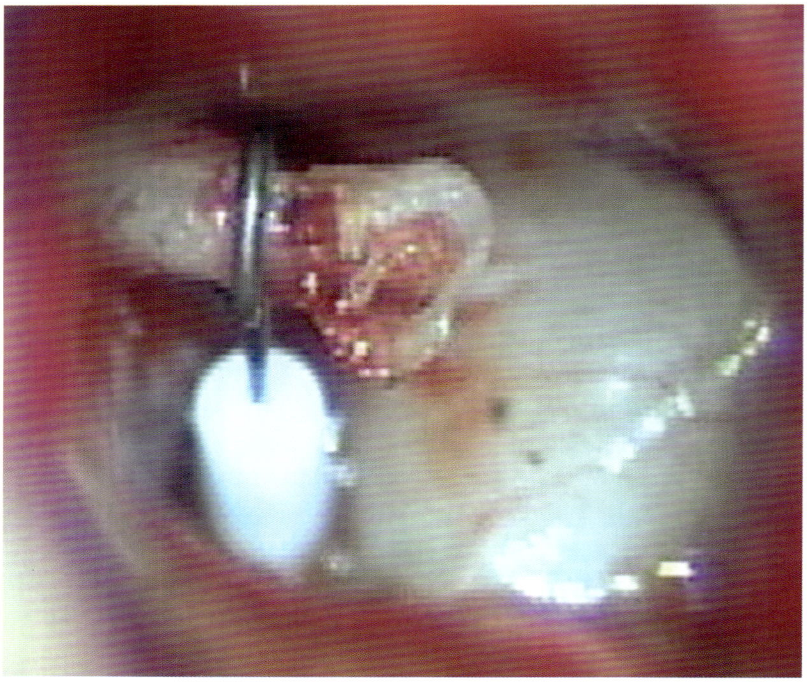

B

Figure 25–19. A–B. Recreation of a 0.7-mm fenestration is performed with the laser in most revision cases. Measurement of the required prosthesis length occurs prior to placing a new prosthesis. (*Right ear*)

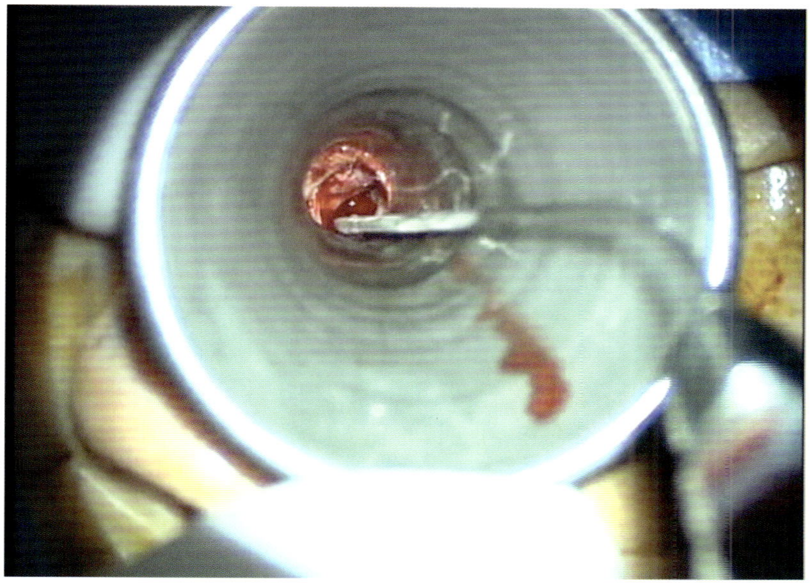

Figure 25–20. Blood is placed within the middle ear space to create a seal at the oval window at the completion of the procedure using a blunt needle and syringe aimed inferiorly into the hypotympanum. (*Left ear*)

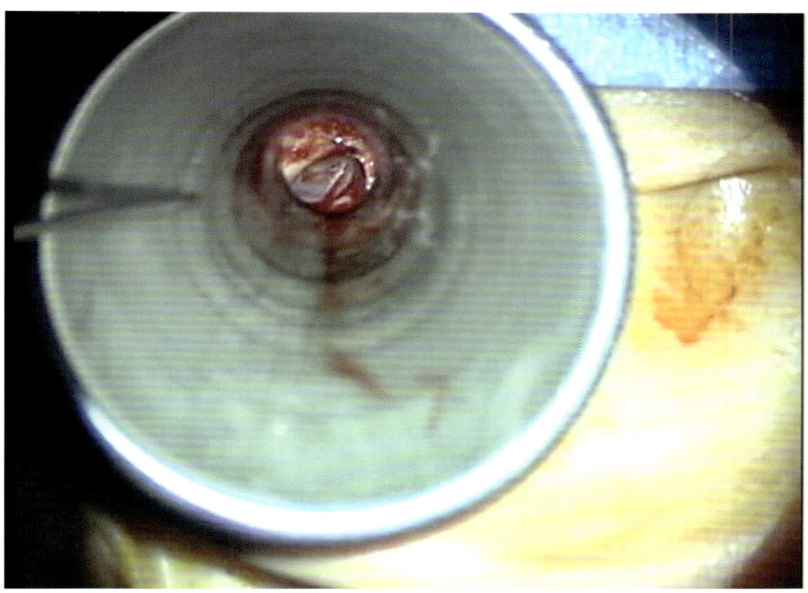

Figure 25–21. The tympanomeatal flap is laid back in position to complete the procedure. Gelfoam® packing is placed along the incision line. (*Left ear*)

CHAPTER 26

Causes of Failure of Stapedectomy

A.G. Pusalkar

The patient who has undergone primary stapedectomy and has not had a good result may need exploration. The purpose of exploration is not limited only to correction of the sound transfer mechanism. Revision surgery is also indicated if the patient experiences severe vertigo. Timing of the surgery is also equally important. In this chapter we discuss a few of the common conditions that can occur following stapedectomy that could result in an unsatisfactory result.

There are some details that the surgeon needs to be aware of when embarking on this surgery:

a. The surgeon needs to have vast surgical experience in stapedectomy and must be familiar with all the nuances, anatomical variations, and their solutions.
b. If the surgeon is contemplating operating on a patient who has been operated on by another surgeon, he must have the details of the primary surgery. Usually these details are missing and thus the surgeon should exercise more caution than he normally would.
c. Revision surgery has the potential to cause worsening of hearing.
d. Patients who have had an unsatisfactory result should be offered the fitting of a hearing aid as one of the options of management of this problem. The operating surgeon must discuss in detail the very real risks of the surgery involved.
e. The prognosis offered to the patient should always emphasize caution. Extravagant claims of success should be avoided.

The following illustrations demonstrate common causes of unsatisfactory surgical outcomes following stapedectomy (Figures 26–1 through 26–9).

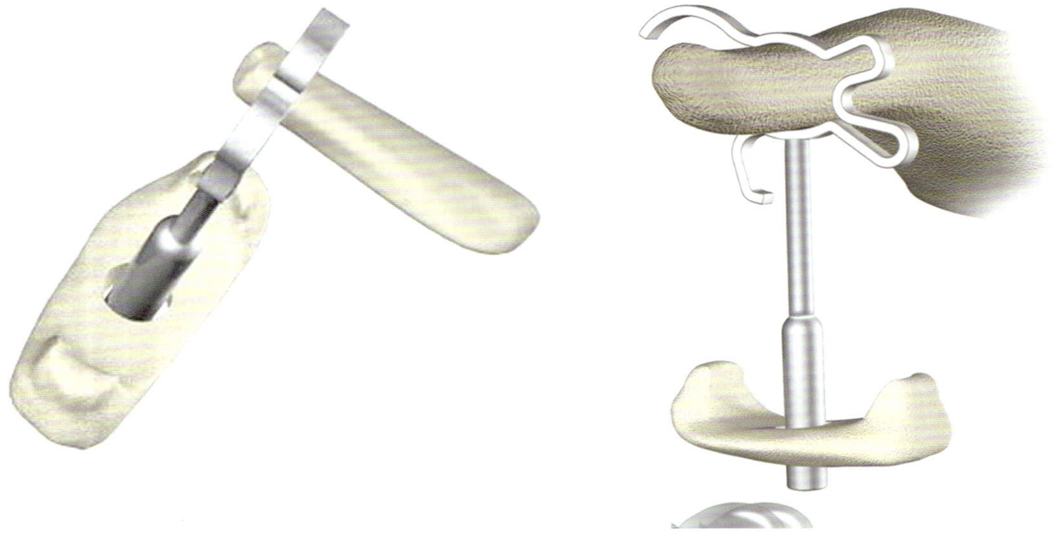

Figure 26-1. Correctly placed implant ("Kurz Clip Piston").

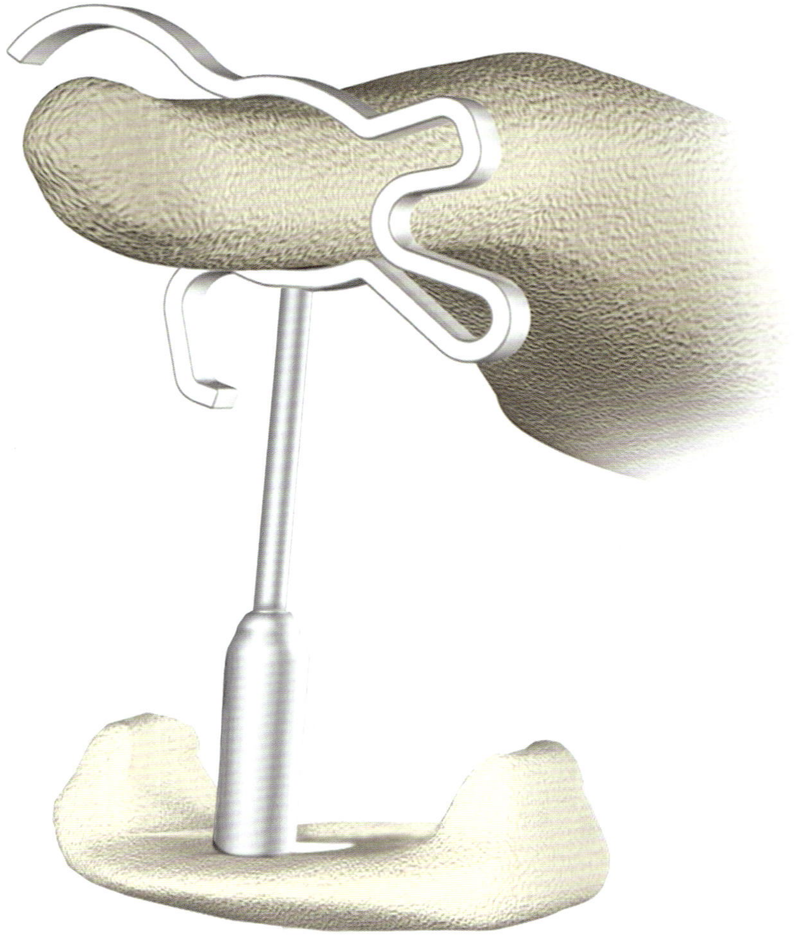

Figure 26-2. Implant resting on the edge of footplate fenestra impairing sound energy transfer.

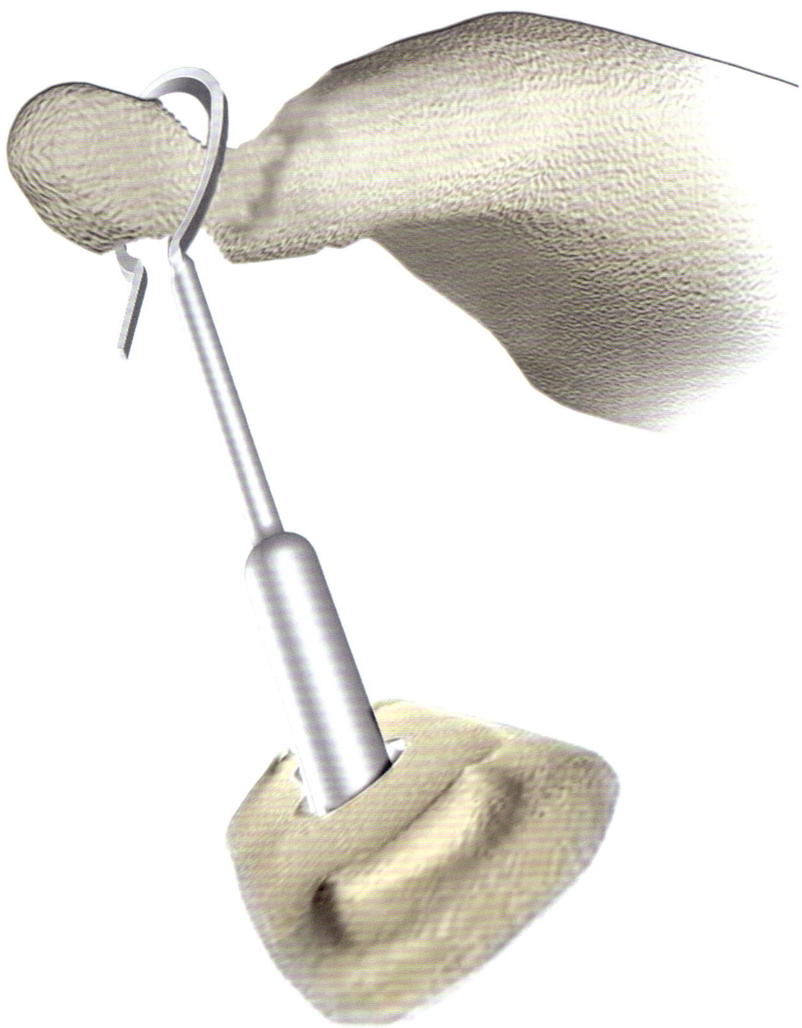

Figure 26–3. Erosion of long process of incus leading to conductive hearing loss.

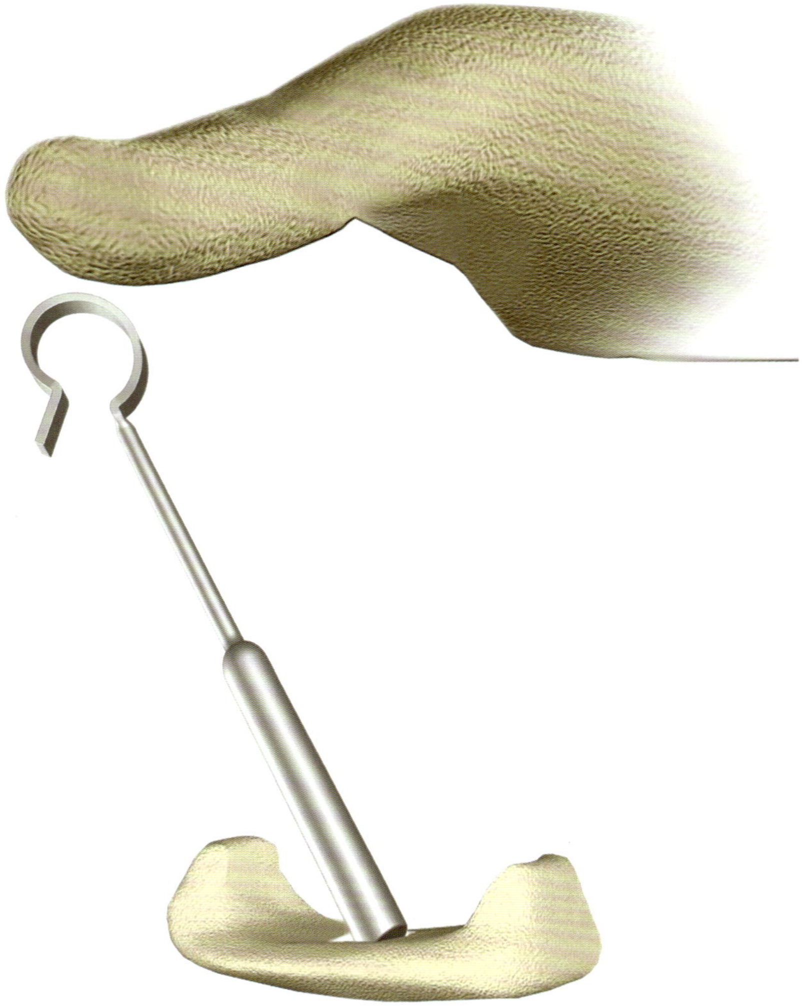

Figure 26-4. Dislodged prosthesis due to prosthesis laying on the edge of the footplate.

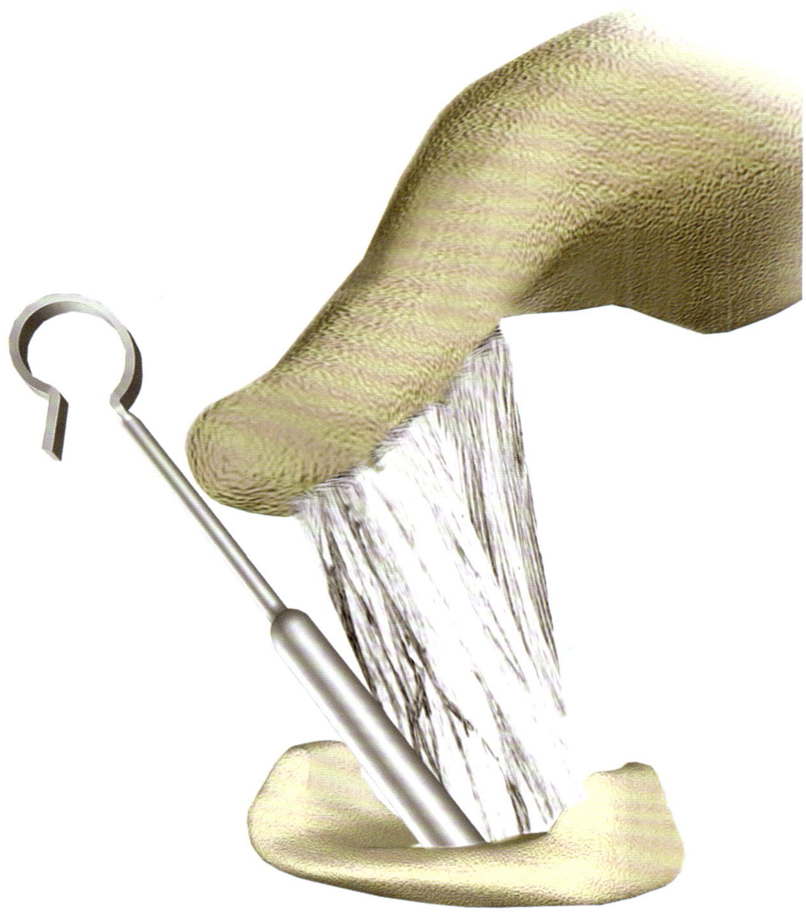

Figure 26-5. Adhesions pulling long process toward promontory causing displacement of implant.

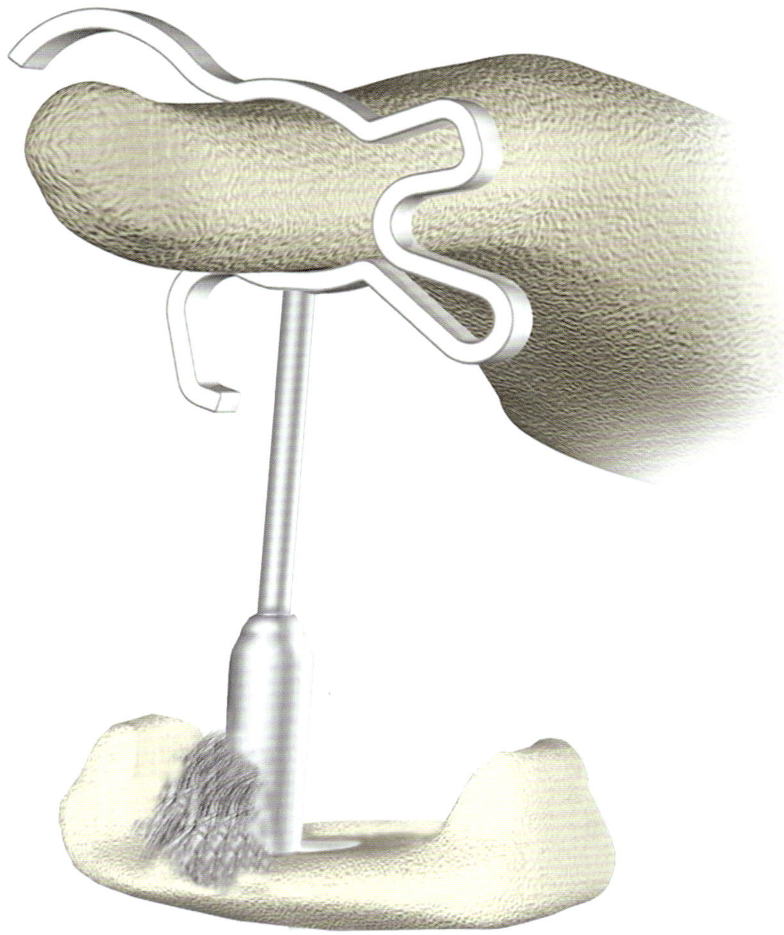

Figure 26-6. Adhesions between implant and stapes curua pulling implant out of fenestra.

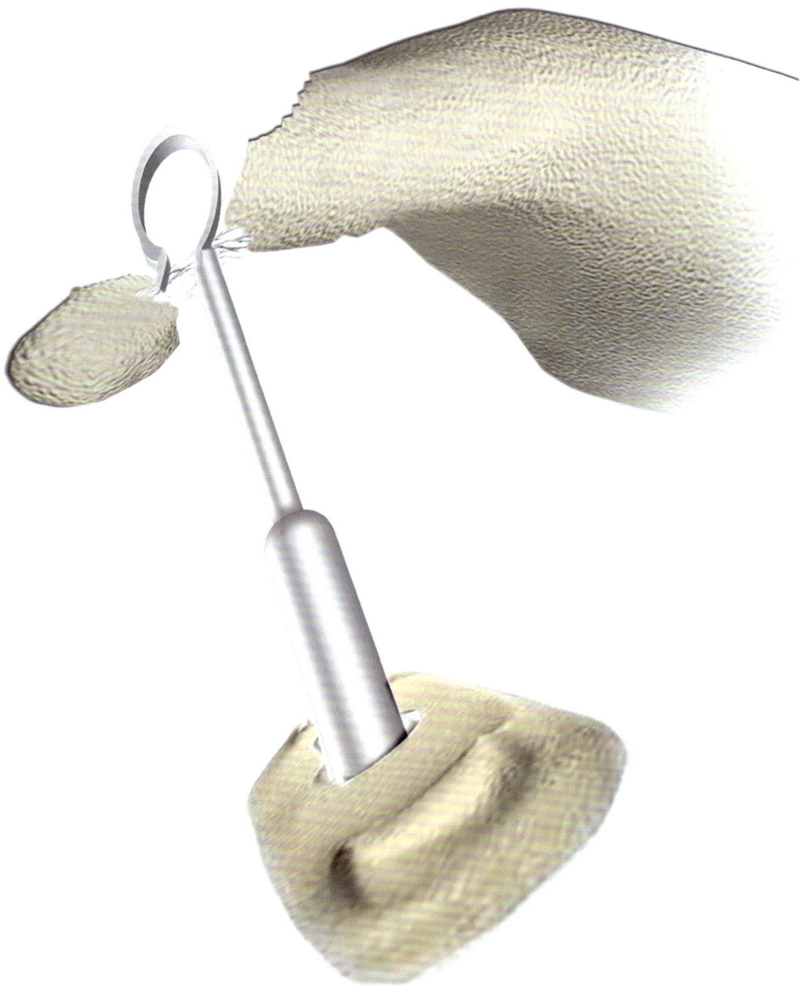

Figure 26-7. Complete necrosis of long process causing dislocation of implant.

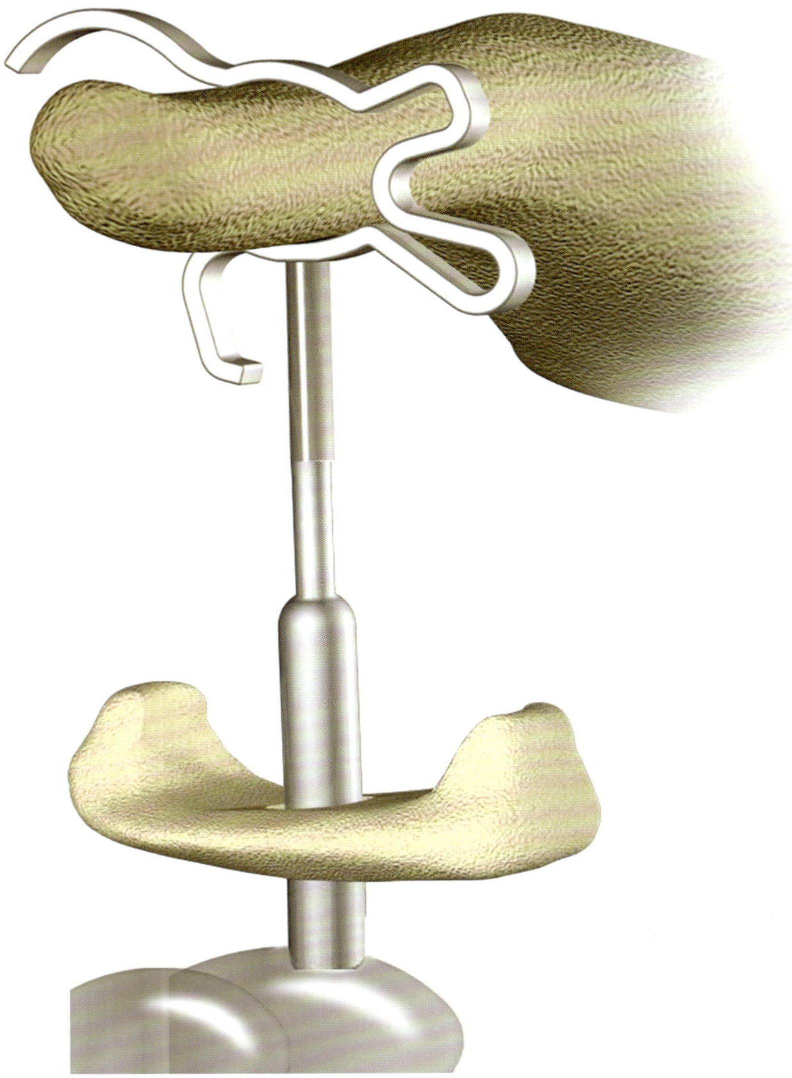

Figure 26-8. Too long prosthesis impinging on utricle or saccule causing vertigo.

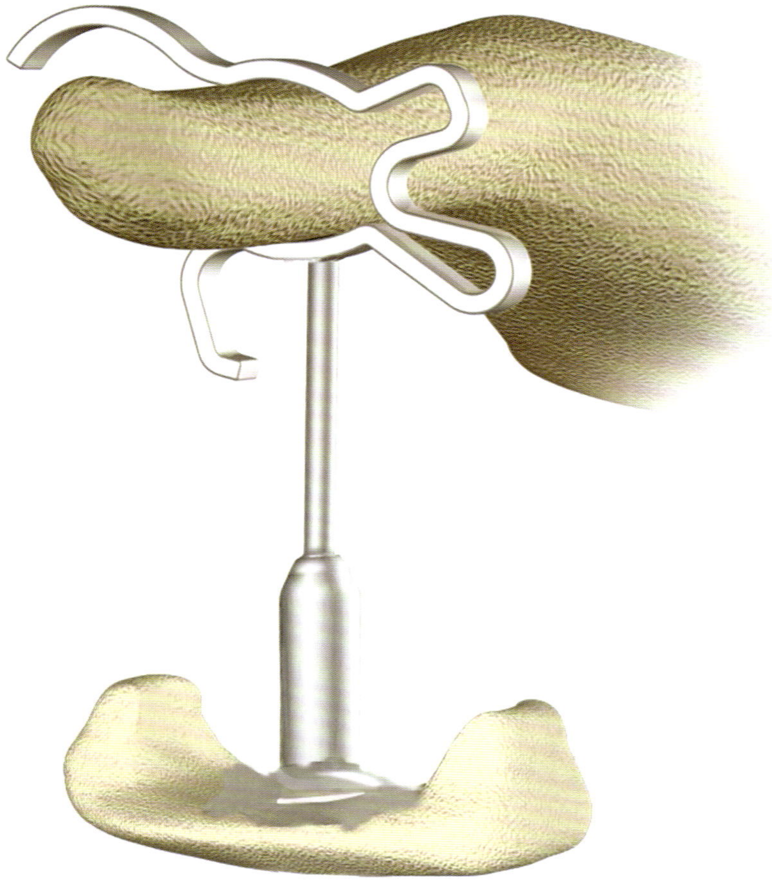

Figure 26-9. Prosthesis is too short.

Index

Note: Page numbers in **bold** reference non-text material

L

M

N

O

P

R

T

U

V

W

Z